Stephen K. Topaz, F.H.
CMDNJ, Rutgers Medical School
Department of Surgery
P.O. Box 101
Piscataway, N.J. 08854

Principles of APPLIED BIOMEDICAL INSTRUMENTATION

Principles of

APPLIED BIOMEDICAL INSTRUMENTATION

L. A. GEDDES and L. E. BAKER

Baylor College of Medicine

JOHN WILEY & SONS, INC., New York · London · Sydney

Dedicated to
HEBBEL EDWARD HOFF
Scientist, Scholar, Teacher, and Physician

Preface

This book has been written primarily for the life scientist who may be engaged in the conduct of a research, teaching, or patient-care program and has recognized the need for additional knowledge of the basic principles underlying many of the physical instruments he employs. It is also intended to satisfy some of the needs of the physical scientist who has just discovered that he has a contribution to make to the life sciences and is relatively unaware of prior work in his new area of interest.

As the title indicates, this is a book that describes the basic principles by which physiological events are measured. As such, it is principle-oriented rather than problem-oriented. Principles cannot be usefully described, however, without examples of their application to the measurement of specific physiological events. Each chapter is therefore richly supplied with examples of the application of the principle discussed. The problem-oriented reader who wants information on all the methods that have been used to measure a particular physiological event is directed to the carefully prepared index, in which he will find this information. We have taken this approach because methods of measuring physiological events change with the passage of time but the basic principles endure. We have also found from experience that the emphasis of principles, rather than the description of specific problems, sparks ideas that produce unique and surprising solutions to new problems and the improvement of established techniques.

Technology in all fields is expanding at an unprecedented rate, and demands on all professions have accelerated to such a point that the qualified specialist hardly has time to peer beyond the boundaries of his chosen field to familiarize himself with techniques and principles that might be of genuine value to him in his work. Even technical papers in his own field have no space for the important and illuminating historical background of a particular problem. As a result, work is often duplicated, and investigaters are unaware that the same problem may have been successfully solved by men in other fields. For these two reasons we have elected to bring together the fields of physiology and engineering and to analyze problems in experimental physiology and medicine in a technical and historical manner. In essence, the topics covered in this book are presented in state-of-the-art expositions in which the emphasis is placed on defining parameters of the problems discussed. Supporting the presentations is an extensive bibliography that will enable the reader to investigate original material in detail and by so doing to evaluate quickly the originality of his own ideas on a given subject.

We wish to recognize the opportunities presented to us by the Administration of Baylor University College of Medicine and the National Heart Institute. It was the support of these two organizations and the continued encouragement and sterling leadership provided by Dr. H. E. Hoff that resulted in the creation of this book. We also acknowledge the contribution of the many medical and graduate students who over a ten-year period clearly indicated the type of information they required to practice better medicine and to conduct research in the life sciences. Because no manuscript of this size comes into existence without the endless typing of rough drafts, we extend our thanks to Miss Lucia Bonno, secretary to the Section of Biomedical Engineering, and to Miss Elaine Peck of the Department of Physiology, Baylor University College of Medicine.

Baylor University College of Medicine
January 1968

L. A. GEDDES

L. E. BAKER

Contents

Principles of APPLIED BIOMEDICAL INSTRUMENTATION

1

The Transduction and Measurement of Physiological Events

Etienne Jules Marey, pioneer physiologist of the last century, called attention to an activity that many believe to be a modern innovation, namely, use of the latest tools of physics and engineering to investigate the phenomena of living organisms. His following statement (1878) was prophetic of the present-day application of these techniques in the biological sciences:

"In effect in the field of rigorous experimentation, all the sciences give a hand. Whatever is the object of these studies, that which measures a force or movement, or electrical state or a temperature, whether he [the investigator] be a physicist, chemist or physiologist, he has recourse to the same method and employs the same instruments."

In the biomedical sciences instrumentation for the purpose of quantification in measurement has not pervaded all areas, and a major task yet to be accomplished is to develop the tools and technology for solving the problems of detection and quantitative measurement of living processes. To do this, transducers must be created. In the chapters that follow many of the current methods for the conversion of physiological events to electrical signals will be described. Although the term transducer is used here to denote the conversion of a physiological event to an electrical signal, it should be recognized that it has a broader meaning—the conversion of one type of energy to another.

When a physiological event is transformed to an electrical signal, there exists the opportunity of deriving the maximum amount of information from it by using appropriate processing and display devices. With the event available as an electrical signal, it is much easier to obtain the advantages

1

of modern computing and display equipment to present the desired information in the most useful form. With an electrical analog of a physiological event, it is possible to store the event on magnetic tape and re-examine it at a later time. Replay and reproduction at different display rates, as by the use of a slow or a fast time scale, permits interrogation of the data for information missed when the event was being measured. This capability offers one means of obtaining the maximum amount of information from a single measurement.

Many methods are employed to convert a physiological event to an electrical signal. The event can be made to vary, directly or indirectly, electrical quantities such as resistance, capacitance, inductance, or the magnetic linkage between two or more coils. The use of piezoelectric and photoelectric transducers is also common. Chemical events can be detected through potentials developed by membrane electrodes or by measurement of current flow through electrolytes. Detectors for radiant energy occupy a prominent place in the detection of physiological events. In some instances changes in the electrical properties of biological material can be employed for transduction purposes. Practical application of the principles of transduction embraces all the phenomena of the flow of electrons or ions through solids, liquids, gases, or a vacuum. In practice, however, it is convenient to use only a few of these possibilities.

Before discussing the various methods employed to convert physiological events to electrical signals, it is important to distinguish between a transducible property and a method or principle of transduction. A transducible property is defined as that singular characteristic of an event to which a principle of transduction can be applied. A principle of transduction is any one of the many methods that can be employed to convert the transducible property to an electrical signal. In essence the transducible property is the characteristic, like a fingerprint, that is singularly different from those of all the others around it; that is, it is the property that makes the event recognizable. The principle of transduction employs the device that recognizes the property and converts it to an electrical signal. For example, if gaseous carbon dioxide is to be detected in a mixture of respiratory air (oxygen, nitrogen, and water vapor), a property which distinguishes carbon dioxide in this mixture is infrared absorption. Carbon dioxide absorbs radiation at wavelengths of 2.7, 4.3, and 14.7 microns. Although water vapor absorbs a small amount of radiation near 2.7 microns, the use of an infrared source operating at either of the other two or all three of the principal absorption bands and a detector sensitive to the same spectrum constitutes a means for detecting carbon dioxide. Thus, with the respiratory air passing between the infrared source and the detector, the output from the latter will decrease in proportion to the amount of carbon dioxide in the respiratory air. In this example the transducible property is infrared absorption, and the principle of transduction employs an infrared source and detector. Parenthetically, it is obvious that the maximum resolution obtainable is intimately related to the singularity of the transducible property and the selectivity of the principle of transduction.

A transducer is in reality the sense organ for the electronic processing equipment. By its very nature it is a highly specialized device ideally possessing sensitivity to but one type of energy. For this reason it is difficult to discuss the merits of these devices in a general manner. Nonetheless, a few characteristics of high-quality transducers can be stated which will serve as a basis for their evaluation.

Irrespective of the event being measured, the transducer, insofar as possible, must obey Kelvin's first rule of instrumentation; that is, the measuring instrument must not alter the event being measured. In biomedical studies this goal is not always realizable, and the degree of alteration must constantly be borne in mind. Frequently, indirect methods are employed which partially isolate the transducer from the event. For this reason it is essential that the transducer exhibit a high degree of selectivity for the phenomenon being measured so that adequate rejection of other events occurs.

The transducer should also obey the three criteria for the faithful reproduction of an event: amplitude linearity, adequate frequency response, and freedom from phase distortion. Because these criteria are discussed in detail in Chapter 14, only brief explanation of their meaning is made here.

Amplitude linearity refers to the ability of the transducer to produce an output signal that is directly proportional to the input amplitude. This requirement is presented graphically in Fig. 1–1 by the solid line $0-A$. If a phenomenon under measurement increases in the opposite direction, the transducer must also linearly indicate this condition, as shown in Fig. 1–1 by the solid line $0-A'$.

Although the input-output characteristic of a transducer is represented as a straight line, careful testing with known inputs usually reveals a small deviation from linearity. In high-quality transducers such a test reveals a series of values which distribute themselves on either side of a straight line. The exaggeration of a typical case is portrayed by the dashed line in Fig. 1–1. In such instances it is customary to describe the degree of linearity in terms of the percentage deviation. For example, a linearity of $\pm 1\%$ means that, within the total operating range of the device, the deviation from linear response will not be greater than $\pm 1\%$.

Another quantity related to the linearity of a transducer is hysteresis, which is a measure of the ability of the transducer to produce an output that follows the input independently of the direction of change in the

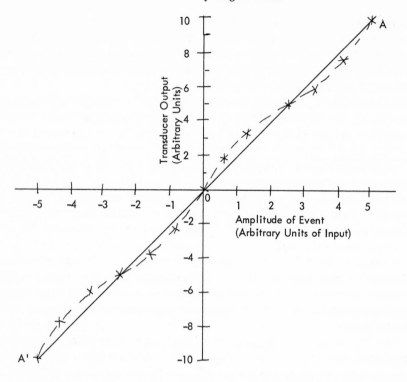

Figure 1–1. The meaning of amplitude linearity.

input. In a linear system with no hysteresis the input-output relationship is a single straight line. If hysteresis is present, an open curve is obtained, as shown in Fig. 1–2. It is customary to express the amount of hysteresis in terms of the percentage of full-scale value. In the exaggerated example shown the hysteresis error is approximately 25%; in a well-designed device it would be less than 1%.

In connection with amplitude linearity it is pertinent to point out that the range of the event to be encountered should not exceed the range specified for the transducer. Large inputs may damage a transducer and hence decrease the linearity and increase the hysteresis error.

The overall *frequency response* and *freedom from phase distortion* refer to the ability of the transducer to provide a signal which will follow rapid and slow changes in the event presented to it. The overall frequency response must be equal to or greater than that dictated by harmonic analysis of the waveform of the event. Freedom from phase distortion requires that the transducer maintain the time differences in the sinusoidal frequency components revealed by harmonic analysis. Examples of the distortion

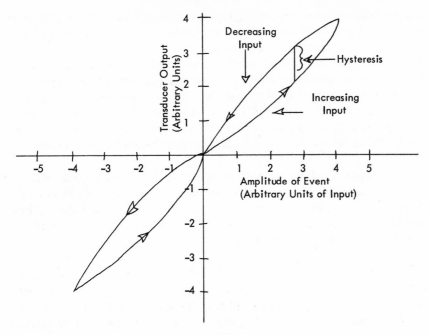

Figure 1–2. Hysteresis errors.

encountered when these criteria are not fulfilled are described in Chapter 14.

Although it is highly desirable to obtain linear signals from all transducers, this is not always possible. Occasionally the transducer develops a signal which is not directly proportional to the event. For example, the resistance change of thermistors is not linear with temperature. Under such circumstances linearizing networks are necessary unless the event can be presented with a nonlinear calibration. Sometimes the signal is nonlinear by the nature of the physiological event itself; for example, the redness of the blood, reflecting the degree of oxygen saturation, is related to a logarithmic ratio of red and infrared transmissions. Under these conditions it is necessary to employ special processing devices to develop a signal linearly related to oxygen saturation.

The means for calibration of a transducer should be examined critically. A transducer which does not lend itself to calibration directly in terms of the physiological event has limited value; it serves to produce data which have meaning in the time domain. For example, waveform and time relation to another event form the basis for analyzing data acquired by transducers that cannot be calibrated.

Transducers can be expensive devices. For this reason selection of a particular type should be based in part on its ability to be incorporated into an existing processing or display system. Fulfilling such a requirement paves the way for the creation of a modular system which can accept a variety of transducers for many purposes.

Ultimately the transduced event is displayed by an indicating device. It is important to call attention to this fact because the type of display and use of the data frequently dictate the degree of precision required. Precision and cost are inextricably linked and often become the basis for bargaining. Perhaps the considerations in this regard were best expressed by Sir Thomas Lewis (1925), the pioneer of clinical electrocardiography, who wrote:

"Coal when weighed for sale is not thrown into a chemical balance, neither is coal placed on a coarse scale when submitted to fine analysis. Like these two machines, both classes of instruments have limitations; these should be recognized and, according to the circumstances of the case, one or the other is employed the more profitably."

In summary, it can be stated that the successful transduction of a physiological event requires the selection of an appropriate transducible property to which a selective principle of transduction is applied. Sometimes there are many suitable transducible properties and principles of transduction for a particular physiological event. In the selection of a principle of transduction a good criterion to bear in mind is Rein's (1940), which, although originally applied to an efficient blood pressure transducer, may be restated as follows: "maximum efficiency in the transducer, a minimum of electronics." In engineering terms the goal is to obtain the highest conversion efficiency, that is, electrical signal per unit of physiological event, while retaining all of the criteria to achieve faithful conversion. Standardization, miniaturization, and financial compatibility with the use of the data are other obvious important considerations.

The field of electronics is replete with devices that will process and display electrical signals, but it has only a meager supply of transducers ideally suited to the measurement of physiological events. For this reason investigators in the biomedical sciences in the past, and to some degree at present, have borrowed and adapted industrial transducers or devised their own. No full-scale program has yet been launched to provide transducers for the biomedical science investigator. It should not be concluded, however, that transduction of the widest variety of physiological events cannot be accomplished. Each physiological event has many transducible properties, and there are several suitable principles of transduction already in existence. That industry has recognized and solved a similar problem can be deduced from a statement made by Carl Berkley (1950): "In nearly twenty years of oscillography, the Allen B. Dumont Laboratories has yet to find a phenomenon which is incapable of being converted to a suitable electrical signal."

Even with all of the channel components (transducer, processor, and reproducer) functioning properly, repeated measurement of the same quantity will not produce exactly the same value. The question logically arising is, "Which is the correct value?" The question should really be rephrased to read "Which is the most representative value?" The answer requires the use of statistical techniques and forces a consideration of the terms precision, accuracy, and error. *Precision* refers to the degree of reproducibility of a measurement, *accuracy* is a measure of the closeness of the measurement to the true value, and *error* is the difference between the measured value and the true value. Although these terms are often used loosely, they convey different messages. For example, if a system has high precision, measurements of the same event under identical conditions differ little, that is, the scatter, spread, or range of values is small. In very many investigations, the accuracy and the error are never known, merely because the true value is not known.

Because a finite body of data contains a limited amount of information, it will be instructive to examine how a series of measurements can yield information about the quantity measured. The point can be well illustrated by the use of an example concerned with the measurement of systolic blood pressure by means of the auscultatory method. The example also illustrates the application of an indirect technique.

Let it be assumed that a human subject has a perfectly uniform heart rate and blood pressure and that an error-free transducer has been connected to the brachial artery just above the arm-occluding cuff. (The reading obtained from it will be taken as true blood pressure.) With the cuff pressure well above systolic pressure, no sound is heard in a stethoscope placed over the brachial artery just distal to the cuff. As the cuff pressure is reduced very slowly, a point is reached at which the arterial pressure exceeds the cuff pressure, the pulse breaks through, and a sound is heard. At the instant the sound occurs the observer reads the cuff pressure and calls this value the systolic pressure. Repeated trials produce the values shown in Table 1–1. The observer naturally wants to know which value to select and how accurate that value is.

Clearly evident is the fact that the measurements exhibit a scatter, spread, or range extending from 124 to 134. It is apparent that the most representative value lies somewhere in this range. Statistical analyses provide several methods to identify the tendency of the readings to cluster about a central value. Whenever data are encountered in this form, it is customary to plot a frequency distribution diagram. In other words, the range of the data is divided into a convenient number of equal steps, called

Table 1-1

Trial Number	Systolic Pressure (mm Hg)
1	131
2	128
3	130
4	131
5	134
6	128
7	130
8	133
9	129
10	132
11	129
12	132
13	130
14	125
15	129
16	130
17	126
18	124
19	127
20	131

class marks or intervals, and the number of values in each interval is tabulated. The width of the intervals is determined by the investigator. In Table 1–2 the data have been divided into intervals of 1 mm Hg, starting with

Table 1-2

Pressure Interval (mm Hg)	Number of Values in Interval
124–125	I
125–126	I
126–127	I
127–128	I
128–129	II
129–130	III
130–131	IIII
131–132	III
132–133	II
133–134	I
134–135	I

124 mm Hg. All values of 124 mm Hg and above (but below 125 mm Hg) are placed in this interval. The process is repeated for pressures up to 135 mm Hg. The number (frequency) in each interval is plotted in Fig. 1–3. When the points are joined by straight lines, the figure is called a frequency polygon: when they are joined by a smooth curve, it is called a curve of distribution. When the points are represented as rectangles (left), the figure is a bar graph; when horizontal lines fill the rectangles, a coin diagram is created; and when the points are displayed as steps (right), the figure is a histogram.

Table 1-3

Pressure (mm Hg)	Deviation from Mean	Deviation Squared
131	+2	4
128	−1	1
130	+1	1
131	+2	4
134	+5	25
128	−1	1
130	+1	1
133	+4	16
129	0	0
132	+3	9
129	0	0
132	+4	16
130	+1	1
125	−4	16
129	0	0
130	+1	1
126	−3	9
124	−5	25
127	−2	4
131	+2	4
TOTAL 2589		TOTAL 138

20| 2589

MEAN   129.4 = 129

STANDARD DEVIATION

$$\sigma = \left(\frac{138}{20}\right)^{1/2} = 2.63$$
$$= 2.6$$

When the frequency-interval technique is employed, it becomes clear that certain values appear more often than others: that is, there is a central value about which the individual measurements appear to cluster. Many

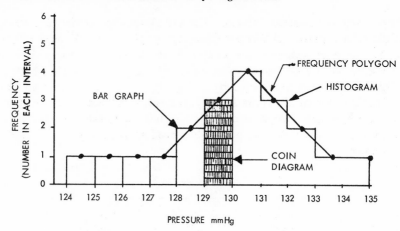

Figure 1–3. Frequency distribution diagram.

terms are used to describe the distribution of data about the central value. Perhaps the most familiar is the mean or arithmetic average, which is simply the sum of the individual values divided by the number of measurements. Useful as the mean is, it does not identify the tendency of the measurements to cluster around a single value. Often the mean and the range are stated. In the example chosen the mean is 129.4 (2589 ÷ 20), which, to the nearest integer, is 129; the range is 124 to 134 or 10 mm Hg. Another term which describes the central tendency is the mode, defined as the value in the table which occurs most frequently. In the example the mode is 130. Another useful term is the median, defined as that value which divides the group into two halves.

Because a vast number of measurement techniques produce data that fit what is called a normal (Gaussian) distribution curve, special terms have been developed to describe data falling into this pattern. The normal distribution curve, which gives equal weight to all measurements and assumes that small errors are more probable than large ones, is shown in Fig. 1–4. Note that the distribution of data plotted in Fig. 1–3 bears a resemblance to this curve.

If the measured data have a normal distribution, there are statistical methods for identifying the most representative value in the presence of a variation (dispersion) in magnitude. A single term that is sometimes used is the average deviation, defined as the sum of the deviations from the mean divided by the number of measurements. In the example cited the average deviation from Table 1–3 is $(+26 - 16) \div 20 = 0.5$. The most frequently used term to indicate variability is the standard deviation. This quantity is a measure of the dispersion of the data and, as will be

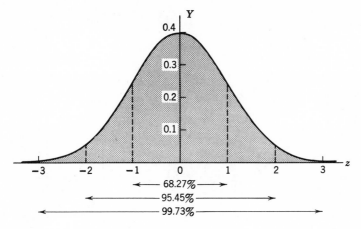

Figure 1–4. The normal distribution curve.

shown, really informs about the reproducibility or precision of the measurement.

The standard deviation (σ) is defined as the square root of the sum of the squares of the deviations from the mean divided by the number of measurements. If the distribution of data points is described by the normal distribution curve, it can be shown that 68.27% of the observations will fall between the mean ± 1 standard deviation. If the limits are widened to $\pm 2\sigma$, 95.45% of the observations will be found; 99.73% of the readings will fall, within the limits of $\pm 3\sigma$.

Applying this information to the example presented, we see (Table 1–3) that the mean value of the blood pressure is 129 mm Hg and the value of one standard deviation is 2.6 mm Hg. Transferring this information to Fig. 1–5, we observe that the most representative value for the blood pressure is 129 mm Hg and that theoretically 68.27% of the readings will fall between 131.6 and 126.4 mm Hg.

It is now pertinent to recall that the true value of systolic blood pressure was measured by using a direct arterial error-free transducer. Thus the error in the blood pressure determined by the indirect method can be taken as the difference between the mean and the true value, bearing in mind that the precision of the measurement is indicated by the spread of values about the mean. If the direct arterial transducer read 134 mm Hg each time a determination was made, it can be stated that the mean of the readings is -5 mm Hg in error.

In this example it was assumed that the direct arterial transducer yielded an accurate measure of systolic blood pressure. To the critical reader it should be apparent that, although the direct arterial transducer measures

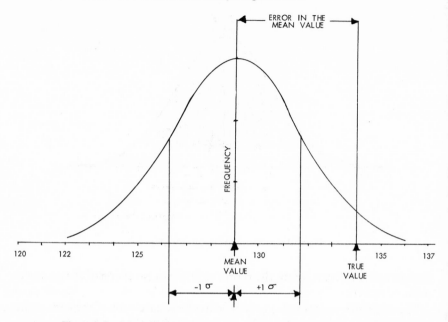

Figure 1–5.   Normal distribution curve of blood pressure measurements.

the event as accurately as possible, it too has its own spread of values to which a statistical treatment must be applied. In connection with this statement there arises the question of ultimate accuracy. In cases in which the readings of a measuring instrument with a high reproducibility (i.e., σ is very small) are compared to an internationally accepted primary standard, the error of the mean can be ascertained and the accuracy of the measuring instrument can be specified. When such an instrument is used to measure a quantity, the standard deviation about the mean of the values obtained is descriptive of the constancy of the event being measured. The mean value of the readings can then be corrected to give the true value of the event.

REFERENCES

Berkley, C. 1950. A review of the design and application of transducers for oscillography. *Oscillographer* (A. B. Dumont Laboratories). **12**:9–22.

Lewis, T. 1925. *The Mechanism and Graphic Registration of the Heart Beat*. London: Shaw & Sons.

Marey, E. J. 1878. *La méthode graphique dans les sciences experimentales et principalement en physiologie et en medicine*. Paris: Masson & Cie.

Rein, H., *A. A. Hampel, and W. A. Heinemann* 1940. Photoelektrische Transmission-manometer zur Blutdruckschreibung. *Arch. Ges. Physiol.* **243**:329–335.

Thompson, S.P. 1910. *The Life of William Thomson, Baron Kelvin of Largs.* London: Macmillan and Co.

2

Resistive Transducers

2–1. THERMORESISTIVE TRANSDUCERS

The variation of resistance has been used extensively to convert temperature and mechanical displacement to electrical signals. The resistance of a conductor, whether solid, liquid, or gas, is dependent on the material, the geometric configuration, and the temperature. Gaseous cells are used for the detection of radiant energy. Most of the transducers that operate on the resistance principle employ solids or liquids; the solid conductors, however, are more common.

Because the resistivity of most metals exhibits a considerable degree of temperature dependence, it is relatively easy to construct a temperature transducer. A resistor designed for such purposes is called a resistance thermometer. Although almost any metallic conductor can be used, choice of the material is based on either the linearity or the sensitivity of its resistance-temperature characteristic. The variation in resistance of most metals is approximately linear over a moderate temperature range near room temperature and is given by the relationship

$$R_t = R_0[1 + \alpha_0(T_t - T_0)],$$

where
R_t = resistance at temperature T_t (measured in °C),

R_0 = resistance at temperature T_0 (measured in °C),

α_0 = temperature coefficient of resistivity at T_0.

Table 2–1 lists the temperature coefficients for some of the commonly encountered metals. From these data it can be seen that most metals exhibit an increase in resistance with rising temperature (positive temperature coefficient), with typical values in the range of a 0.3 to 0.5%

change in resistance per degree centigrade temperature change. Plantinum has a temperature coefficient of 0.37% per degree centigrade and is frequently used because of its wide linear resistance-temperature relationship.

Table 2-1   Resistivities and Temperature Coefficients *

Material	Resistivity† (micro-ohm cm)	α = Temperature Coefficient† (ohms/ohm/°C)
Copper (annealed)	1.724	0.0039
Copper (hard drawn)	1.77	0.0038
Aluminum (commercial)	2.828	0.0036
Silver	1.629 (18°C)	0.0038
Platinum	10	0.00377
Nichrome	100	0.0004
Iron	10	0.005
Mercury	98.5 (50°C)	0.00089
Carbon	3500 (0°C)	−0.0005

Handbook of Chemistry and Physics, Chemical Rubber Publishing Co., Cleveland, Ohio, 1962.
†At 20°C.

Resistance thermometers are usually low in resistance, varying from a few ohms to a few hundred ohms. Because of their low thermal sensitivity, it is necessary to use a Wheatstone bridge (Fig. 2–1a) with a sensitive indicator to show the temperature of the thermal element (R_D). The bridge can be operated from either direct or alternating current.

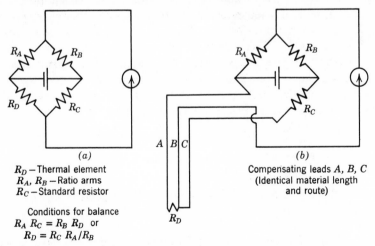

(a)

R_D —Thermal element
R_A, R_B —Ratio arms
R_C —Standard resistor

Conditions for balance
$R_A R_C = R_B R_D$ or
$R_D = R_C R_A/R_B$

(b)

Compensating leads A, B, C
(Identical material length and route)

Figure 2–1.   Wheatstone bridge (a) and compensated bridge; (b) circuits.

To eliminate errors caused by changes in resistance of the wires connecting the resistance thermometer to the bridge it is necessary to employ compensating leads. The method of obtaining temperature compensation is shown in Fig. 2–1b. Initially R_D and R_C are made equal at the reference temperature. When R_D is then used to measure an unknown temperature and the temperature of the wires connecting R_D to the bridge changes, an equal amount of resistance is added to R_C and R_D, thereby minimizing errors caused by thermal gradients which exist along the wires. When this technique is employed, a temperature can be measured with an accuracy of a few hundredths of a degree centigrade. Miniature resistance elements that have a small thermal capacity and a short response time can be made. Once calibrated, such detectors are remarkably stable.

Several precautions must be taken when using a resistance thermometer. If it is immersed in electrolytes, electrical shunting and fluid absorption must be prevented. Also, if the resistance of the thermal element is affected by magnetic fields (as is the case with some materials), its use in such environments may lead to error in temperature measurement. These effects are described in detail later. Perhaps the most important precaution to be observed is to avoid heating the resistance thermometer by the current employed to measure its resistance.

The thermistor is also widely used to measure temperature. It is a hard ceramic-like device composed of a compressed and sintered mixture of metallic oxides of manganese, nickel, cobalt, copper, magnesium, titanium, and other metals. Molded into beads, rods, disks, washers, and many other forms, thermistors exhibit temperature coefficients many times larger than those of pure metals. Furthermore, the coefficient is negative; that is, with increasing temperature, the resistance of a thermistor element decreases considerably. With most thermistors the temperature coefficient approximates a 4 to 6% change in resistance per degree centigrade change in temperature. Figure 2–2 compares the variation for copper with that for a typical thermistor. The resistance-temperature relationship of the thermistor is exponential; the usual form of the relationship is given by the following equation [Victory Engineering (1955)]:

$$R_t = R_{t_0}\, e^{\beta(1/T - 1/T_0)},$$

R_t = temperature at $T°K$,

R_{t_0} = temperature at $T_0°K$,

β = temperature coefficient (typical values 3000 to 4000),

$e = 2.71828$.

Most of the thermistors used in biomedical studies are very small in size, thus minimizing the thermal mass and reducing the response time

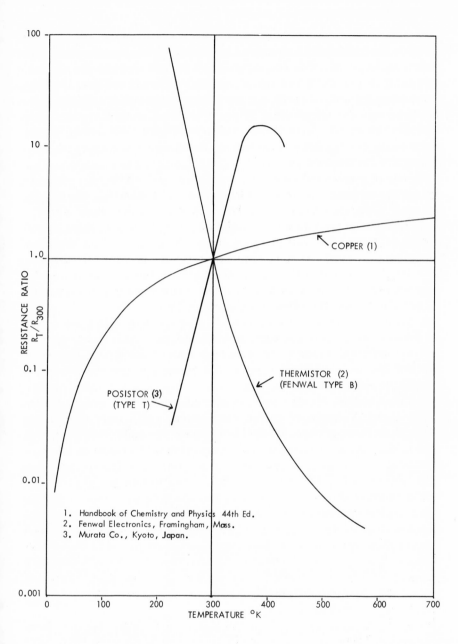

Figure 2–2. Resistance-temperature characteristics of copper, a typical thermistor, and a posistor.

correspondingly. Typical resistance ranges extend from a few hundred ohms to approximately a megohm. As with the resistance thermometer, great care must be exercised to limit the current through the thermal element in order to reduce errors resulting from self-heating. In many of the standard units, if the power dissipation is kept to the milliwatt level, measurement of a temperature differnce of 0.01°C or smaller is possible without difficulty. Because of the large temperature coefficient, compensating leads are not usually required with thermistors when making routine temperature measurements.

The thermistor is not, however, without its limitations; for example, the resistance-temperature characteristic of some of the earlier thermistors exhibited hysteresis. In addition, unlike pure metallic resistance elements, some thermistors tend to show a slight degree of long-term aging, which manifests itself as a small change in nominal resistance at a particular temperature. A comprehensive report on precautions in the use of thermistors in physiology was made by Fleming (1958). Modern manufacturing methods and improved quality control techniques have largely eliminated the defects present in the first thermistors.

A survey of the characteristics of many typical thermistors was presented by Van Dover and Bechtold (1960). In their comprehensive article they tabulated resistance range, maximum wattage dissipation, operating temperature, time constant, temperature coefficient, and dimensions of a variety of configurations.

The high thermal coefficient is in part offset by the nonlinear nature of the resistance change, which becomes noticeable when large temperature changes are encountered. If a linear temperature scale is desired, it is necessary to employ linearizing techniques. One of the easiest methods of obtaining a linear scale is to connect a resistor of the appropriate value in parallel with the thermistor. A review of this technique was presented by Cornwall (1965).

One manufacturer[1] has devised a method of overcoming the nonlinear characteristics of thermistors by developing temperature sensors which contain pairs of thermistors. With these sensors employed in the circuits shown in Fig. 2–3, a linear voltage-temperature or resistance-temperature characteristic can be obtained over a range of temperature change of about 100°C. With these thermilinear[1] sensors the maximum departure from linearity is less than 0.2°C.

Recently a new series of thermistors, called posistors,[2] has been announced. These devices, made from barium titanate ceramic, have

[1] Yellow Springs Instrument Co., Yellow Springs, Ohio 45387.

[2] Murata Manufacturing Co., Ltd., Kyoto, Japan.

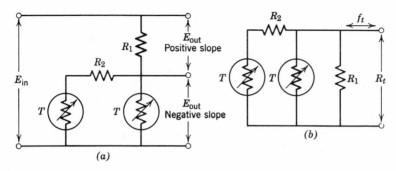

Figure 2–3. Circuits for obtaining linear temperature characteristics with thermilinear thermistors: (*a*) linear voltage versus temperature; (*b*) linear resistance versus temperature. (Courtesy Yellow Springs Instrument Co., Yellow Springs, Ohio.)

remarkably high positive thermoresistive coefficients in the temperature range of -50 to $+100°C$. In one model the resistance at room temperature is multiplied tenfold by an increase in temperature of $60°C$. The characteristics of the type T posistor are shown in Fig. 2–2.

Both resistance thermometers made of pure metals and thermistors have a variety of applications in biomedical studies. Quite apart from their obvious use as electrical transducers for measuring the temperature of the skin and of many regions inside the body, they see other service. Occasionally, heated thermistors are employed as hot-wire anemometers to measure volume flow. Heated thermistors have been placed in the respiratory air stream to detect respiration and give a biphasic signal for a single breath being cooled by both inspiration and expiration. Simons (1962) employed an unheated thermistor to determine the respiratory frequency of aircraft pilots and obtained a unidirectional change in resistance with each breath.

Ledig and Lyman (1927) used platinum resistance thermometers for transduction of carbon dioxide and oxygen to electrical signals by measurement of the thermal conductivities of these gases. By means of the same system, Lamson and Robbins (1928) measured the amount of carbon tetrachloride in respiratory air when a known amount of this substance was injected into the lumen of the gut.

There have been several applications of the thermoresistor that demonstrate the response time attainable. Hill (1920) showed that when an 11-micron heated filament was laid across the lumen of a tube connected to a conical receiver placed over a pulsating vessel the rapid pulsations of the air stream modulated the temperature of the wire, hence its electrical resistance. The response time was short enough to show the notched transient (dicrotic wave) in the pulse curve. This pulse detector was used by Bramwell et al. (1923) in pulse wave velocity studies. The principle was later improved by Tucker and Paris (1921) to construct a hot-wire microphone having a resonant frequency of 200 cps. Anrep et al. (1927) used a hot wire to show the changes in coronary blood flow during the cardiac cycle. Blood collected in a reservoir displaced air which passed over and cooled a heated thermal element. A somewhat different blood flow velocity transducer was described by Katsura *et al.* (1959); it used two thermistors, one mounted at the tip of a catheter and the other farther up the catheter. One thermistor detected the temperature of the blood, whereas the other was maintained slightly above the blood temperature. A change in flow cooled the hotter thermistor, and more current was sent through it to restore its temperature. A record of the increase in current to maintain the temperature difference was related to blood flow. An improved isothermal blood flowmeter was described by Mellander and Rushmer (1960). The improvement consisted of a spring arrangement which held the probe in the center of the vessel.

One manufacturer[3] has announced the availability of single- and double-lumen medical grade catheters in which thermistors have been embedded. Standard units with nominal resistances of approximately 1250 ohms at body temperature (37°C) can be employed to measure temperatures in blood vessels, ducts, and hollow organs. In addition, the response times listed (0.1 to 4 seconds) are short enough to follow rapid changes in temperature such as those encountered when the thermodilution method is used to determine cardiac output.

2–2. METALLIC STRAIN GAUGES

A more popular use of the resistance change principle is in the detection of a small mechanical displacement from which the force producing the displacement can be determined directly. Tomlinson (1876–1877) found that when conducting wires were stretched the length increased and the diameter decreased and that these dimension changes were effective in increasing the resistance. The opposite situation obtains when conductors are compressed. Resistance elements constructed from specially prepared alloys, which change their resistance more than an amount attributable to elongation or alteration in cross-sectional area, are called strain gauges. Although virtually any metallic conductor can be used as a strain gauge, highly desirable

[3] Victory Engineering Corp., Springfield Ave., Springfield, N. J.

characteristics for the material are (a) a high resistance-elongation coefficient, (b) a low value of resistance change and dimension change per unit change in temperature, and (c) a high sensitivity to strain in the direction measured and a low sensitivity to perpendicular strain.

Two types of strain gauge are in popular use. One is the bonded gauge (Fig. 2–4), in which the resistance element is cemented to a backing approximately the size of a postage stamp.[4] In the other type (unbonded) the resistance wire is stretched between supporting members. The bonded gauge was patented by Simmonds (1942). With both types the deformation to be measured is coupled to the strain gauge element so that tension in the resistance wire is altered.

Strain gauges are usually made of wire approximately 0.001 inch in diameter. The term customarily employed to denote the change in resistance of the strain gauge material when stretched is the gauge factor,

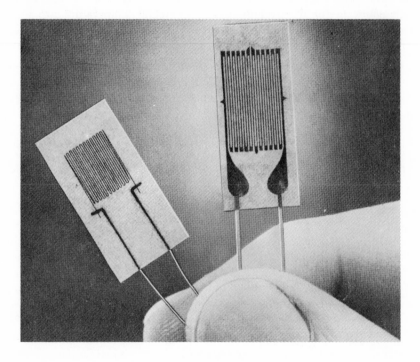

Figure 2–4. Bonded strain gauges. (Courtesy of BLH Electronics, Inc., a subsidiary of Baldwin-Lima-Hamilton Corporation, Waltham, Mass.)

[4]The methods of attaching strain gauges are described in *Bulletin* 4311A, Baldwin-Lima-Hamilton Corp., Waltham Mass.

defined as the fractional change in resistance divided by the fractional change in length; that is,

$$G = \frac{\Delta R/R}{\Delta L/L}$$

where R and L are the resistance and the length, respectively. Although this ratio was discussed by Tomlinson, the term gauge factor is of more recent origin.

The gauge factors of various materials are shown in Table 2-2. From these data it can be seen that the gauge factor of most metals is approximately 2.0 whereas that of silicon is 60 times larger. For silicon the gauge factor depends entirely on the method of preparation and can be higher or lower than that shown; however, the slightly higher temperature coefficient often makes it difficult to take advantage of the high gauge factor if extremes in environmental temperature are to be encountered. In addition to the change in resistivity, Sanchez (1961) reported a slight decrease in gauge factor with increasing temperature.

Table 2-2   **Characteristic of Strain Gauge Materials** [*]

Material	Gauge Factor G	Temperature Coefficient[†] (ohms/ohm/°C)
Advance	2.1	0.00002 (25°C)
Constantan	2.0	0.000002 (25°C)
Isoelastic	3.5	0.00047
Manganin	0.47	0.0000 (25°C)
Monel	1.9	0.002
Nichrome	2.5	0.0004
Nickel	12.1 to -20	0.006
Phosphor bronze	1.9	0.003
Platinum	6.0	0.003
Silicon	120	0.005–0.007 (25°C)

[*]From LeGette (1958), Mason and Thurston (1957), Smith (1954), and Sanchez (1961); see also: *Shock and Vibration Handbook*, C. M. Harris and C. E. Crede, Eds., McGraw-Hill, New York, 1961, Vol. 1, Table 16.5.

[†]Values are for 20°C unless stated otherwise.

In physiologic language the strain gauge is an isometric device, permitting measurement of only small displacements. The extension permissible is dependent on the material from which the strain gauge is made and can be calculated from the following expression:

$$\frac{\Delta L}{L} = \frac{f}{E},$$

where f is the tensile strength of the material, and E is Young's modulus.

Table 2-3   Mechanical Characteristics of Strain Gauge Materials

Material	Ultimate Tensile Strength (f) (psi = force/area $\times 10^3$)	Young's Modulus (E) (psi $\times 10^6$)	Reference
Constantan	60–125	24	International Nickel Co.
Isoelastic	85–155	26	International Nickel Co.
"R" Monel	85–100	26	International Nickel Co.
Nichrome	100–200	27	Driver Harris Co.
Nickel	60–135	30	Wilbur B. Driver Co.
Phosphor Bronze	130	16	International Nickel Co.
Platinum	50–100	22	Wilbur B. Driver Co.
Silicon (P)	90	27	Kulite Semiconductor Prods.
479 (Pt-Rh)	200–300	34	Sigmund Cohn

Table 2–3 lists typical values for Young's modulus and the tensile strengths for various materials. If large displacements are to be measured, their amplitudes must be reduced by suitable mechanical transformation.

Strain gauge elements are small and stiff; these characteristics together yield a rapid response time. In practice, the speed of response is more often determined by the device to which the strain gauge is affixed. The resistance of strain gauges is relatively low, ranging from about 100 to 2000 ohms. The resistance change is small with extension. By combining the expressions for length and gauge factor we can express the change in resistance as follows:

$$\frac{\Delta R}{R} = \frac{Gf}{E}.$$

The values for Young's modulus of elasticity E and the safe tensile stress f given in Table 2–3 can be used to calculate the maximum extension and resistance change expected. In practice, however, the change in resistance produced by the maximum safe extension is usually less than 1%.

Because temperature errors may be encountered, the use of a single strain gauge element is uncommon. To reduce temperature errors pairs of strain gauges are usually employed in a bridge circuit, with strains in the opposite directions applied to adjacent arms of the bridge, as shown in Fig. 2–5a. When strain gauges are employed in double pairs, strain in the

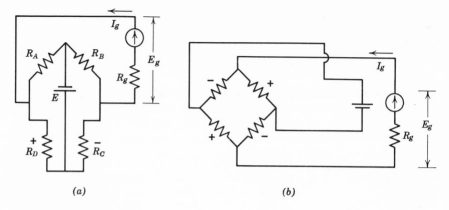

(a)   (b)

Figure 2–5. Strain gauge bridge circuits: (a) two strain gauge elements; (b) four strain gauge elements.

same direction is applied to diagonal arms of the bridge, as shown in Fig. 2–5b. If a direct voltage is employed to energize the bridge, a galvanometer of resistance R_g is used, and the change in resistance of each gauge (ΔR) is small with respect to R ($= R_A = R_B = R_C = R_D$); the galvanometer current I_g for an applied strain is given by the following expression:

$$I_g = \frac{\Delta R}{R} \left(\frac{E}{R + R_g} \right).$$

If, instead of a galvanometer, an a-c or d-c voltage-indicating device of very high-resistance is employed in a bridge with two active strain gauges, as shown in Fig. 2–5a, the voltage obtained (E_g) for an applied strain is

$$E_g = E \frac{(\Delta R)}{2R}.$$

When two active strain gauges are employed, as indicated above, temperature compensation is achieved. With four active gauges the voltage obtained is doubled. With either two or four strain gauges, alternating or direct current can be employed to energize the bridge, and signals in the low millivolt range are obtained in typical applications.

The strain gauge is frequently used in biomedical studies. One of the earliest applications appears to have been made by Grundfest and Hay (1945) who mounted one on a stiff lever to create a nearly isometric myograph. Strain gauge elements were used by Lambert (1947) to construct a transducer in which the motion of a stiff diaphragm exposed to blood pressure was detected to obtain transduction of this physiological event. Many commercially available blood pressure transducers operate on this principle.

Physiologists have long been concerned with the force of contraction of cardiac muscle. To measure this parameter of cardiac function on an excised papillary muscle, Garb (1951) developed and employed a strain gauge myograph. Boniface et al. (1953) devised an ingenious strain gauge arch (Fig. 2–6a) which, when sutured to the wall of the left or right ventricle, (Fig. 2–6b), provided an *in situ* means of continuously recording the

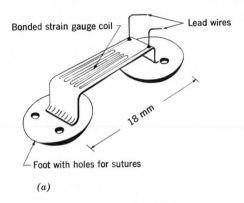

(a)

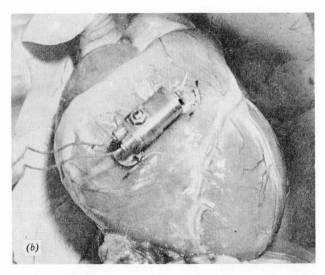

(b)

Figure 2–6. Strain gauge transducers for the measurement of contractile force of cardiac muscle fibers: (a) strain gauge arch; (b) encapsulated strain gauge arch attached to ventricular wall. [From Brown, *Anesthesia Analgesia Current Res.* **39**: 487–488 (1960).]

force developed by the cardiac fibers between the "feet" of the gauge unit. Encapsulated versions of the strain gauge arch have been permanently implanted in experimental animals to study the response of the heart to imposed workloads and to drugs. A larger transducer for measurement of the same parameter of cardiac activity was described by Cotten (1957). With this device (Fig. 2–7) it is possible to prestress the cardiac muscle fibers to investigate the response to what is called diastolic loading, that is, the effect of an increased stretch to increase the force of contraction. This response is referred to as Starling's law of the heart.

Recognizing the potential of the strain gauge in biomedical studies, one manufacturer[5] has developed a universal transducer (Fig. 2–8) containing strain gauge elements, which, with interchangeable attachments, can be used as a pressure transducer, a sensitive and a stiff myograph. The compatibility of this device with basic strain gauge recording instruments should make it a useful general purpose transducer for events which can be converted to pressure or force.

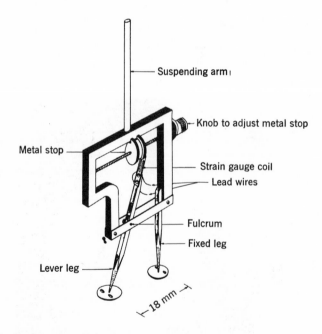

Figure 2–7.   Strain gauge which permits the application of an initial stress to muscle fibers. [From M. deV. Cotten, *Am. J. Physiol.* **189**: 580–586 (1957).]

[5] Statham Instruments, Los Angeles, Calif.

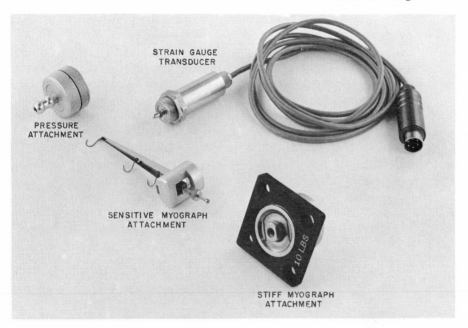

STRAIN GAUGE
TRANSDUCER

PRESSURE
ATTACHMENT

SENSITIVE MYOGRAPH
ATTACHMENT

STIFF MYOGRAPH
ATTACHMENT

Figure 2–8. Universal strain gauge element with attachments. (Courtesy Statham Industries, Los Angeles, Calif.)

In Figs. 2–9 and 2–10 are shown several strain gauge pressure transducers employed in biomedical research. Figures 2–9a illustrates one of the popular strain gauge bridge transducers employed for blood pressure measurement in man and animals; Fig. 2–9b shows a miniature version mounted in a stopcock. Figure 2–9c illustrates a strain gauge pressure-sensing element mounted in the plunger of a 20-cc syringe. To measure pressures in the heart chambers, a catheter-tip strain gauge transducer shown in Fig. 2–10 is available. A unique feature of this device permits the withdrawal of blood from the region where the pressure is being measured.

Recently the semiconductor materials (silicon and germanium) have been employed in transducers. Despite the high thermoresistive coefficient of silicon, Angelakos (1964) was able to construct a practical four-element strain gauge microtransducer, which he affixed to the tip of a No. 7 catheter. Because of the small size of the device the mass was low. The high gauge factor permitted use of a mounting possessing high stiffness. The net result was a frequency response in excess of 2000 cps. This demonstration of a solution to the thermal drift problem will undoubtedly stimulate others to employ semiconductor strain gauge elements.

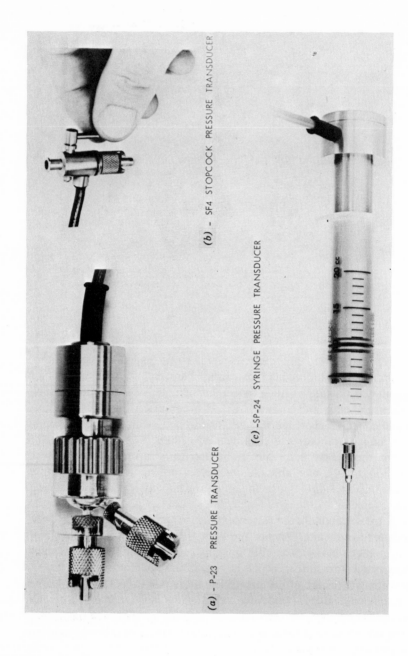

(a) - P-23 PRESSURE TRANSDUCER

(b) - SF4 STOPCOCK PRESSURE TRANSDUCER

(c) -SP-24 SYRINGE PRESSURE TRANSDUCER

Figure 2–9. Strain gauge pressure transducers: (*a*) P-23 pressure transducer; (*b*) SF4 stopcock pressure transducer; (*c*) SP-24 syringe pressure transducer.

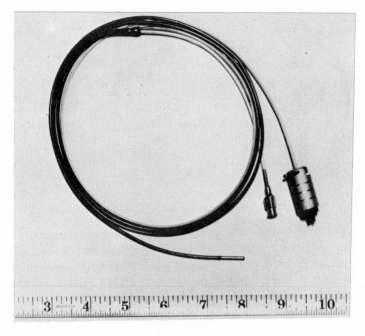

Figure 2–10. Catheter-tip strain gauge pressure transducer. (Courtesy Statham Medical Instruments, Los Angeles, Calif.)

2–3. POTENTIOMETER TRANSDUCERS

Wire-wound or carbon rotary or rectilinear potentiometers can be employed as high-efficiency transducers to detect movement when the moving object can develop a moderate force and when the movement is not rapid. Although there are few physiological applications of this type of transducer at present, the unusually high efficiency attainable will no doubt encourage wider application. Respiration was detected by Adams (1962), who measured changes in thoracic circumference by connecting a rotary potentiometer to a chest band on a monkey. Geddes et al. (1961) converted the rotation of a spirometer pulley to an electrical signal by using a low-torque potentiometer (Fig. 2–11). A device for recording the contraction of skeletal muscle *in situ* was also described by Geddes et al. (1966). In this transducer (Fig. 2–12), a low-torque potentiometer serves as the pivot for the caliper arms, which embrace the belly of the muscle. Contraction of the muscle causes the arms to be driven apart, and their motion is measured by the potentiometer.

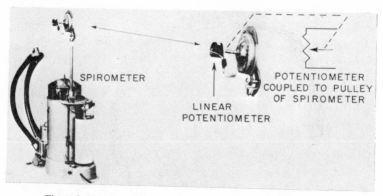

Figure 2–11.   Potentiometer transducer applied to a spirometer.

A truly isotonic myograph for slowly contracting muscles could be constructed by passing a cord over a pulley mounted on the shaft of a low-torque potentiometer. One end of the cord could be connected to the muscle, the other to a weight. Contraction of the muscle would move the same weight through a height measured by the rotation of the pulley.

As previously stated, the unusually attractive feature of the potentiometer transducer is its high efficiency. With a large voltage applied across the potentiometer, the voltage appearing between the moving contact and one end terminal is related to the position of the moving contact. The amount of voltage that can be applied is limited by the wattage rating of the resistance element. Linear, logarithmic, sine, cosine, etc., resistances proportional to rotation are available. Rotary units are available with 360-degree rotations, and rectilinear models can be obtained with strokes from a fraction of an inch up to almost 1 foot. With the rectilinear models a resistance-motion linearity of 1 to 2% is attainable. If the resistance element

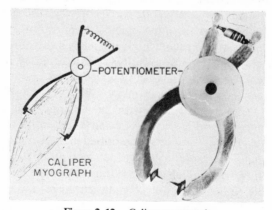

Figure 2–12.   Caliper myograph.

is a carbon film, the output is continuously related to the movement of the sliding contact. If the resistance element is wire-wound, the output versus movement is stepped; that is, the voltage changes abruptly with movement of the sliding contact as it passes from one wire to the next. With high-resistance units the number of wires is large and the steps are fine.

The force required to move the sliding contact depends on the design of the potentiometer. Between 0.2 and 0.5 ounce inch is needed to move low-torque rotary potentiometers, compared to 0.5 to 6 ounce inches for conventional potentiometers. The starting torque is slightly higher than the running torque.

In practical application the response time of a potentiometer transducer is difficult to describe quantitatively because it is intimately related to the mass, elasticity, and damping of the member to which the device is coupled. Nunn (1959) quoted a frequency response of up to 4 cps for a potentiometer coupled to a Bourdon tube. In the experience of the authors, potentiometric transducers can function at high efficiency for events which change at rate less than a few cycles per second.

2–4. MAGNETORESISTIVE TRANSDUCERS

Many substances exhibit a change in resistivity when exposed to a magnetic field. For example, most metals increase their resistivity with increasing field strength; with ferromagnetic metals the resistivity decreases. The magnetoresistive effect is small in most metals. For example, the resistivity of copper is increased by only 0.25% when exposed to a field of 200 kilogauss. When bismuth is exposed to a magnetic field, however, a considerable increase in resistivity occurs. At room temperature a field of 20 kilogauss doubles the resistivity. If the temperature is lowered, the effect is much more pronounced. If the same field is presented to bismuth at the temperature of liquid air, the resistivity is multiplied by 250. The relationship of increase in resistivity with increasing magnetic field strength for 0 and − 50°C is shown in Fig. 2–13.

The phenomenon of resistivity change with a change in magnetic field has been employed in detectors for field strength. It was used by Hampel (1941) in a blood pressure transducer. On an elastic diaphragm exposed to blood pressure was mounted a double resistance coil, one half of which entered a field while the other half moved out of the field when the diaphragm was deformed. Thus the two coils became resistors that varied in response to pressure. A record of the variation in resistance, as measured by a Wheatstone bridge and galvanometer, reproduced the blood pressure wave. A similar method was employed by Holzer (1940), who constructed a myograph in which four coils (two of copper and two of bismuth) were

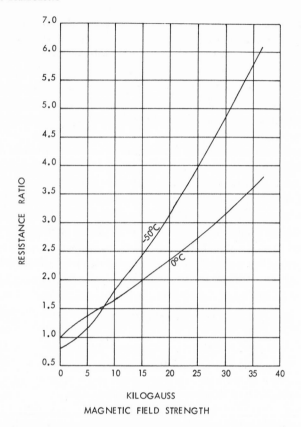

Figure 2–13. The effect of magnetic field intensity on the resistance of Bismuth. (Redrawn from data by Graetz, Handbuch der Elektrizität, 1920).

employed in a bridge circuit. The coils were mounted on a tube and connected so that with movement the bismuth coils were pulled out of the magnetic field. The bismuth coils constituted one diagonal pair of the bridge resistors; the copper coils, the other. The stiffness of the system and the strength of the magnetic field combined to yield a rapid response time and a high efficiency. To illustrate these characteristics, Holzer recorded the twitch of a frog gastrocnemius muscle.

2–5. THE HALL EFFECT

The Hall effect, discovered in 1879, is another interesting phenomenon associated with conductors exposed to magnetic fields. It cannot be better described than in Hall's own words: "If the current of electricity in a fixed conductor is itself attracted by a magnet, the current should be drawn to one side of the wire and therefore the resistance experienced should be increased." With this as his thesis, Hall proceeded to test the theory experimentally, using at first a thick conductor and finally a strip of gold leaf. Success rewarded his efforts, and he concluded, "It is perhaps allowable to speak of the action of the magnet as setting up in the strip of gold leaf a new electromotive force at right angles to the primary electromotive force."

To understand the nature of the Hall effect, consider a thin rectangular film of conducting material equipped with four electrodes, two at the ends (M, N) and two on the middle of the sides (P, Q). When current is led into and out of electrodes M and N, as shown in Fig. 2–14, there will be no potential E measured between the side electrodes P and Q. If a magnetic field B is caused to pass through the conducting film at right angles to the plane of the film, the moving charges will be deflected toward the top or bottom of the film, depending on the directions of the field and current. Deflection of the charge carriers causes a potential to appear across electrodes P and Q, the magnitude and polarity of which depend on the direction and intensity of the magnetic field, the current, the type of charge carrier, and the dimensions of the film. The usual form of the relationship is

$$E = KIB/t,$$

where E = the Hall voltage,
  I = the current in amperes through the film,
  B = the field strength in gauss,
and t = the thickness of the film in centimeters.

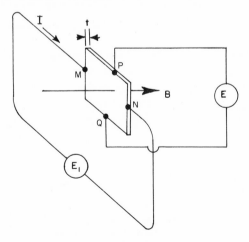

Figure 2–14. The Hall effect.

The Hall coefficient K depends on the material and temperature. It is small for most metals; the constants for bismuth, tellurium, and silicon, however, are approximately one hundred thousand times larger. N-type germanium, indium antimonide and indium arsenide Hall devices are employed to obtain high outputs (Star, 1963), and are most frequently in Hall effect detectors for a-c or d-c magnetic fields. The outputs available are in the range of millivolts per kilogauss for typical models with rated current. Although a linear voltage-field strength relationship can be obtained, with some materials the linearity is poor when low-intensity fields are used; with other materials the reverse is true. In addition, although it would appear that with a given field B the Hall voltage can be increased by decreasing the thickness of the film t and increasing the current I, a limit is soon reached at which the current density in the film is such that excessive heat is produced and the film changes its characteristics.

The output impedance of Hall effect generators depends on the resistivity and dimensions of the film. In commercially available probe detectors for magnetic fields it extends from a few to a few hundred ohms.

Figure 2–15 illustrates two typical Hall effect devices produced by one manufacturer.[6] The transverse type is useful for measuring the field strength in a thin gap. The axial device finds application in measuring the field strength inside a coil. The triaxial type contains three Hall devices mounted to be mutually perpendicular and serves for mapping magnetic fields.

Hall effect devices can be used in a variety of ways. Figures 2–16a,b,c illustrate their application in transducers for displacement. In Fig. 2–16a(1) the Hall device occupies the null position; that is, each side is subjected to the same field intensity. Movement of either the magnets or the Hall device will produce a Hall voltage. In Fig. 2–16a(2) a field of varying strength exists between the magnets. The output of the Hall device is dependent on its position in this field. Thus, movement along the direction of the arrow will give rise to an increase in the Hall voltage. In

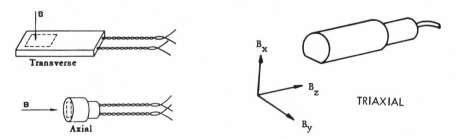

Figure 2–15.   Typical configurations of Hall effect devices.

[6] Bell, Inc., Columbus, Ohio.

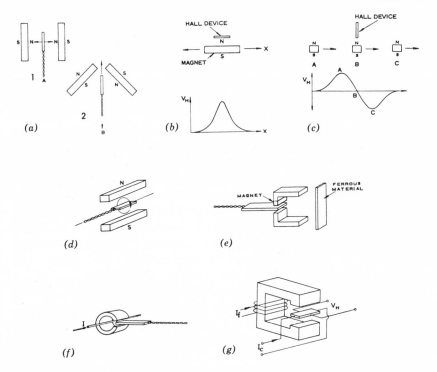

Figure 2–16. Applications of Hall effect devices. (Courtesy Bell, Inc., B56 North Ave., Columbus, Ohio.)

Fig. 2–16*b,c* movement of the magnets past the Hall device produces a position-dependent voltage as shown. Use of the Hall device to detect rotary position is shown in Fig. 2–16*d*. Because the presence of ferromagnetic material alters the magnetic field passing through the Hall device, the assembly shown in Fig. 2–16*e* can serve as a detector for such materials. Figure 2–16*f* indicates how a Hall device can be used to measure alternating or direct current by measurement of the magnetic field surrounding the current-carrying conductor.

Figure 2–16*g* diagrams the full potential of the Hall effect device as a circuit element. In reality, two variables, current and field strength, are related in the operation of the device. The variables may be alternating current or direct current or combinations thereof. The Hall voltage is proportional to the product of the two; thus the device functions as a multiplier.

Hall effect devices have been used relatively little in biomedical studies. They have obvious application in mapping the magnetic field produced by current from externally applied electrodes in studies of electroanesthesia and ventricular defibrillation. It is expected that Hall effect devices will find use in magnetobiology studies such as those reported by Valentinuzzi (1961, 1962) and Barnothy (1964) which describe the effects of magnetic fields on living specimens. Probably the magnetic fields that accompany biological action currents will be detected by Hall effect transducers.

2–6. GRANULAR STRAIN GAUGES

Another type of resistor used for transduction purposes consists of a capsule loosely packed with carbon granules. On one side of the capsule is a fixed electrode, and on the other is a movable one. When a force is applied, the granules are compacted and the resistance is reduced. Such capsules originated with the carbon button telephone transmitter, in which the diaphragm is coupled to the moving electrode. Small movements of the diaphragm change the resistance considerably and result in a high-efficiency conversion of sound pressure to an electrical signal.

In experimental physiology, the carbon button (granule) microphone was one of the first transducers to convert human heart sounds to an electrical signal. In 1895 Hurthle connected one in series with a battery and an inductorium, the secondary of which was connected to electrodes on a muscle attached in turn to a tambour that activated a writing lever. When the heart sounds occurred, the muscle was stimulated and the ensuing muscle twitches were recorded. Simultaneously, the movements of the chambers of the heart were detected and recorded by another tambour placed over the cardiac apex. The record did not illustrate the heart sound frequencies but did identify their temporal location in the cardiac cycle. About the same time Einthoven and Geluk (1894) recorded the heart sounds directly by connecting the carbon button microphone to a capillary electrometer. They were the first to record human, rabbit, and dog phonocardiograms. When electron tube amplifiers became available, the first amplifying stethoscopes used carbon button microphones.

To illustrate how efficient the carbon button microphone is in detecting feeble sounds, it was used by Falls and Rockwood (1923) to detect fetal heart sounds. Because of its high conversion efficiency, it is still employed in telephones today but is infrequently used for research in acoustics because of its inferior frequency response and variable sensitivity. Perhaps the most serious defects in the carbon granule capsule are the inherently high hysteresis and high internal electrical noise, making it an unreliable device for the faithful registration of acoustic events.

Because of its high efficiency the carbon granule capsule still enjoys some popularity in biomedicine for detecting changing events. Using a carbon button in contact with an artery, Waud (1924) and Turner (1928) recorded the human pulse. No amplifier was employed in either study; the carbon button served to drive a recording pen directly in the former study and a string galvanometer in the latter. Gallagher and Grimwood (1953) included it in their indirect blood pressure-measuring system to detect the pulse in the caudal artery of the rat.

A variant of the carbon granule capsule was described by Clynes (1960). This device consisted of a distensible rubber tube filled with graphite. When wrapped around the chest, transduction of the respiratory movements was obtained.

Carbon-packed capsules are characterized by resistances in the hundreds of ohms and exhibit an appreciable and inconstant change in resistance with dimension change. High currents can be passed through them, resulting in high outputs—often sufficient to drive recorders directly. These devices, however, exhibit a poor baseline stability and, on occasion, tend to "freeze"; that is, the granules compact and must be loosened by vibration. If a high-gain system is employed with carbon granule capsules, the no-signal noise is quite high, a factor which caused the carbon button microphone to be abandoned in the early days of broadcasting.

2–7. ELASTIC RESISTORS

By the appropriate addition of conducting material to rubber or to certain plastic materials, it is possible to make a resistor which alters its value in response to strain. The addition of carbon to latex, which is then appropriately cured, produces a rubber with conducting properties which permit its use for the construction of elastic strain gauges. Badamo (1964) reported that one product, S-2086 electrically conducting carbon black loaded Silastic,[7] has been made to have a volume resistivity ranging from 8 to 60 ohm cm. Another manufacturer[8] reported a standard product (UK 3032) with a resistivity of 7 ohm cm. By varying the mixture, resistivities from 7 to 10^{16} ohm cm were obtained. The elongation factor for UK 3032 is given as 2.1. The S-2086 conducting Silastic can be elongated by factors ranging from 1.4 to 2.5; the resistance of this material increases almost as an exponential function of elongation. The manufacturer reports that a 25% elongation more than triples the relaxed resistance. Figure 2–17 illustrates the resistance-elongation characteristic of a piece of this material measured by one of the authors. It shows that linearity is attainable only over a limited range of extension (10 to 20%). Although larger extensions can be tolerated by some conducting elastomers, with others, elongations greater than 25 to 30% result in appreciable resistance hysteresis.

[7] Dow Corning Center for Aid to Medical Research, Midland, Mich.

[8] Minor Rubber Co., Inc., Bloomfield, N. J.

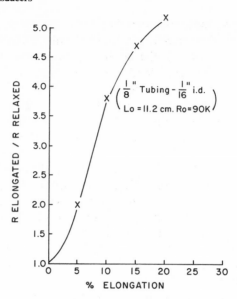

Figure 2–17.   Elastic resistor-resistance versus elongation.

The attractive characteristics of elastic resistors recommend their use for the transduction of events associated with an appreciable dimension change. In practical applications, however, it is frequently difficult to establish a stable electrical contact with the material. Conducting paints, clamps, nuts and bolts have all been employed. One of the authors has had success in making contact with conducting tubing by forcing the ends over short metal rods or tubes that served as electrodes.

2–8. ELECTROLYTIC STRAIN GAUGES

Elastic strain gauges which employ liquid conductors are used to a limited extent in biomedical studies. As far back as the turn of the century Grunbaum (1898) described the first of such devices, an aqueous electrolytic pressure capsule 5 mm in diameter and 12.5 mm in length mounted on the end of a catheter. On the side of the capsule was a thin rubber window carrying an electrode. The other electrode was mounted on the inside wall of the capsule, which was filled with zinc chloride. Pressure applied to the distensible window decreased the interelectrode distance, thereby reducing the resistance between the electrodes. This device was certainly one of the first catheter-tip pressure transducers and must have produced blood pressure records of high fidelity for that time. However, no such records produced by this instrument have been found to date.

Successors to Grunbaum's transducer were described by Schutz (1931) and Wagner (1932). Schutz employed platinum electrodes and a copper sulfate solution as the electrolyte. Wagner's instrument also consisted of a capsule filled with copper sulfate solution mounted at the end of a catheter. Using this device, which exhibited a resonant frequency of approximately 60 cps, he presented some of the earliest electrically transduced records of the pressures in the right ventricles of rabbits.

For some reason the electrolytic strain gauge fell into disuse for many years, being revived by Muller (1942) and Dalla-Torre (1943) to record human digital volume pulses. Their strain gauges consisted of rubber tubing, a fraction of a millimeter in diameter, filled with an electrolyte. The ends of the tubing were plugged by the electrodes. When such tubes are stretched, the length increases and the diameter decreases, thereby raising the resistance appreciably.

Aqueous electrolyte strain gauges are lightweight, easy to make, and inexpensive. They are medium to high in resistance. Muller's units were 0.2 mm in diameter and 5 to 6 cm long. When filled with diluted Electroargol the strain gauge had a resistance of 1 megohm. After an initial elongation the resistance increased nearly linearly with extension over a fairly wide range. Figure 2–18 presents the equation for the resistance increase and the degree of linearity that can be expected. Elongations to 50% of the relaxed length are often used to permit measurement of the large changes in circumference or length experienced by many organs and members. Although a large signal per unit of extension can be obtained, this advantage

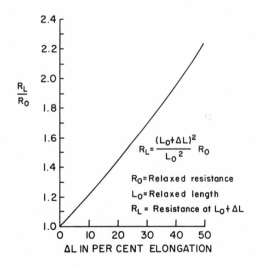

$$R_L = \frac{(L_0 + \Delta L)^2}{L_0{}^2} R_0$$

R_0 = Relaxed resistance

L_0 = Relaxed length

R_L = Resistance at $L_0 + \Delta L$

ΔL IN PER CENT ELONGATION

Figure 2–18.   Electrolytic resistor-resistance versus elongation.

is partly offset by the errors introduced by temperature changes. The temperature coefficient for many aqueous electrolytes is -2% per degree centigrade but can be as high as -10%. Hence temperature compensation is necessary.

An interesting electrolytic resistor strain gauge was described by Waggoner (1965). In this device the electrolyte was an electrode paste contained in a rubber tube. Waggoner reported that the resistance of such gauges depends on the dimensions, and in practice with tubing 0.2 to 3 mm in diameter resistances varying between 1 and 400 kilohms were observed. The change in resistance varied as L^2/V, where L is the length and V the volume of the gauge. A small negative resistance-temperature coefficient was noted. Waggoner reported successful use of these strain gauges for recording respiration, cardiac contraction, kidney volume, and thumb pulse.

Aqueous electrolytic strain gauges usually have a relatively short life because electrolytic decomposition of the electrodes proceeds even when the devices are not in use. When direct current is passed through the element, the lifetime is further reduced. For maximum life, alternating current should be employed for excitation.

2–9. MERCURY STRAIN GAUGE

Whitney (1949) described the construction of strain gauges using small-bore rubber tubing filled with mercury. Like the aqueous electrolytic types, these gauges permit the measurement of small or large changes in elongation. Because they are lightweight, easy to construct, inexpensive, and available commercially,[9] they see considerable service in biomedical studies; for example, Whitney (1949, 1953, 1954) and Greenfield et al. (1963) employed them to measure the volume changes in body segments as blood entered and left the region encircled by the gauge. Rushmer (1955, 1965) measured the changes in circumference, hence the volume changes of the rapidly beating canine left ventricle and aorta, by means of similar gauges. Lawton and Collins (1959) used the mercury strain gauge to measure the pulsatile changes in aortic circumference. Maulsby and Hoff (1962) sutured similar strain gauges to the right ventricles of dogs and continuously measured the dimension changes that reflected the volume changes in that cardiac chamber. Shapiro et al. (1964) encircled the chests of human subjects with mercury-in-rubber gauges to detect the changes in thoracic circumference which accompany respiration.

When mercury is employed in small-bore (approximately 0.5 mm I.D.) elastic tubing, the resistance of typical gauges is in the vicinity of

[9]Parks Electronics Laboratory, Box 35, Beaverton, Ore.

0.02 to 0.20 ohm per centimeter of length. The force necessary to elongate a typical 35-mm gauge 6 mm was given by Lawton and Collins (1959) as 20 grams. The force-extension curve exhibited a slight nonlinearity. Rushmer (1955) noted that good linearity was obtained beyond a small initial extension. He also reported that his gauges performed satisfactorily with extensions up to 100% of the relaxed length.

The change in resistance with elongation can be determined from Fig. 2–18, which was calculated from perfect elasticity and constant-volume considerations, that is, an increase in length results in a corresponding decrease in diameter, the total volume remaining constant. For small extensions the coefficient is approximately 2% increase in resistance for a 1% increase in length. This value was quoted by Whitney, who employed rubber tubing. In a typical application, in which a low voltage was applied to a Wheatstone bridge containing a 3.5-cm gauge, a signal of 0.24 mv was obtained per millimeter change in length per volt applied to the bridge (Lawton, and Collins 1959). Most investigators employ 2 to 6 volts to energize the bridge.

Elsner et al. (1959) described a method of eliminating many of the difficulties encountered in using the mercury strain gauge with direct current. By coupling the gauge to a step-up transformer placed in one arm of an impedance bridge and by connecting balancing resistors to a transformer placed in the adjacent arm, they were able to operate the bridge on alternating current and obtain practical ease in balancing the bridge. The alternating current also permitted the use of conventional R-C coupled or carrier amplifiers to process the signal for ultimate recording. With this system these investigators reported obtaining an overall sensitivity of 1 mm of recorder deflection for 2 microns of extension of a mercury gauge 5 cm in length.

In practical applications a rapid response time is attainable with the mercury strain gauge. Rushmer (1955) reported a value (0 to 100%) of less than 0.01 second with his 35-mm gauges, and Lawton and Collins (1959), by applying a sinusoidal stretching force, carefully measured the frequency response and phase shift of similar gauges at various elongations. They found that the sine wave frequency response curve was essentially 100% to 20 cps, increasing to 110% at approximately 50 cps and reaching 150% at 100 cps. The phase shifts at these frequencies were 10, 25, and 45 degrees, respectively.

Because of its practical features, the mercury strain gauge will see continued application, despite its defects. As is the situation with the aqueous electrolyte strain gauge, temperature changes constitute a source of error in many applications. Although the temperature coefficient of resistivity for mercury is considerably less than that of the copper wires employed with the gauge, Whitney described the need for compensating resistors when mercury strain gauges are employed for peripheral plethysmography on human subjects. In biothermal plethysmographic studies the thermal resistance variation becomes objectionable. Eagan (1961) reported that a 22.5°C change in temperature is equivalent to a 2% change in resistance or a 1% change in length. Honda (1962) stated that a 25°C change in temperature of the mercury is equivalent to a 1% change in length. To compensate for this change he mounted a compensating resistor made of copper wire in a rubber tube adjacent to the mercury strain gauge element. The compensating resistor was connected to the adjacent arm of the bridge. By using alternating current on the bridge and transformer coupling to the gauge and compensating resistor, he was able to adjust the bridge for full compensation for a 25°C temperature change.

A nother factor worthy of attention is the short-term creep reported by Lawton and Collins (1959). However, they felt that this was unimportant in dynamic studies.

Perhaps one of the chief drawbacks to prolonged use of mercury gauges involves the corrosive nature of mercury. Some types of rubber tubing are attacked by mercury, and in nearly every case the electrodes deteriorate after a period of time. Copper, brass, and platinum electrodes have been employed with some success. All who have made mercury strain gauges called attention to the need to use clean mercury, preferably triply distilled.

Although latex rubber tubing was employed in the early gauges, silicone rubbers are now universally employed. Whitney in the United Kingdom employed No. 1 surgical drainage tubing[10] (0.7-mm bore, 0.7-mm wall) and latex tubing[10] (0.5-mm bore, 0.8-mm wall). In the United States silicone[11] tubing can be readily obtained.

REFERENCES

Adams, R. 1962. Personal communication. School of Aerospace Medicine, Brooks AFB, Texas.

Angelakos, E. T. 1964. Semiconductor pressure microtransducers for measuring velocity and acceleration of intra-ventricular pressures. *Am. J. Med. Electron.* **3**: 260–270.

Anrep, C. V., E. W. H. Cruickshank, A. C. Downing, and A. S. Rau. 1927. The coronary circulation in relation to the cardiac cycle. *J. Physiol.* **14**: 111–134.

Badamo, D. J. 1964. The silicones as bioengineering materials. *Proc. 17th Ann. Conf. Eng. Biol. Med.* Washington, D. C., McGregor and Werner, 129 pp.

Barnothy, M. 1964. *Biological Effects of Magnetic Fields.* New York, Plenum Press, 324 pp.

Boniface, K. H., D. J. Brodie, and R. P. Walton 1953. Resistance strain gauge arches for direct measurement of heart contractile force in animals. *Proc. Soc. Exp. Biol. Med.* **84**: 263–266.

[10]Dunlop Special Products, England.

[11]Dow Corning Center for Aid to Medical Research, Midland, Mich.; Huntingdon Rubber Mills, Box 70, Portland, Ore.; Becton Dickinson (Vivosil 7002–012), Rutherford, N. J.

Bramwell, J. C., A. V. Hill, and B. A. McSwinney. 1923. The velocity of the pulse wave in man. *Heart.* **10**: 233–256.

Brown, J. M. 1960. Anesthesia and the contractile force of the heart. *Curr. Res. in Anesth. Analg.* **39**: 487–498.

Clynes, M. 1960. Respiratory control of heart rate. *IRE Trans. Med. Electron.* ME-7: 2–14.

Cornwall, J. B. 1965. The matching and linearising of thermistor probes. *World Med. Electron.* **3**: 233–234.

Cotten, M. de V., and H. M. Maling. 1957. Relationships among stroke work, contractile force and fiber length changes in ventricular function. *Am. J. Physiol.* **189**: 580–586.

Dalla-Torre, L. 1943. Utilization d'une nouvelle méthode pour l'inrégistrement du sphygmogramme des artères digitales. *Helv. Physiol. Pharmacol. Acta.* **1**: C14–15.

Eagan, C. J. 1961. The mercury gauge method of digital plethysmography. U.S.A.F. Tech. Note AAL-TN-60-15 (Feb. 1961), TN,60-16 (Mar. 1961), TN-60-17 (Feb. 1961). Alaskan Air Command.

Einthoven, W., and M. A. Geluk. 1894: Die Registreirung der Herstöne. *Arch. Ges. Physiol.* **57**:617–639.

Elsner, R. W., C. H. Eagan, and S. Andersen. 1959. Impedance matching circuit for mercury strain gauge. *J. Appl. Physiol.* **14**: 871–872.

Falls, F. H., and A. C. Rockwood. 1923. Use of microphone stethoscope in demonstration of fatal heart sounds. *J. Am. Med. Assoc.* **81**: 1683–1684.

Fleming, D. G. 1958. Precautions in the physiological application of thermistors. *J. Appl. Physiol.* **13**: 529–530.

Gallagher, D. J. A., and L. H. Grimwood. 1953. A simple method for measuring blood pressure in the rat tail. J. Physiol. **121**: 163–166.

Garb, S. 1951. The effects of potassium, ammonium, calcium, strontium, and magnesium on the electrogram and myogram of mammalian heart muscle. *J. Pharmacol. Exp. Therap.* **101**: 317–326.

Geddes, L. A., H. E. Hoff, A. G. Moore, and M. Hinds. 1966. An electrical caliper myograph. Am. J. Pharm. Educ. **30**: 209–211.

Geddes, L. A., H. E. Hoff, and W. A. Spencer. 1961. The Center for Vital Studies—A new laboratory for the study of bodily functions in man. *IRE Trans. Bio-Med. Electron.* **BME-8**: 33–45.

Greenfield, A. D. M., R. J. Whitney, and J. F. Mowbray. 1963. Methods for the investigation of peripheral blood flow. *Brit. Med. Bull.* **19**: 101–109.

Grunbaum, O. F. F. 1898. On a new method of recording alternations in blood pressure. *J. Physiol.* **22**: 49–50.

Grundfest, H., and J. J. Hay. 1945. A strain gauge recorder for physiological volume, pressure and deformation measurements. *Science* **101**: 255–256.

Hall, E. H. 1879. On a new action of the magnet on electric currents. *Am. J. Math.* **2**: 287–292.

Hampel, A. 1941. Elektrisches Transmissionmanometer auf der Grundlage elektrischer Widerstandsänderungen des Wismuts im Magnetfeld. *Arch. Ges. Physiol.* **244**: 171–175.

Hill, A. V. 1920–1921a. An electrical pulse recorder. *J. Physiol.* **54**: lii–liii.

Hill A. V. 1920–1921b. The meaning of records made with the hot wire sphygmograph. *J. Physiol.* **54** cxvii–cxix.

Holzer, W. 1940. Über die Anwendung des galvano-magnetischen Longitudinal-effektes des Wismuts zur elektrischen Fernübertragung von Bewegungsvorgängen. *Arch. Ges. Physiol.* **244**: 176–180.

Honda, N. 1962. Temperature compensation for mercury strain gauge used in plethysmography. *J. Appl. Physiol.* **17**: 572–574.

Hurthle, K. 1895. Beiträge zur Hämodynamik. *Arch. Ges. Physiol.* **60**: 263–290.

Katsura, S., R. Weiss, D. Baker, and R. F. Rushmer. 1959. Isothmeral blood flow velocity probe. *IRE Trans. Med. Electron.* **ME-8**: 283–285.

Lambert, E. H., and E. H. Wood. 1947. The use of resistance wire strain gauge monometer to measure intra-arterial pressure. *Proc. Soc. Exp. Biol. Med.* **64**: 186–190.

Lamson, P. D., and B. H. Robbins. 1928. Thermal conductivity methods of gas analysis in the study of pharmacological problems. *J. Pharm. Exp. Therap.* **34**: 325–331.

Lawton, R. W., and C. C. Collins. 1959. Calibration of an aortic circumference gauge. *Appl. Physiol.* **14**: 465–467.

Ledig, P. C., and R. S. Lyman. 1927. An adaptation of the thermal conductivity method to the analysis of respiratory gases. *J. Clin. Invest.* **4**: 494–565.

Le Gette, M. A. 1958. Strain gauge principles. *Instr. Automation* **31**: 447–449.

Mason, W. P., and R. N. Thurston. 1957. Use of piezoresistive materials in the measurement of displacement, force and torque. *J. Acousti. Soc. Am.* **29**: 1096–1101.

Maulsby, R. L., and H. E. Hoff. 1962. Hypotensive mechanisms of pulmonary insufflation in dogs. *Am. J. Physiol.* **202**: 505–509.

Mellander, S., and R. F. Rushmer. 1960. Venous blood flow recorded with an isothermal flowmeter. *Acta Physiol. Scand.* **43**: 13–19.

Muller, A. 1942. Über die Pulsform und Wellengeschwindigkeit in den Fingerarterien. *Arch. Krieslaufforsch* **11**: 198–206.

Nunn, H. E. 1959. A guide to static pressure transducers that have a diaphragm, bellows or Bourdon pressure cell. *Prod. Eng.* **30**: 48–49.

Rein, H., A. A. Hampel, and W. A. Heinemann. 1940. Photoelektrische Transmissionmanometer zur Blutdruckschreibung. *Arch. ges. Physiol.* **243**: 329–335.

Rushmer, R. F. 1965. Pressure circumference relations in the left ventricle. *Am. J. Physiol.* **186**: 115–121.

Rushmer, R. F. 1955a. Pressure circumference relations in the aorta. *Am. J. Physiol.* **183**: 545–549.

Rushmer, R. F. 1955b. Length-circumference relations of the left ventricle. *Circ. Res.* **3**: 639–644.

Sanchez, J. C. 1961. Semiconductor strain gauges—a state of the art summary. *Str. Gauge Readings.* **4**: 3–16.

Schutz, E. 1931. Konstruktion einer manometrischen Sonde mit elektrisher Transmission. *Z. Biol.* **91**: 515–521.

Shapiro, A., H. D. Cohen, E. Maher, and W. J. McAveney. 1964. On-line analog computation of volume of respired air. *Proc. 17th Ann. Conf. Eng. Med. Biol.* Washington D. C., McGregor and Werner, 129 pp.

Simmonds, E. E. 1942. U. S. Pat. 2,292,549.

Simons, D. G. 1962. Personal communication. School of Aerospace Medicine, Brooks AFB, Texas.

Smith, C. S. 1954. Piezoresistive effect of germanium and silicon. *Phys. Rev.* **94**: 42–49.

Star, J. 1963. Hall effect transducers. *Instr. Control Systems* **36**: 113–116.

Swanson, C. A., and A. C. Emslie. 1954. Low temperature electronics. *Proc. IRE* **42**: 402–413.

Tomlinson, H. 1876–1877. On the increase in resistance to the passage of an electric current produced on stretching. *Proc. Roy. Soc. (London)* **25**: 451–453.

Tucker, W. S. and E. T. Paris. 1921. A selective hot-wire microphone. *Phil. Trans. Roy. Soc. London Ser. A* **221A**: 389–430.

Turner, R. H. 1928. A sphygmograph using a carbon grain microphone and the string galvanometer. *Bull. Johns Hopkins Hosp.* **43**: 2–13.

Valentinuzzi, M. 1961. Magnetobiology. Los Angeles, Calif., North American Aviation, 74 pp.

Valentinuzzi, M. 1962. A theory of magnetic growth inhibition. Chicago, Ill., Committee on Math. Biol., 58 pp.

Van Dover, J. and N. F. Bechtold. 1960. Survey of thermistor characteristics. *Electronics* **33**: 58–60.

Victory Engineering Corp., Union, New Jersey. 1955. *Thermistor Data Book.*

Waggoner, W. C. 1965. High-impedance elastic force gauge. *A. J. Med. Electron.* **4**: 175–177.

Wagner, R. 1932. Die Beeinflussung des Druckablaufes in verschiedenen Herzabschnitten bei wechselnden Bedingungen der Herztätigkeit. *Z. Biol.* **92**: 55–86.

Waud, R. A. 1924. An electric polygraph. *J. Am. Med Assoc.* **82**: 1203.

Whitney, R. J. 1949. The measurement of changes in human limb-volume by means of a mercury-in-rubber strain gauge. *J. Physiol.* **109**: 5P-6P.

Whitney, R. J. 1953, 1954. The measurement of volume changes in human limbs. *J. Physiol.* 1953, **121**: 1–27; 1954, **125**: 1–24.

3

Mechano-Electronic Transducer Tube

The mechano-electronic transducer tube (RCA 5734) converts mechanical displacement to a current change. This ingenious device, developed originally by Olson (1947) for use in phonograph pickups and microphones and illustrated in Figs. 3–1 and 3–2, is a triode vacuum tube in which the protruding anode is movable. Electron emission from the heated cathode is attracted to the anode and produces a current flow. When deflected, the protruding anode pin moves either closer to or farther away from the cathode, resulting in an increase or a decrease in anode current.

Because of its high conversion efficiency in detecting small mechanical displacements, this device is sensitive to thermal gradients and sometimes difficult to employ. With careful design these difficulties can be overcome, and this transducer therefore enjoys some popularity in biomedical studies. It was an early favorite of those who sought a myograph with a short response time. Among them was Curtis (1949), who used it to record the development of tension in isolated turtle cardiac muscle fibers, thereby establishing the precise relationship between the ECG and muscular contraction. The time relations of the development of tension in frog and toad muscle fibers were investigated by Hill (1951), who employed a 5734 transducer tube in a system with a natural resonant frequency of 2800 cps. Hakansson (1957), in studies that investigated the time relationship between the action potential and the development of tension in frog skeletal muscle, was able to obtain a system resonant frequency of 800 cps with a 5734 transducer. In these studies of muscular contraction, the existence of such high resonant frequencies indicates that the rise times were short and that the tension-time records were faithfully reproduced.

Talbot et al. (1951) in an exhaustive investigation listed the characteristics of the 5734 transducer tube and described its use in ballistocardiography and in the construction of an isometric myograph. Brown et al. (1952), like Talbot, coupled the protruding pin to a ballistocardiograph table to derive

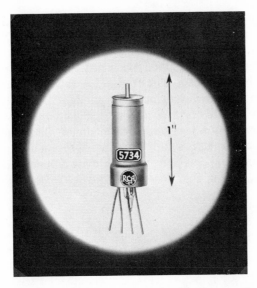

Figure 3–1. RCA 5734 mechano-electronic transducer tube. (Courtesy Radio Corporation of America, Harrison, N.J.)

an electrical signal from the movements of the body produced by cardiac action. Curtis (1949) and Clamann (1951) detected peripheral pulses by means of the 5734 tube. Silverman (1950) employed it to sense the deflection of a diaphragm exposed to small air pressure changes in his pneumotachograph. Also with the 5734, Arnott et al. (1951), Ainsworth and Eveleigh (1954), and Clemedson et al. (1959) detected the deflection of a small

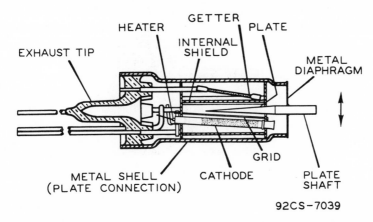

92CS–7039

Figure 3–2. RCA 5734 mechano-electronic transducer tube. (Courtesy of Radio Corporation of America, Harrison, N.J.)

diaphragm exposed to pressure. High sensitivity and rapidity of response were obtained in all these studies. Brecher and Praglin (1953) chose the 5734 to construct a rapidly responding flowmeter in which a bristle connected to the protruding anode was deflected in proportion to the velocity of the blood stream. The transducer tube was incorporated into an ultrasensitive isometric myograph by Ranney (1954) for use on extracted muscle fibers. A similar device is now available commercially.[1]

Because the maximum permissible deflection of the protruding anode is only ± 0.5 degree, precaution must be taken to prevent unexpected transient forces from exceeding this safe limit. A type of mounting suitable for myography is shown in Fig. 3–3. With this holder the protruding anode

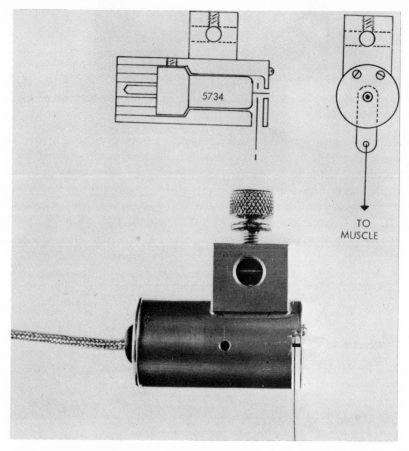

Figure 3–3. Mechano-electronic transducer tube used as a myograph.

[1] W. H. Niclas, 148–25, 89th Ave., Jamaica, N.Y.

cannot exceed the safe operating range. The 5734 is mounted in a brass rod which is drilled down the center and milled on the side to permit access to the protruding anode pin. To the end of the holder is screwed a plate with a hole (0.047 inch), mounted concentric with the anode pin. This diameter of hole prevents the anode from exceeding the maximum permissible deflection. Deflection of the anode pin is achieved by placing a link of metal over the pin as shown. A small V-shaped notch prevents the link from changing position on the anode pin. With this arrangement (which compromises the sensitivity of the tube slightly), the maximum load that can be applied safely is about 50 grams.

The outstanding characteristics of the mechano-electronic transducer tube are its high conversion efficiency and rapidity of response. The manufacturer gives a figure of ± 20 volts for a deflection of ± 0.5 degree (Fig. 3–4a) and a natural resonant frequency of 12,000 cps. The moment of inertia of the movable anode is 3.4 mg cm², and the deflection compliance is 0.075 degree/gm cm. The small moment of inertia and high resonant frequency make the device very useful for the measurement of rapidly changing forces of low intensity.

Various circuits have been employed with the 5734 transducer. The possible configurations are restricted partly by the electrode connections already present in the device. Although there is access to the anode, grid, cathode, and heater terminals, the movable anode terminal is connected to the metallic case of the transducer tube. In practice, safe operation requires that the case be grounded, a precaution that in turn necessitates the use of a floating power supply (Fig. 3–5a). The voltage of this supply is in part dictated by the maximum ratings of the device: 5 ma maximum plate current and 90 volts maximum heater-cathode voltage. Usually the grid is connected to the cathode, and the device functions as a deflectable anode diode. The manufacturer suggests the use of a 300-volt anode supply with a 75,000-ohm anode load resistor. With this load resistor [Fig. 3–4b (1)] there occurs a ± 20-volt change across the anode resistor for a deflection of the anode of ± 28 minutes.

Although these conditions provide a satisfactory mode of operation, they require that the cathode be at a large voltage negative with respect to the grounded anode and that a filament supply connected to a voltage not greater than 90 volts with respect to the cathode be available. This requirement often creates practical difficulties since most filament supplies are at ground potential. If such a filament supply is to be used, it is advisable to operate the transducer tube with a 150-volt anode-cathode supply. Under these conditions the operating characteristics are as shown in Fig. 3–4b (2). This mode of operation underrates the transducer tube, reduces the heat production, prolongs the life, and lowers the deflection sensitivity by 60%.

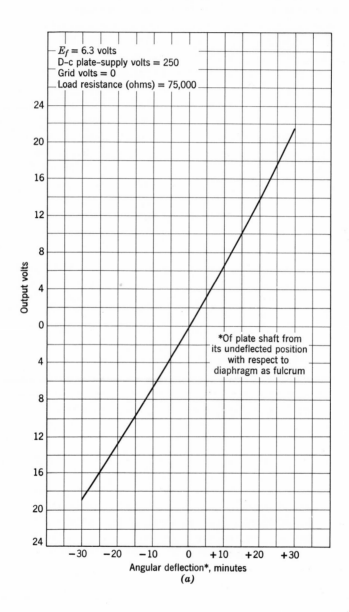

Figure 3–4. Characteristics of RCA 5734. (Courtesy Radio Corporation of America, Harrison, N.J.)

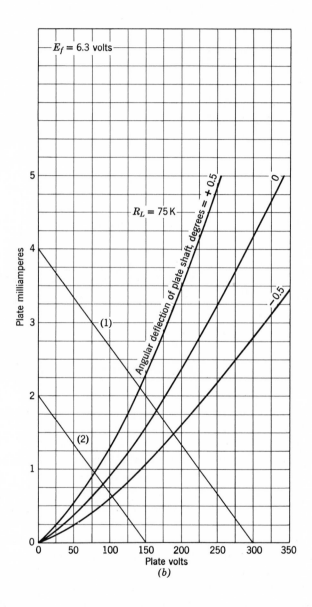

Figure 3-4. (*continued*)

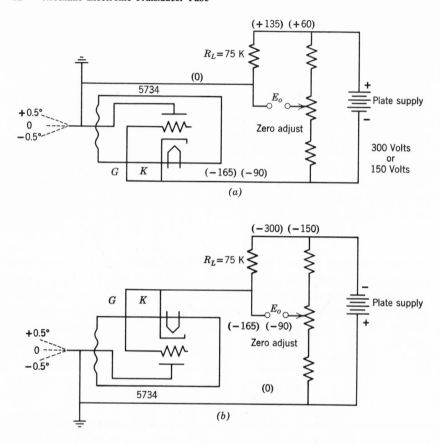

Figure 3–5. Circuits for use with the RCA 5734 transducer tube: (*a*) anode load; (*b*) cathode load.

Although a 90-volt heater-cathode potential is permissible, it is advisable to maintain the smallest possible heater-cathode voltage.

In the circuit just described (Fig. 3–5*a*) one side of the output E_o is at ground potential but the power supply must be free of any connection to ground. An alternative method of operating the RCA 5734 is shown in Fig. 3–5*b*. In this circuit the 75,000-ohm resistor is placed in the cathode circuit. This configuration permits grounding the movable anode and the positive side of the power supply. Under these conditions the output E_o is referenced to approximately 165 volts below ground potential if a 300-volt anode supply is used and to 90 volts below ground potential for a 150-volt anode supply.

With the circuit shown in Fig. 3–5*b*, it is also necessary to maintain a potential difference of less than 90 volts between cathode and heater. If an unreferenced heater supply is available, the cathode can be connected to it; but if the heater supply is connected to ground, it is necessary to reduce the anode supply to 150 volts to avoid exceeding the maximum heater-cathode rating of the tube.

As mentioned previously, the stability of the RCA 5734 is increased if it is operated with reduced plate voltage and current. An ingenious method of achieving this goal and obtaining a signal that is more easily amplified than that produced by the normal mode of operation was described by Clemedson et al. (1959), who used the transducer tube as an oscillator by connecting a tuned circuit to the grid and a feedback winding to the plate. Thus, with no deflection of the anode pin, the circuit provided a high-frequency sinusoidal voltage across the feedback coil in the plate circuit. Deflection of the anode pin by blood pressure applied to the stiff membrane changed the tube parameters (μ, r_p, g_m) and hence the feedback in the circuit, which in turn altered the amplitude of the high-frequency sinusoidal voltage across the feedback winding. Thus the change in amplitude of the high-frequency voltage was proportional to pressure.

In commenting on the characteristics of the circuit, Clemedson and his associates reported that the plate voltage and current were 65 volts and 300 μa, respectively. When coupled to the membrane used to measure blood pressure, it was possible to detect a movement as small as 10^{-5} mm. The total volume displacement of the blood pressure transducer was 0.33 $\times$ 10^{-2} mm^3/100 mm Hg.

REFERENCES

Ainsworth, M., and J. W. Eveleigh. 1954. A simple electromanometer. *J. Sci. Instr.* **31**: 471–472.

Arnott, W. M., G. Cumming, P. Davison, and A. C. Pincock. 1951. A high-frequency mechano-electronic transducer manometer. *J. Physiol.* **113**:31P–32P.

Brecher, G. A., and J. Praglin. 1953. A modified bristle flowmeter for measuring phasic blood flow. *Proc. Soc. Exptl. Biol. Med.* **83**:155–157.

Brown, H. R., de Lalla, M. A. Epstein, and M. J. Hoffman. 1952. *Clinical Ballistocardiography*. New York: The Macmillan Co.

Clamann, H. G. 1951. Simultaneous recording of pulse contours on central and peripheral arteries with mechano-electronic transducers. *Proc. Soc. Exptl. Biol. Med.* **78**:50–52.

Clemedson, C–J., C–E. Englund, and H. Pettersson. 1959: A mechano-electronic transducer blood pressure recorder. *Acta Physiol. Scand.* 47, Supp. **162**:1–20.

Curtis, H. J. 1949. Action potential of heart muscle. *Am. J. Physiol.* **159**: 499–504.

Curtis, H. J., and J. L. Nickerson. 1949. Application of the transducer tube to the recording of the peripheral pulse. *Proc. Soc. Exptl. Biol. Med.* **70**:383–384.

Hakansson, C. H. 1957. Action potential and mechanical response of isolated cross-striated frog muscle fibers at different degrees of stretch. *Acta Physiol. Scand.* **41**:199–216

Hill, A. V. 1951. The earliest manifestation of the mechanical response of striated muscle *Proc. Roy. Soc. (London)* **138**B:339–348.

Olson, H. F. 1947. Mechano-electronic transducers. *J. Acoust. Soc. Am.* **19**:307–319.

Ranney, R. E. 1954. A myograph for measurement of isometric tension developed by extracted muscle fibers. *J. Appl. Physiol.* **6**:513–516.

Silverman, L. 1950. A direct writing pneumotachograph, *J. Lab. Clin. Med.* **36**:158–162.

Talbot, S. A., J. L. Lillienthal, J. Besser, and L. W. Reynolds. 1951. A wide range mechano-electronic transducer for physiological applications. *Rev. Sci. Instrs.* **22**:233–235.

4

Inductance Transducers

4–1. SINGLE INDUCTOR

The inductance of a coil depends upon its geometry, the number of turns, and the magnetic permeability of the medium in which it is located. The low-frequency inductance in microhenries of a single-layer air-core coil can be calculated by the following approximate formula due to Wheeler (1928):

$$L = \frac{r^2 n^2}{9r + 10l},$$

where r and l are the radius and length in inches, and n is the number of turns. This expression is accurate when the length of the coil is much greater than the diameter. Wheeler stated that the accuracy is within 1% when l is greater than 0.8 times the radius. Although there are many other expressions for the inductance of single-layer coils in which a form factor (dependent on the ratio of length to diameter) is present, the important fact is that the inductance varies with the square of the number of turns and the geometry of the coil. Thus distortion of the coil, as by stretching or compressing, will alter its inductance. This method of inductance change is seldom used because of the small inductance and the even smaller inductance change occurring in coils that can be distorted. If a coil spring happens to be present in a system in which it is desired to detect motion, the changing dimensions of the spring can serve as an inductance transducer. If the spring is of ferromagnetic material, the inductance will be somewhat greater than that expected from calculations on the basis of coil geometry. If the coil surrounds a material having a magnetic permeability greater than that of air, the inductance is increased considerably.

Practically, control of the inductance can be gained by altering the magnetic permeability of the medium. A considerable increase in inductance can be obtained by inserting a magnetically permeable core into the coil. Under these conditions the inductance will depend on the amount of core inside the coil, thereby affording a method of translating displacement to an inductance change.

Single inductors have frequently been employed to measure physiological events which can be converted to movement. One such transducer was described by Fuller and Gordon (1948). They fitted the diaphragm of a Marey tambour with a ferromagnetic ring. Inside the tambour was an iron-cored coil, the inductance of which was changed when the diaphragm was displaced by pressure. Müller et al. (1948) described a simple flowmeter consisting of a variable-inductance differential pressure transducer connected to a Pitot tube. Their transducer consisted of an iron-cored coil placed close to an elastic diaphragm which carried a small soft iron disk. Movement of the disk, in response to pressure changes across the diaphragm, altered the inductance and unbalanced a 5-kc bridge circuit, thereby producing an alternating voltage proportional to pressure, which was in turn proportional to blood flow. Rushmer (1954) described a truly remarkable application of the variable-inductance technique to measure continuously the diameter of the left ventricle of a dog as the heart was beating. He was able to suture a small coil to one ventricular wall and the core to the septum. As the diameter changed with each heart beat, the core moved within the coil, causing inductance changes that, when recorded in the unanesthetized dog, indicated alterations in the size of the ventricle during a variety of experimental conditions.

A commercially available[1] catheter-tip single-inductance blood pressure transducer is shown next to a sailmaker's needle in Fig. 4–1. A cutaway diagram of the variable-inductance sensor is shown on the left. Pressure applied to the elastic membrane alters the position of the core in the inductor, which forms part of the frequency-determining circuit of an oscillator. As the core is displaced the inductance is changed, giving rise to a frequency-modulated signal, which is recorded after suitable processing.

4–2. MUTUAL INDUCTANCE

The principle of mutual inductance, which employs two coils, is also used in the measurement of physiological events. When two coils are joined in series and their fields link, the inductance L is equal to $L_1 + L_2 \pm 2M$, where L_1 and L_2 are the inductances of the individual coils, and M, the

[1]Carolina Medical Electronics, Winston-Salem, N. C.

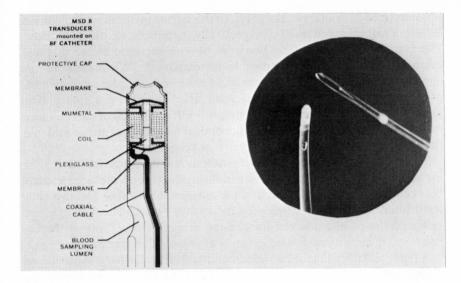

Figure 4–1. Catheter-tip inductance pressure transducer. (Courtesy Carolina Medical Electronics, Winston-Salem, N.C.)

mutual inductance between them, is dependent on the coupling between the coils. The coupling can be altered by inserting a magnetically permeable core or by moving one coil with respect to the other.

If the two coils are not joined electrically and an oscillator is connected across one of them, a voltage will be induced in the other. The arrangement constitutes a transformer. The two windings are designated the primary and the secondary. The primary is the winding to which the energy source is connected. The magnitude of the voltage appearing across the secondary coil is dependent on the coupling, which can be varied by the insertion of a magnetically permeable core or by moving one coil with respect to the other.

There are many practical applications of two inductances connected in series opposition in which the coupling between them is altered by changing the position of a centrally mounted core. One such application is that of Gauer and Gienapp (1950), who built a unique catheter-tip blood pressure transducer. A diaphragm having the diameter of the catheter actuated a small ferromagnetic core, which, moving in response to the pressure changes, altered the coupling between the coils and produced proportional changes in inductance. This early catheter-tip pressure transducer had a resonant frequency of 1000 cps in fluid and for a considerable time stood alone as the highest-fidelity blood pressure transducer.

A larger two-inductance pressure transducer, the "Clark Capsule," was described by Motley et al. (1947). In this device two coils were mounted on either side of a distensible, magnetically permeable, elastic diaphragm. The two coils constituted the two arms of an inductance bridge that was balanced with no pressure applied to the diaphragm. When pressure was applied, the diaphragm was deformed and the bridge became unbalanced, producing a signal that was recorded after suitable processing. The performance was reported to be only slightly inferior to that of the Hamilton manometer, one of the highest-quality optical manometers and considered the standard instrument for blood pressure recording.

Scher et al. (1953) constructed an interesting inductance transducer for blood flow in which a ferromagnetic paddle in a flow tube was placed midway between two coils wrapped around the outside of the tube. The two coils constituted the arms of a balanced inductance bridge. The flow of blood deflected the paddle and unbalanced the bridge. A recording of the unbalance voltage was calibrated in terms of volume flow per minute.

A pulse pickup using the two-winding variable transformer was developed by Benjamin et al. (1962). In their transducer the two coils were mounted in a small chamber which was affixed to the skin over a pulsating artery. In the chamber facing the artery a rubber diaphragm carried the movable coil and the frame of the capsule carried the fixed coil. The coil on the rubber membrane was energized by a 100-kc oscillator, and its position was modulated by the pulse. Amplification, rectification, and graphic recording of the signal produced a pulse tracing of high fidelity.

Blood flow was recorded by Pieper (1958), who constructed a catheter-tip velocity flowmeter employing the variable transformer. In this device a ferromagnetic sleeve carrying a small flange was displaced by the velocity of the blood stream. The displacement altered the coupling between the coils, thereby producing a recordable signal. A unique expandable, umbrella-type fixture was provided to maintain the transducer in the center of the vessel. Pieper reported a linear output with flow up to a velocity of 45 cm per second and a frequency up to 25 cps.

4-3. LINEAR VARIABLE DIFFERENTIAL TRANSFORMER (LVDT)

When three coils are used, the device is designated a differential transformer and takes many forms, the commonest being an arrangement of two identical coils placed on either side of a third energizing coil (Fig. 4–2). This configuration was introduced by Schaevitz (1947) and is used extensively by industry. The central coil of the LVDT is excited by alternating current, which produces a field that induces equal voltages in the two adjacent coils. The outer coils are connected in series opposition so that the voltage generated in one cancels that from the other. In practice the

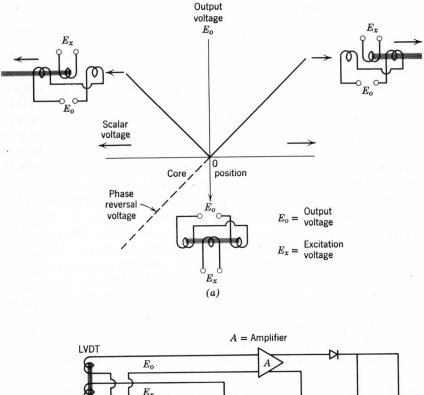

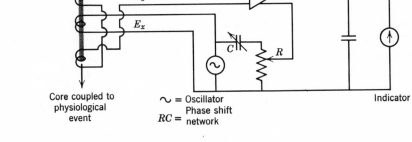

Figure 4–2. The Linear Variable Differential Transformer (LVDT): (*a*) output versus core position; (*b*) phase-sensitive detector for LVDT.

residual voltage is in the order of 1% of the maximum output voltage. Insertion of a core unbalances the system so that the voltages generated in the outer coils are no longer equal. The imbalance voltage is proportional to the core position. The relationship between the output voltage and the position of the core in the differential transformer is shown in Fig. 4–2*a*. In comprehensive articles, Shaevitz (1947) and Heath (1958) have further analyzed the operation of the LVDT under a variety of practical measurement conditions.

It is to be noted that an output of the same magnitude is produced if the core is displaced an equal amount in either direction from its central position. The phase of the output differs, however, by 180 degrees on either side of the neutral position. To obtain direction sensitivity with the LVDT, two techniques are available. In one, the core is offset and operation is centered around a position other than the one that moves the core through the central point. Thus a signal of increasing or decreasing magnitude is obtained with movement of the core. The other method of operation is illustrated in Fig. 4–2*b*. This circuit arrangement constitutes a phase-sensitive detector in which the oscillator voltage and that derived from the LVDT are added before rectification. With the core in its central position, the oscillator voltage, corrected for phase shifts in all of the circuitry by adjustment of C, is fed to the indicator to bring it to midscale by adjustment of R. As the core is displaced from the central position, the voltage E_o, after amplification, adds to or subtracts from the oscillator voltage, depending on the magnitude and phase of E_o, which in turn depend on the magnitude and direction of the displacement. Thus the indicator can be calibrated for the full range of core motion.

The first catheter-tip blood pressure transducer incorporating one type of LVDT was described by Wetterer (1943). In this device the oscillator was connected to two primary coils and the detecting system to the two secondary coils, connected in series opposition. At the tip of the 3.5-mm catheter was an elastic diaphragm coupled to a movable core that altered the coupling between the primary and the two secondary coils when pressure was applied. The small mass and high stiffness of the moving parts resulted in a high resonant frequency (515 cps), thereby producing a rapid response time.

Small movements were detected by Tucker (1952), using a three-coil transformer transducer. His device was accurate to 0.005 cm over a 1-cm range and provided enough power to drive a pen recorder without amplification.

The relatively high efficiency of the commercially available[2] three-coil LVDT's has stimulated many investigators to employ them for the measurement of physiological events. A blood pressure transducer which employed a differential transformer was described by Shafer and Shirer (1949). In this device the core was affixed to a small circular elastic diaphragm exposed to blood pressure. The whole assembly was mounted in a 2-cc syringe. The natural frequency of this transducer was 600 cps; when

[2]Schaevitz Engineering Co., Camden 1, N. J.

it was connected to a 20-gauge needle a frequency response flat to 100 cps was obtained.

Erdos et al. (1962) described a truly isotonic myograph incorporating the LVDT. In this device the muscle specimen under study was connected to a beam-type balance. The motion of the balancing weight, which occurred with contraction of the muscle, was measured by variations in the position of the core in the LVDT.

Figure 4–3 illustrates the use of the LVDT to construct an efficient pressure transducer.[3] In this device movement of the tip of a Bourdon tube is detected by an LVDT. Linearity, rapidity of response and a small volume displacement are achieved by means of a very stiff, short Bourdon tube. A very interesting electrical caliper incorporating the LVDT was described by Gow (1966). Employed for the continuous measurement of pulsatile arterial diameter changes, this device consisted of a jeweled-bearing, scissor-like, lightweight caliper, one end of which embraced the artery, while the other end was affixed to the LVDT. The small pulsatile changes in the artery modulated the position of the embracing ends of the caliper to provide (after four stages of amplification) an output of 1 to 1.5 volts for changes in the diameter of the thoracic aorta and of the femoral artery, amounting to 500 and 80 microns, respectively. The low mass of the instrument resulted in a sinusoidal frequency response essentially uniform to 20 cps measured on a segment of rubber tubing. When the device was tested for transient response, the natural resonant frequency was found

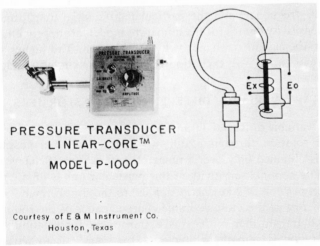

PRESSURE TRANSDUCER
LINEAR-CORE™

MODEL P-1000

Courtesy of E & M Instrument Co.
Houston, Texas

Figure 4–3. LVDT pressure transducer. Linear Core. Model P-1000. (Courtesy E & M Instrument Co., Houston, Tex.)

[3] E & M Instrument Co., Houston, Tex.

to be in excess of 180 cps, dramatically indicating the rapid response time available.

Because of the small size and low mass of the core of an LVDT, an insignificant load is imposed on the event being measured. With the core in the null position, no electromagnetic pull is imposed on it. In practical units very little pull is encountered when the core is displaced from the null position. Although the transduction efficiency is moderate, the differential transformer is rugged and relatively insensitive to temperature changes, the sensitivity alteration being almost entirely due to the resistance change of the coils. Its ability to detect rapid changes is good, being limited to the characteristics of the moving system, the frequency of the excitation voltage, and the characteristic of the magnetic material. If extremely rapid rates of change are to be measured, high-frequency excitation and powdered magnetic materials must be used in the construction of the core.

Linear variable differential transformer units are relatively low in impedance and can be constructed to have almost any dimensions. Although many component manufacturers provide a standard line, they will construct special units to meet almost any particular need. *Engineering Bulletin* A2 of the Schaevitz Co. lists transformers having linear displacement ranges of ± 0.005 to ± 1.000 inch, with a residual output (at balance) of 0.5% of that obtained with maximum displacement. The excitation voltage of many differential transformers is 3 to 10 volts at frequencies ranging from 60 cps to 20 kc. The output per unit of displacement is dependent on the excitation voltage, its frequency, and the particular differential transformer model. Typical sensitivity figures for the miniature models are approximately 0.2 to 5 mv per thousandth inch per volt of excitation. The higher sensitivity figures are obtained with excitation voltages in the kilocycle range.

4-4.   ROTARY VARIABLE DIFFERENTIAL TRANSFORMERS

Rotary variable differential transformers are also available commercially. Although rotation through a full 360 degrees is often possible, ± 1% linearity is obtained only over a range of ± 40 degrees (Schaevitz R3B 1 S model). The nominal sensitivity of this particular unit is 1.8 mv per degree of rotation per volt of 2 ke energy applied to the transformer.

Perhaps one of the most desirable characteristics of the rotary variable differential transformer is that, as a transducer for rotation, its output versus rotation is smooth or stepless. However, it is to be noted that in many models the maximum rotation is approximately 90 degrees. When continuous rotation is possible the output voltage varies as the sine or cosine of the angle of rotation.

REFERENCES

Benjamin, F. B., E. Mastrogiovanni, and W. Helveig. 1962. Bloodless method for continuous recording of pulse pressure in man. *J. Appl. Physiol.* **17**:844.

Erdos, E. G., V. Jackman, and W. C. Barnes. 1962. Instrument for recording isotonic contractions of smooth muscles. *J. Appl. Physiol.* **17**:307–8.

Fuller, J. T., and T. M. Gordon. 1948. The radio inductograph. *Science* **108**:287–8.

Gauer, O. H., and E. Gienapp. 1950. A miniature pressure-recording device. *Science* **112**:404–5.

Gow, B. S. 1966. An electrical caliper for measurement of pulsatile arterial diameter changes *in vivo. J. Appl. Physiol.* **21**:1122–1126.

Heath, J. H. 1958. The differential transformer as a sensitive measuring device. *Electron. Eng.* **30**:631–633.

Motley, H. L., A. Cournand, L. Werko, D. Dresdale, A. Himmelstein, and D. W. Richards. 1947. Intravascular and intracardiac pressure recording in man: Electrical apparatus compared with the Hamilton manometer. *Proc. Soc. Exptl. Biol. Med.* **64**:241–244.

Müller, A., L. Laszt, and L. Pircher. 1948. Über ein Manometer mit elektrischer Transmission zur Druke und Geschwindigkeitmessung. *Helv. Physiol. Acta* **6**:783–794.

Pieper, H. P. 1958. Registration of phasic changes of blood flow by means of a catheter type flowmeter. *Rev. Sci. Instrs.* **29**:965–967.

Rushmer, R. F. 1954a. Heart size and stroke volume. *Minn. Med.* **37**:19–29.

Rushmer, R. F. 1954b. Continuous measurements of left ventricular dimensions in intact unanesthetized dogs. *Circulation Res.* 1954, **2**:14–21.

Schaevitz, H. *Engineering Bulletin* A2 and R38. Shaevitz Co., Box 505, Camden 1, N. J.

Schaevitz, H. 1947. The linear variable differential transformer. *Proc. Soc. Stress Anal.* **4**:79–88.

Schafer, P. W., and H. W. Shirer. 1949. An impedance gauging system for measurement of biologic pressure variables. *Surgery* **26**:446–451.

Scher, A. M., T. H. Weigert, and A. C. Young. 1953. Compact flowmeters for use in the unanesthetized animal, an electronic version of Chauveau's hemodrometer. *Science* **118**:82–84.

Tucker, M. J. 1952. A linear transducer for the electrical measurement of displacement. *Electron. Eng.* **24**:420–422.

Wetterer, E. 1943. Eine neue manometrische Sonde mit elektrischer Transmission. *Z. Biol.* **101**:333–350.

Wheeler, H. A. 1928. Simple inductance formulas for radio coils. *Proc. IRE* **16**:1398–1400.

5

Capacitive Transducers

5–1. SINGLE CAPACITOR

A capacitor or condenser consists of two conducting surfaces separated by a dielectric, which can be solid, liquid, gaseous, or a vacuum. The capacitance (coulombs per volt) is measured in farads. The magnitude of the capacitance depends on the nature of the dielectric and varies directly with the area of the conducting surfaces and inversely with their separation. The capacitance can be altered by changing any of these three factors.

A parallel-plate capacitor has identical plates, each of area A cm², which are separated by a distance d cm; between them is placed a material of dielectric constant K. The capacitance is given by the following formula:

$$C\mu\mu f = 0.0885 \, \frac{A}{d} \, K.$$

Because the dielectric constant of air is only very slightly higher than that of a vacuum, K can be given the value of unity for air condensers. Thus a practical figure for rapid calculation of the capacitance of an air condenser can be derived. A condenser consisting of two plates 1 cm² in area separated by 1 mm has a capacitance of 0.885 $\mu\mu$f, that is, slightly less than 1 $\mu\mu$f. In inch dimensions a capacitor having plates 1 sq inch in area separated by 0.1 inch exhibits a capacitance of 2.17 $\mu\mu$f, or slightly more than 2 $\mu\mu$f. Although the equation for a parallel plate capacitor indicates that the capacitance varies inversely with the distance between plates, this relationship holds only for distances which are small in comparison to the size of the plates. If the separation between the plates is large compared to their size, the capacitance-distance relationship deviates from that of a hyperbola.

Alternating current is usually employed to obtain a signal which reflects the value of a capacitance. Depending on the application, the voltage proportional to the static value of the capacitance is disregarded, and only the change is processed for ultimate reproduction. This method is illustrated in Fig. 5–1a. In this circuit the capacitance transducer is in series with a large resistance R. A small change in capacitance will produce a proportional change in the voltage across the capacitor and resistor.

A more convenient method of employing capacitance involves placing the capacitance transducer in a bridge circuit as shown in Fig. 5–1b. Frequently it is possible to create a differential capacitance transducer, each half being placed in adjacent arms of a bridge. The event being detected is caused to increase the capacitance of one side of the bridge and to decrease that of the other side. When this method is employed, the output signal is twice that obtainable by varying one capacitive element. This technique is characterized by a high degree of temperature stability.

When capacitance transducers are employed in bridge circuits, two methods are available to obtain direction sensitivity. Either the bridge is operated slightly off balance, or a phase-sensitive detector is employed. With the first method the output of the bridge increases or decreases with a change in capacitance. The amount of initial unbalance chosen is dictated by the maximum expected change in C required to drive the bridge toward the balance point. With a phase-sensitive detector direction sensitivity is automatically obtained.

Occasionally a single-element capacitive transducer is placed across a tuned circuit which is detuned by the change in capacitance, thereby causing a current change in the associated circuitry. Sometimes the tuned circuit constitutes the frequency-determining component in an oscillator. A change in the capacitance of the transducer alters the frequency of the oscillator, giving rise to a frequency-modulated signal that is detected and displayed with the aid of appropriate circuitry.

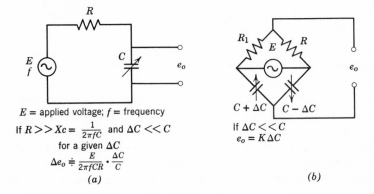

E = applied voltage; f = frequency

If $R \gg Xc = \dfrac{1}{2\pi fC}$ and $\Delta C \ll C$

for a given ΔC

$$\Delta e_o \doteq \frac{E}{2\pi fCR} \cdot \frac{\Delta C}{C}$$

(a)

If $\Delta C \ll C$

$e_o = K\Delta C$

(b)

Figure 5–1. Capacitive transducer circuits: (a) series circuit; (b) bridge circuit.

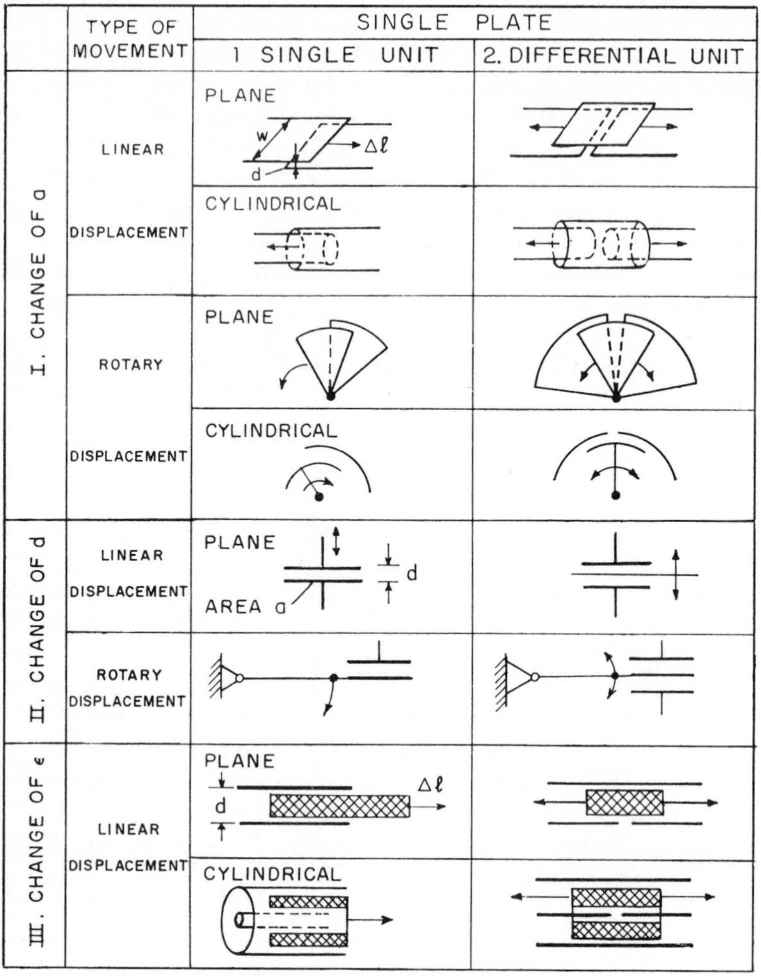

TYPE OF MOVEMENT		SINGLE PLATE	
		1 SINGLE UNIT	2. DIFFERENTIAL UNIT
I. CHANGE OF a	LINEAR DISPLACEMENT	PLANE	
		CYLINDRICAL	
	ROTARY DISPLACEMENT	PLANE	
		CYLINDRICAL	
II. CHANGE OF d	LINEAR DISPLACEMENT	PLANE AREA a	
	ROTARY DISPLACEMENT		
III. CHANGE OF ε	LINEAR DISPLACEMENT	PLANE	
		CYLINDRICAL	

Figure 5–2. Synopsis of capacitive displacement transducers. [From Foldvari and Lion, Instr. Control Systems **37**:77–85 (1964).]

Capacitive transducers are frequently employed to detect mechanical displacement by movement of one or both of the condenser plates, thereby producing a change in separation or effective area. Figure 5–2, composed by Foldvari and Lion (1964), illustrates many of the methods in which the capacitance change principle can be employed.

The capacitance method has often been applied to the measurement of physiological events, particularly the determination of blood pressure, for which the capacitive transducer has been extensively employed since the late

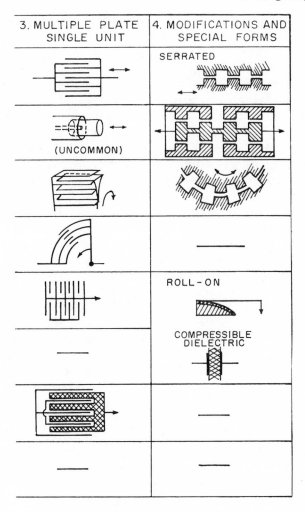

Figure 5–2. (*continued*)

1930's. This transducer was developed because higher fidelity and sensitivity were needed than were available from optical manometers, which had been perfected to a remarkably high degree by reducing mass, increasing stiffness, and recovering the lost sensitivity by increasing the distance to the photographic recording surface. The practical inconvenience of the optical systems was a major factor which stimulated application of electrical transduction systems.

In the application of the capacitance method to measure blood pressure an elastic member exposed to blood pressure constitutes one plate of the capacitor; the other plate is nearby and fixed. For high sensitivity each investigator using this technique has placed the distensible plate as close as possible to the fixed plate. To obtain a rapid response time the elastic member is made as small and as stiff as possible. This combination guarantees that only a small amount of fluid will be displaced when pressure is applied. The displacement is usually expressed in terms of cubic millimeters of fluid entering the transducer per 100 mm Hg of applied pressure. In practical terms this figure describes the ability of the transducer to measure transient pressure changes applied to interconnecting catheters and needles. Transducers having low volume displacement figures can be employed to record faithfully pressure transients with small-bore inter-connecting tubing.

Schutz (1937) appears to have been one of the first to use the capacitance method to measure blood pressure. In his transducer the elastic member was a silvered glass membrane. The smallness and stiffness of the membrane he employed produced a natural frequency of 207 cps. Following his lead, many other investigators constructed pressure transducers. Among these were Lilly (1942), Frommer (1943), Buchtal and Warburg (1943), and Hansen and Warburg (1947). In all these transducers the elastic members were small and stiff, providing a short response time and a small volume displacement. In all, the fixed and movable plates were in very close proximity. Ratios of area to separation varying from ten to ten thousand have been employed.

An interesting application of the capacitive method to measure blood pressure is due to Beyne and Gougerot (1939), who converted the height of mercury in a U-tube manometer to an electrical signal. One "plate" of the condenser was the mercury itself, whereas the other consisted of tin foil wrapped around the outside of the glass tube forming the manometer. As the mercury column rose, the capacitance between the mercury and the tin foil increased, causing a change in the current flowing through the condenser. Although application of the principle in no way improved the fidelity of the manometer, it permitted remote location of the pressure-indicating device. It is to be noted that the fluid in such a manometer need not be mercury. Any solution of lower specific gravity can be used to produce a sensitive manometer or fluid level transducer. Beyne also used the same principle to convert small air pressure changes in the respiratory system of a dog to an electrical signal by fitting the diaphragm of a Marey tambour with an electrode of tin foil which became the movable plate of a condenser.

The condenser microphone has seen service in physiology for the detection of heart sounds. Asher (1932) recognized its potentialities and used it to detect human heart sounds, which, after amplification, were converted to variations in light intensity. A photographic record of the light beam produced phonocardiograms of high fidelity.

Liston (1950) employed a capacitive transducer to detect infrared radiation in his analyzer for gaseous carbon dioxide. The detector, sometimes referred to as a gas microphone, consisted of two carbon dioxide-filled chambers, each with a window for the admission of infrared radiation. Between the chambers was a distensible diaphragm which constituted one plate of the capacitive transducer. A second fixed plate was placed nearby. When carbon dioxide, which strongly absorbs infrared energy of characteristic wavelengths, is enclosed in a chamber, the pressure will rise in proportion to the amount of infrared radiation absorbed. The window of each detector was exposed to an infrared source. In front of one window was placed an infrared transparent tube containing the gas to be analyzed. Thus, when a gas sample containing carbon dioxide was present, the amount of infrared radiation reaching one detector was reduced, creating an unbalance in the pressure in the two cells and a deflection of the diaphragm between them. The change in capacitance so produced was calibrated in terms of the amount of carbon dioxide in the gas sample.

Adams et al.(1960) described the construction of a miniature capacitance microphone which they used as a high-fidelity pulse pickup. This device consisted of a small chamber containing a fixed electrode. Covering the chamber (and a short distance from the fixed electrode) was a metalized Mylar film, which constituted the other plate of the capacitor. In use the device was placed with the Mylar film applied to the skin over a pulsating vessel. The film tracked the skin motion and thereby modulated the capacitance. By means of a suitable processing apparatus a recordable electrical signal was developed.

Calibration of the capacitance transducer applied to the radial artery was achieved first by occluding the artery at a point central to the transducer. This procedure established zero pressure. With the occlusion removed, the sensitivity was calibrated by requesting the subject to raise his arm 33.8 cm, which is equivalent to a change in pressure of 25 mm Hg.

5-2. BIOLOGICAL CAPACITORS

An unusual application of the capacitance change principle employs the dielectric property of the living tissue itself as a part of the capacitor. A few examples are noteworthy, Cremer (1907) inserted a beating frog heart between the plates of a condenser and recorded the capacitance change as the heart filled with blood and emptied of it. A similar system was described by Joseph (1944), who placed electrodes over the thoraxes of human beings. Using a 90-volt battery in series with a 2-megohm resistor, he was able to detect pulsatile changes in capacitive current. A simultaneous record of the ECG showed that the capacitive changes were associated with cardiac activity, but calibration was not attempted.

In blood flow studies Atzler and Lehman (1932) and Atzler (1935) applied a capacitance change method to human beings by placing one electrode above the chest and one in contact with the back. Using an ultrahigh-frequency current which was modulated by respiration and the systolic discharge from the heart, they detected the capacitance changes, calling their method "Dielektrographie." Whitehom and Pearl (1949) carried out studies similar to those of Atzler and his associates. Their electrodes were 15 cm square and were placed before and behind the thorax. The pulsatile changes in capacitive reactance frequency modulated a 10.7-mc oscillator. Calling these records "cardioelectrograms," they attempted calibration of the tracings and stated, "Values for stroke volumes, cardiac output and cardiac indices, calculated from such records on the basis of preliminary calibration of the instrument by introduction of known volumes of saline between the plates, fall within the range of accepted normal values but conclusions as to the validity of this method are not yet possible."

Another application of the capacitance method was made by Fenning (1936–37), who described an instrument which he later called the "Oscilla-tocapacitograph." A rat was laid on one plate of the condenser, and the other plate, 1 cm square in size, was placed 5 mm above the thorax of the animal. These plates were connected across the tuned circuit of a Hartley oscillator. Respiratory movements, changing the capacitance by varying the area, separation, and distribution of the dielectric, altered the anode current of the oscillator tube. By monitoring this current, a good record of respiration in the rat was obtained. In the hands of Fenning and Bonnar (1936–37) the same instrument was used to record maternal respiration, uterine contractions, and fetal respiration in the rat. Employing a slight modification of this technique, Tomberg (1963, 1964) detected human respiration by placing electrodes on the thorax without making ohmic contact with the chest wall. Frequencies between 50 and 300 mc were employed.

Heart sounds have been detected in an ingenious application of the capacitance change principle. For example, Yamakawa et al. (1954) placed a metal electrode near the tip of a closed catheter, which was then advanced into the hearts of dogs and human subjects. When the changes in capacitive reactance, measured between the catheter tip and the body of the subject, were recorded, heart sounds were clearly identified. So sensitive was their system that the sounds of vocalization were clearly recordable.

A similar investigation of heart sounds was carried out by Groom et al. (1957, 1964), who constructed a monopolar electrode condenser microphone consisting of a chamber in contact with the thorax. Inside the chamber was the other electrode, mounted concentrically so that it did not contact the thoracic wall. Thus the heart sounds and all cardiac vibrations communicated to the thorax modulated the capacitance. The frequency response they attained extended from 0 to 50,000 cps. In all probability cardiac vibrations had never been detected previously with such a large bandwidth.

When the capacitive method is applied by placing electrodes in, on, or near living tissue, it is often difficult to know whether capacitance changes are the only ones measured. Usually the circuit contains both resistive and reactive components, and what is measured is in reality an impedance change. The various physiological events which have been measured by impedance change are described in Chapter 10.

5-3. DIFFERENTIAL CAPACITOR

An ingenious application of the differential capacitance principle (Fig. 5–1b) was described by Boucek et al. (1959), who used it to construct a myograph for recording the contractions of the chick embryo heart at the 72-hour stage. At this time the heart is in a dynamic stage of development, changing from a tube to a four-chambered organ that a little while later exhibits an adult electrocardiogram. It is, however, incapable of exerting much force. To detect these feeble movements, Boucek and his colleagues placed the heart in a drop of plasma or saline. One end of a light lever was made to rest on the part of the heart from which movement was to be recorded; to the other was affixed a metal plate centrally placed between two other fixed plates. The assembly thus constituted a differential capacitor. As the heart beat, the lever was moved and its recorded motion described the mechanical activity of the organ. The lever also constituted one of the electrodes for the ECG; the other electrode was a wire dipping into the plasma or saline solution. Thus these investigators were able to record and correlate the embryo ECG with the movement of the various chambers of the heart.

An interesting differential capacitor pneumotachograph was described by Krobath and Reed (1964). This device consisted of a circular aluminized Mylar membrane 0.0001 inch thick in which six equally spaced cuts were made, creating leaflets which moved backward and forward as air passed through. On either side were placed two circular plates having hexagonal holes. The metalized membrane constituted the movable plate; the plates with the hexagonal holes were fixed. When respiratory air was caused to flow through the assembly, the capacitance changed in proportion to the flow velocity. With a 200-kc voltage applied to the capacitor in a bridge configuration, a substantial signal reflecting the velocity of respiratory air was obtained. Time integration of the velocity signal produced an output reflecting the volume of air per breath.

5-4. DIODE TWIN-T CAPACITIVE TRANSDUCER

An ingenious method of employing the capacitance method has been described by Lion (1964). He pointed out that in a bridge circuit either the transducer or the oscillator must be operated above ground potential and that meeting this requirement frequently presents difficulties, surmountable only by the addition of special components and circuits. Instead of a bridge circuit he proposed the use of the diode twin-T circuit shown in Fig. 5–3. With this circuit configuration one side of the oscillator, transducing capacitor, and output signal are all at the same potential which can be ground.

In Lion's circuit S is a radio-frequency oscillator producing sine or square waves of an amplitude E_i. During the positive half cycle diode D_1 conducts and charges C_1. During the next negative half cycle D_1 does not conduct and C_1 discharges through R_1 and R_L and also through R_2 and D_2. Similarly, during the first positive half cycle D_2 does not conduct, but during the second negative half cycle D_2 conducts and charges C_2. During the following half cycle C_2 discharges through R_2 and R_L and also through R_1 and D_1. If diodes D_1 and D_2 are identical, $C_1 = C_2$ and $R_1 = R_2$ the currents through R_1 and R_2 are equal in magnitude and opposite in sign, and when flowing through R_L the output circuit, the net current is zero. Any variation in C_1 and C_2 causes current to flow through R_L, the load, which can be a resistor or a direct-reading microammeter. If display by a rapidly responding recorder is desired, the voltage across R_L can be amplified and displayed appropriately.

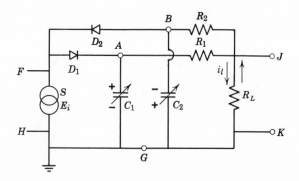

Figure 5–3. Diode twin-T circuit.

Lion (1964) and Foldvari (1964) gave the following expression, in which $R = R_1 = R_2$, for the current through R_L:

$$I = E_i \frac{R + 2R_L}{(R + R_L)^2} \text{Rf}(C_1 - C_2 - C_1 e^{-k_1} + C_2 e^{-k_2}),$$

where $\quad k_1 = \dfrac{R + R_L}{2\text{Rf}C_1(R + 2R_L)} \quad$ and $\quad k_2 = \dfrac{R + R_L}{2\text{Rf}C_2(R + 2R_L)}.$

Maximum sensitivity of the circuit occurs when $1/k_1 = 1/k_2 = 0.57$. In commercially available transducers[1] consisting of a two-plate capacitor with a separation of 0.005 inch, a sensitivity on the order of 1000 volts per inch can be obtained.

The output impedance of the diode twin-T circuit is determined by the choice of R_1 and R_L and is virtually independent of C_1 and C_2. By suitable choice of R_1 and R_2 an output impedance of 1 kilohm to 100 kilohms can be obtained. Optimum selection of these components will permit display of the capacitance change with a microammeter. If the output is to be displayed by means of a rapidly responding indicator, the rise time available is also dependent on the load resistance R_L and the oscillator frequency. With an R_L of 1000 ohms and an oscillator frequency of 1.3 mc, for an instantaneous change in capacitance a rise time of 20 μs is attainable.

Foldvari and Lion (1964) called attention to some of the highly desirable characteristics of their interesting circuit. Because the diodes operate at high level and in the linear portion of their characteristic, selection of matched diodes is not necessary. Another attractive feature is that changes in oscillator frequency do not adversely affect the sensitivity of the circuit; for example, a 10% change in frequency results in only a 1% alteration in sensitivity to capacitance change. Extremely desirable also is the fact that the output is remarkably high. For example, with 46 volts (rms sinusoidal) for E_i at a frequency of 1.3 mc, a capacitance change from -7 to $+7$ $\mu\mu$f produces an output of -5 to $+5$ volts across a 1-megohm load (R_L).

5-5. CHARACTERISTICS OF CAPACITIVE TRANSDUCERS

The extreme flexibility of capacitive transducers is perhaps their most attractive feature. In many applications they can be employed to detect dimension change without direct mechanical contact with the moving member. For this reason capacitive transducers, which are often called proximity detectors, are free from loading, frictional, and hysteresis errors.

[1]Lion Research Corp., Cambridge, Mass.

By careful design of the capacitive element, extremely small or relatively large displacements can be measured. Another attractive feature of the capacitive transducer is the fact that the capacitance does not depend on the conductivity of its plates. Thus temperature errors from this source are extremely small, although not entirely absent since the dimensions of the plates depend on temperature. The variation in the dielectric constant of air with temperature is small. Stability is achieved through the mechanical design of the capacitive transducer and the electrical circuitry connected to it. With efficient mechanical and electrical design these sources of error can be reduced to insignificant levels.

Because the output impedance of a capacitive transducer is usually high, shielding is necessary and a coaxial cable is frequently required to connect the transducer to the electronic processing equipment. In many applications the type of cable employed merits special consideration because its capacitance is in parallel with that of the transducing capacitor. Therefore a mechanically stable low-capacitance coaxial cable is required. Often movement of the cable produces an undesirable capacitance change resulting from a slight displacement of the outer shield relative to the inner conductor, which produces a signal indistinguishable from that made by the transducer. The use of special coaxial cables, in which a layer of conducting powder has been applied to the dielectric directly below the shielding and in contact with it, greatly attenuates this source of error. In many instances the problems presented by the high output impedance can be eliminated by locating some of the processing circuitry at the capacitive transducer. With this technique it is usually possible to incorporate an impedance transformer which provides a low output impedance, permitting location of the transducer at a distance from the processing equipment.

REFERENCES

Adams, R., B. S. Corell, and N H. Wolfesboro, 1960. Cuffless; noncannula, continuous recording of blood pressure. *Surgery* **47**:46–54.

Asher, A. G. 1932. Graphic registration of heart sounds by the argon glow tube. *Arch. Internal Med.* **50**:913–920.

Atzler, E. 1935a. Dielektrographie. *Handbuch der biologischen Arbeitsmethoden* **5**:1073–184.

Atzler, E. 1935b. Neues Verfahren zur Funktionsbeurteilung des Herzens. *Deut. Med. Wochschr.* **59**:1347–1349.

Atzler, E., and G. Lehman. 1932. Über ein neues Verfahren zur Darstellung der Herztätigkeit. (Dielektrographie) *Arbeitsphysiologie* **5**:636–680.

Beyne, J., and L. Gougerot. 1939. Une méthode de transmission électrique et d'enregistrement à distance de la pression artérielle et du débit respiratoire. *Compt. Rend. Biol.* **131**:770–774.

Boucek, R. J., W. P. Murphy, and G. H. Paff. 1959. Electrical and mechanical properties of chick embryo heart chambers. *Circulation Res.* **7**:787–793.

Buchtal, F., E. Warburg. 1943. A new method for direct electrical registration of intra-arterial pressure in man with examples of its application. *Acta Physiol. Scand.* 5:55–70.

Cremer, H. 1907. Über die Registrierung Mechanischer Vorgänge auf Menschen. *Med. Wochschr.* 54: 1629.

Fenning, C. 1936–37. A new method for recording physiologic activities. I. Recording respiration in small animals. *J. Lab. Clin. Med.* 22:1279–1280.

Fenning, C., and E. B. Bonnar. 1936–37. A new method of recording physiologic activities II. The simultaneous recording of maternal respiration, intrauterine fetal respiration and uterine contractions. *J. Lab. Clin. Med.* 22:1280–84.

Foldvari, T., and K. Lion. 1964. Capacitive transducers. *Instrs. Control Systems* 37:77–85.

Frommer, J. C. 1943. Detecting small mechanical movements. *Electronics* 16:104–105.

Groom, D., and Y. T. Sihvonen. 1957a. High sensitivity pickup for heart sounds and murmurs. *IRE Trans. Med. Electron* PGME-9:35–40.

Groom, D., and Y. T. Sihvonen. 1957b. A high sensitivity pickup for cardiovascular sounds. *Am. Heart J.* 54:592–601.

Groom, D., L. H. Medena, and Y. T. Sihvonen. 1964. The proximity transducer. *Am. J. Med. Electron.* 3:261–265.

Hansen, A. T., and E. Warburg. 1947. An improved manometer for measuring intra-arterial and intra-cardiac pressures. *Am. Heart J.* 33:709–710.

Joseph, N. R. 1944. Direct current dielectrograph for recording movements of the heart. *J. Clin. Invest.* 23:25–28.

Krobath, H., and C. Reed. 1964. A new method for the continuous recording of the volume of inspiration and expiration under widely varying conditions. *Am. J. Med. Electron.* 3: 105–109.

Lilly, J. C. 1942. The electrical capacitance diaphragm manometer. *Rev. Sci. Instrs.* 13:34–37.

Lion, K. 1964. Non-linear twin-T network for capacitance transducers. *Rev. Sci. Instrs.* 35: 353–356.

Liston, M. 1950. Performance of a double-beam infra-red recording spectrophotometer. *J. Opt. Soc. Am.* 140:93–101.

Schutz, E. 1937. Konstruktion einer manometrischen Sonde mit elektrischer Transmission. *Z. Biol.* 91:515–521.

Tomberg, V. T. 1963. The high frequency spirometer. *Proceedings of the International Congress Medical Electronics*, Liege, Belgium.

Tomberg, V. T. 1964. Device and a new method of measuring pulmonary respiration. *17th Annual Conference on Engineering in Biology and Medicine* Washington, D.C. McGregor and Werner.

Whitehorn, W. V., and E. R. Pearl. 1949. The use of change in capacity to record cardiac volume with human subject. *Science* 109:262–263.

Yamakawa, K., Y. Shionoya, K. Kitamura, T. Nagai, T. Yamamoto, and S. Ohta. 1954. Intracardiac phonocardiography. *Am. Heart. J.* 47:424–431.

6

Photoelectric Transducers

In the measurement of physiological events in living subjects photoelectric transducers are employed in two ways. The photosensor functions in the first method as a detector of the changes in the intensity of light of a given wavelength, as in conventional colorimetry or spectrophotometry, and in the second method as a detector of changes in the intensity of light in which wavelength is relatively unimportant. There are numerous applications in both categories.

There are three basic types of photoelectric transducers: (1) the photoemissive (phototube), in which electrons are released from a metallic surface (usually alkali), (2) the photovoltaic (barrier-layer cell), in which a potential difference is produced between two substances in contact, and (3) the photoconductive (photoresistor), in which a change in conductivity occurs. Although there is some overlap in applicability, each has its own spectral response, light sensitivity, output current, and voltage characteristics that recommend it for certain tasks. The following sections describe the principles of operation, characteristics, and applications of each type.

6–1. PHOTOEMISSIVE TUBES

The photoemissive tube consists of an evacuated or gas-filled bulb with two electrodes. On one, the cathode, is a coating of a specially prepared material that releases electrons when illuminated. The other electrode, the anode, usually consists of a thin rod or loop of wire. For electron emission to occur there are certain restrictions on the type of surface and the wavelength of the impinging light. Electron emission is possible only if the wavelength is shorter than a certain threshold value which depends on the amount of energy required to release an electron from the metal (work function). Thus there is a long-wave limit of sensitivity.

The electrode materials most frequently employed for the emissive surface are cesium, antimony, silver, and bismuth in combination with trace amounts of other substances. Each type of surface exhibits its own spectral characteristics. Some surfaces are designed to be highly sensitive to narrow spectral regions; others are designed to have a fairly broad spectral sensitivity.

Photoemissive tubes come in a variety of configurations and sizes. In general they, like other photodetectors, are described in terms of the direction of the light with respect to the location of the terminals connected to the internal electrodes. For example, if the terminals are on one end or on both ends of the device and the light enters at right angles, the device is designated as a side-on photodetector. If the electrode terminals are on one end or on both ends and the light enters at one end, the term end-on photodetector is employed. Typical configurations for the photoemissive tube are illustrated in Fig. 6–1, in which a, b, c illustrate side-on types, and d, e, end-on types.

With the photoemissive detector a relatively high voltage (0 to 200 volts) must be applied between the two electrodes. The electrons released by the

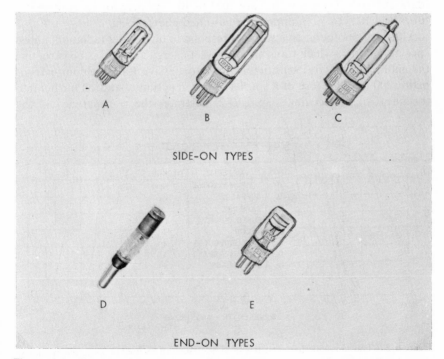

SIDE-ON TYPES

END-ON TYPES

Figure 6–1. Photoemissive tubes: (a), (b), (c) side-on types; (d), (e) end-on types. (Courtesy Radio Corporation of America, Lancaster, Pa.)

light quanta are attracted to the anode. The electron flow constitutes a current which is linearly proportional to the intensity of the incident light. In the vacuum type the current produced is small and is not used to operate an indicator directly; it is usually led through a high resistance, and the voltage thus developed is applied to an amplifier having a high input impedance.

When higher currents are required, gas mixtures are often incorporated into the photoemissive detector. With this technique the primary electrons released by the incident light collide with gas molecules and produce secondary electrons and positive ions, thereby increasing the available current. To avoid the occurrence of a glow discharge, lower anode-to-cathode voltages must be employed. Although the current intensity is increased about tenfold, the linear current-light relationship is compromised at higher intensities.

Both vacuum and gas-filled photoemissive photodetectors respond quickly to changes in light intensity. The response time of the former is approximately 10^{-9} second, whereas that of the latter is much longer, approximating 10^{-3} second. Both exhibit a small current flow with no light (dark current). Typical values are 10^{-8} to 10^{-9} ampere for vacuum phototubes and 10^{-7} to 10^{-8} ampere for gas-filled phototubes.

Although photoemissive surfaces respond to ultraviolet radiation, unless special materials which transmit ultraviolet energy are used in constructing the bulb, the spectral sensitivity of photoemissive tubes seldom extends below 200 mμ. The use of a special bulb will permit operation further into the ultraviolet spectrum. Figure 6–2 illustrates the transparency of the

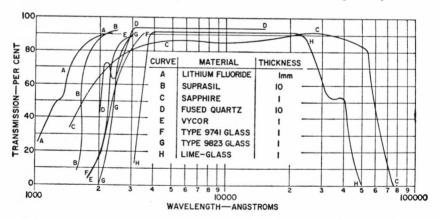

Figure 6–2. Transmission characteristics of various substances used in phototube windows. (From "RCA Phototubes and Photocells." Radio Corporation of America, Lancaster, Pa., 1963. By permission.)

various materials used as windows in photodetectors.

Most photoemissive tubes are sensitive to visible light, and a few respond to infrared radiation down to 800 mμ. The spectral sensitivity of a photoemissive surface is designated by the letter S and a number. This designation refers to a spectral curve recognized by all manufacturers. Data showing some of the spectral characteristics described by the various S-numbers are presented in Fig. 6–3 and Table 6–1.

Table 6–1   Spectral Characteristics of the S-numbers

Spectral Designation	Wavelength For Maximum Response (mμ)	50% Points
S1	800	620– 950
S3	420	350*– 640
S4	400	320– 540
S5	340	230–*510
S8	370	320– 540
S9	480	350– 580
S10	450	350– 590
S11	440	350– 560
S12	500	Narrow Band
S13	440	260– 560
S14	1500	760–1730
S15	580	500– 660
S17	490	310– 580
S19	330	190– 460
S20	420	325– 595
S21	450	260– 560

*Interpolated Values

Data derived from RCA Photosensitive Devices and Cathode Ray Tubes, 1960 – Radio Corp. of America, Electron Tube Division, Harrison, New Jersey.

By incorporating additional anodes (dynodes), each at a higher potential, a current amplification can be obtained through secondary electron emission. Photoelectrons emitted from the photoelectric surface are drawn to and strike the first dynode, releasing secondary electrons which are attracted to the second anode at a higher potential (75 to 150 volts); there the process is repeated. With ten or more stages a current amplification of several million can be obtained.

The spectral sensitivity of such a device, called a photomultiplier, is determined by the emitting surface. The response curves for typical tubes are S1, 4, 5, 8, 10, 11, 13, 17, 19, 20. Thus photomultipliers are available for

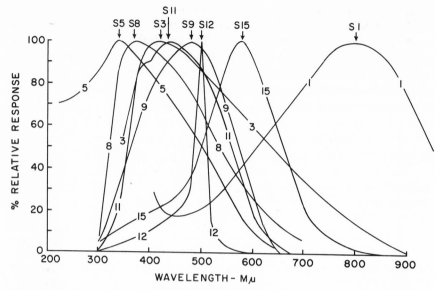

Figure 6–3. The S-Curves.

practically the whole of the visible region and parts of the ultraviolet and infrared regions.

As with other members of its family, the photomultiplier tube has a small dark current of about 10^{-7} ampere. The response time is extremely short, on the order of 10^{-8} to 10^{-9} second. Because of its very high sensitivity and short response time, the photomultiplier is an ideal detector for brief flashes of light of low intensity, such as those produced when radiation strikes the specially prepared crystals employed in scintillation counters.

6–2. PHOTOVOLTAIC CELLS

The photovoltaic (photogalvanic) cell is encountered very frequently in biomedical studies. Unlike the photoemissive tube, which requires a relatively high voltage and produces a small current when illuminated, the photovoltaic cell develops a voltage which can drive a substantial current through a galvanometer or other low-impedance circuit.

One of the most popular of the photovoltaic cells consists of a sandwich of a thin coating of selenium on an iron or steel backing. Above the selenium is a thin transparent film of metal. The film and selenium are insulated from each other, and this region constitutes the barrier layer. When the barrier layer is illuminated, light quanta are absorbed, electrons are released, and a potential difference appears across the barrier. The transparent metal film becomes negative and the selenium positive. Completion of a circuit between the two electrodes causes a current to flow. It is interesting to note that the resistance between the electrodes decreases with illumination. This feature makes it possible to parallel photovoltaic cells: only those that are illuminated will supply current; those not illuminated do not load the others. In the solar power supplies used on board satellites, a diode is placed in series with each group of photodetectors to eliminate possible loading by partially illuminated photocells. This technique guarantees unidirectional flow of current (Acker et al., 1960).

Other substances are used in voltaic cells. Cuprous oxide in contact with gold or platinum is sometimes employed in barrier layer cells. Although these devices are available, they are not common because, compared to the selenium cell, they have low sensitivity to light. The spectral peak of the cuprous oxide cell is around 560 mμ. Diffused-junction silicon photovoltaic cells are now available with a peak at 800 mμ at room temperature. Diffused-junction indium-antimonide photovoltaic cells exhibit a peak sensitivity at 4.9 microns when operated at a temperature of approximately $-200°$C.

Selenium photocells cover the visible spectrum (300 to 700 mμ) with a spectral sensitivity curve peaking around 550 to 570 mμ. With an inexpensive filter it is easy to obtain a spectral curve closely resembling that of the human eye. For this reason these devices are used in illumination meters, exposure meters, and simple colorimeters, all of which operate without electronic amplification. The spectral sensitivity curves of many of the photovoltaic cells commercially available are shown in Fig. 6–4.

The silicon photovoltaic cell is a *P-N* junction device which can produce a relatively large current and is employed to power a variety of mechanisms. The high efficiency of the silicon cell in producing power from sunlight has earned this device the name "solar battery." When such cells are illuminated by daylight, powers of 30 to 90 mw per square inch of light-sensitive surface can be obtained.

The relationship between light intensity and the voltage developed by the photovoltaic sensor is not linear if the device is operated without a resistive load. At saturation a typical open-circuit voltage is in the vicinity of 200 to 600 mv. If a resistive load is placed across the device, the current flow becomes more linearly related to light intensity as the resistance is decreased. Hence it is necessary to employ a low-resistance galvanometer or measuring circuit to indicate light intensity if a linear scale is to be obtained. When a galvanometer having an internal resistance of approximately 100 ohms is employed, a current of 0.5 ma can be obtained from many standard photovoltaic cells when adequately illuminated.

Because of the large capacitance of the barrier layer, the response

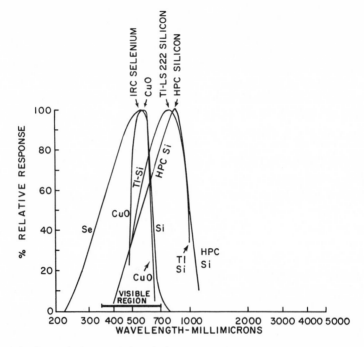

Figure 6-4. Spectral characteristics of photovoltaic cells. (Redrawn from data in manufacturers' bulletins.) TI = Texas Instruments; HPC = Hoffman Electronics Corp.; IRC = International Rectifier Corp.

time of a typical photovoltaic cell is seldom less than 5 ms, although a few miniature types exhibit response times of 0.1 ms. Perhaps the most undesirable feature of the photovoltaic cell in biomedical application is its sensitivity to temperature changes as the load resistance is varied. With many cells there is an optimum value for the resistance which can be connected across the device to minimize the sensitivity change with temperature. This resistance value is not necessarily the one that yields the maximum power transfer or linearity of current with light intensity.

6-3. PHOTOCONDUCTIVE CELLS

The photoconductive or photoresistive cell consists of a thin film of a material such as selenium, germanium, silicon, or a metal halide or sulfide. When exposed to certain types of radiant energy, it exhibits the photoconductive phenomenon, that is, a decrease in resistance. When light quanta are absorbed by the material, electrons are released into the conduction band and, if a voltage is applied to the film, a current will flow. The resistance change with illumination is considerable. In most photoconductive cells the conductance is nearly linear with high intensity. Resistance therefore varies reciprocally with intensity. Most photoconductive cells will exhibit a drop in resistance from many megohms in the dark to a few hundred ohms when illuminated. Such devices are extremely sensitive photodetectors and are often employed as light-controlled switches.

Figure 6–5 illustrates a few of the standard configurations of photoconductive cells. A wide range of diameters is available: some card-reading cells are as small as 5 mm; others used in photoelectric relays are as large as 25 mm. Many manufacturers supply the same photosensitive material in side-on and end-on models.

Many of the photoconductive cells show good sensitivity to visible light, and a few are sensitive to the ultraviolet and x-ray spectra. A large number, however, are exquisitely sensitive to the infrared region, a characteristic which prompted their development for spectroscopy and self-guiding, infrared-seeking missiles. The sensitivity peaks of many units can be shifted by cooling; for example, Moss (1949) showed that the spectral peaks of lead sulfide, lead selenide, and lead telluride can be shifted farther into the infrared region by cooling to 20°K. The spectral characteristics of several of the photoconducting surfaces operated at room temperature are shown in Fig. 6–6. Jacobs (1960) has listed the characteristics of many of the commercially available photoconductors when operated at reduced temperatures.

The response and decay times vary widely with the type of material and are not independent of the illumination level. In general, the response time is shorter with a high light level. Typical response times for photoconductors operated at room temperatures vary between 0.1 and 30 ms.

6-4. COMPARISON OF PHOTODETECTORS

With such an array of different photodetectors, it is worthwhile reviewing the prominent characteristics of each type. From the viewpoint of linearity and rapidity of response to incident radiation, the photoemissive tube is superior to the photovoltaic cell and photoconductor. Its spectral characteristics lie predominantly in the visible region with few types showing a sensitivity to infrared radiation. Only a small output current is produced for a high anode voltage. However, when the small current is passed through a high resistance, a large output voltage is obtained. The frigility of the glass envelope restricts operation of the device to situations in which only small acceleration forces are encountered.

The photovoltaic cell offers the advantage of a high output current and low voltage which can energize a rugged galvanometer, relay, or other low-impedance circuit without requiring an external source of voltage. The

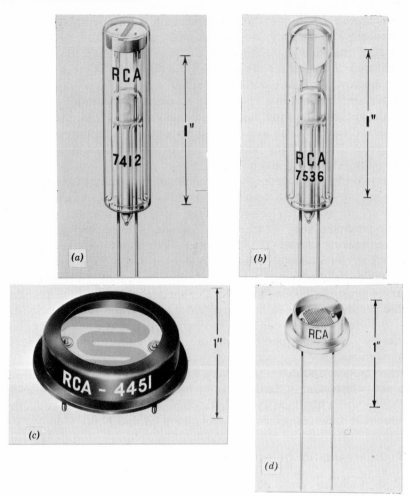

Figure 6–5. Photoconductive cells: (*a*) CdS end-on; (*b*) side-on; (*c*) CdS end-on; (*d*) end-on. (Courtesy Radio Corporation of America, Lancaster, Pa.)

slow response to a flash of light limits its application when light modulation techniques are employed. Photovoltaic cells are temperature sensitive and rugged. The spectral sensitivity of some types strongly resembles that of the eye, and for this reason they are extremely practical for illumination meters.

The photoconductive transducer is a sensitive, relatively high-resistance photoresistor which requires the use of an external voltage to obtain a current related to the intensity of radiant flux. Although the device is sensitive to visible light, the peak spectral sensitivity of most types lies in

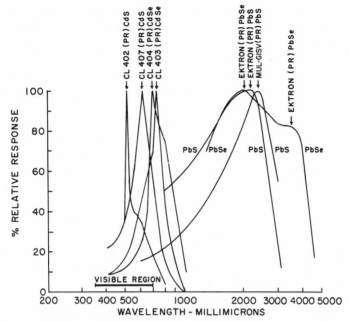

Figure 6–6. Spectral characteristics of photoconductive cells: PR = Photoresistive; CL = Clairex Corp.; EKTRON = Kodak Corp.; MUL = Mullard Corp.

the red and infrared regions. The large change in resistance makes the photoconductive transducer useful as a light-sensitive switch that can be employed to operate a variety of devices. The response time varies from a fraction of a millisecond to several tens of milliseconds. The photoconductive cell is rugged, small, usually inexpensive, and available with a reasonably wide variety of spectral sensitivities.

6–5.   COLORIMETRIC APPLICATIONS

Apart from their use in colorimeters and spectrophotometers to analyze biological fluids, photoelectric transducers see service in the measurement of physiological events in the living subject. Two applications are determination of the oxygen saturation in the blood as it circulates and measurement of cardiac output by the dye-indicator method. In both applications photodetectors are employed with appropriate filters to detect color density changes.

The determination of oxygen saturation by measuring the "redness" of the blood in the living subject is accomplished by transillumination of a web of tissue richly endowed with a capillary bed, such as the lobe or pinna of the ear. The emergent light is detected by two photovoltaic detectors, each of which is covered with a filter. The first detects radiation in the red portion of the spectrum at 640 mμ and the second in the infrared at 800 mμ. The red channel provides a signal which contains information on the amount of oxygen in the blood and the amount of blood and tissue in the optical path. The infrared channel signal is independent of oxygen saturation and carries information on the amount of the blood and tissue in the optical path.

Figure 6–7 illustrates the spectral characteristics of fully oxygenated blood (HbO$_2$) and blood without oxygen (Hb). Also shown are the spectral response of the bloodless ear (Elam et al., 1949) and the approximate bandpass characteristics of the red and infrared channels of a typical oximeter earpiece employing iron-selenium photovoltaic cells covered by appropriate red and infrared filters.

Oxygen saturation is determined by calibrating the photodetector against chemically analyzed blood samples. The calibration curve is a plot of oxygen saturation versus the ratio of the logarithm of the transmission in the red to the logarithm of the transmission in the infrared band. When such a calibration curve has been constructed on a well-flushed ear, 95% of the readings can be expected to fall within ±5% of the true value (Wood and Geraci, 1949).

The first practical oximeter was developed by Millikan (1942). In it the photodetectors were mounted in a small fixture which fitted over the pinna of the ear. In an improved instrument described by Wood and Geraci (1949) the photocell assembly was equipped with a pressure capsule that permitted

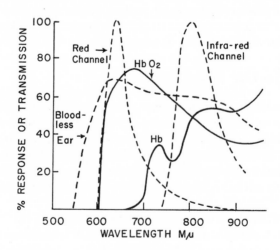

Figure 6–7. Spectral data employed in oximetry.

rendering the optical path bloodless to make initial settings. Figure 6–8 shows a commercial version[1] of the Wood-Geraci ear oximeter.

It has been possible to determine oxygen saturation by reflectance colorimetry. After finding that the amount of light in a narrow band in the red spectrum reflected from a film of blood 3.5 mm or more in thickness was proportional to oxygen saturation, Zijlstra (1951) set about to construct a reflectance-type oximeter for human use. He employed a barrier layer photocell in which was mounted concentrically a small lamp covered by a red filter transmitting light of 600 to 680 mμ. A small box held the photocell and light bulb a short distance from the forehead of the subject. To obtain adequate stability in his first model, Zijlstra had to cool the photocell with a water chamber mounted behind it. In a second model two photocells were used and a differential circuit was employed, thereby eliminating the need for a cooling chamber. In a later model two spectral bands (red and green) were utilized and a third photocell was added for compensation purposes.

The output of the photocells was calibrated in terms of oxygen saturation by chemically analyzed blood samples. Zijlstra stated that, if the oximeter was employed without calibration, the output of the photocells reflected only changes in saturation. He recommended use of the device for monitoring saturation during surgery.

An outstanding intravascular reflectance oximeter using fiber optics was described by Enson et al. (1962). It was applicable to the measurement of oxygen saturation or cardiac output by means of the dye-indicator method. In this device beams of red (660 mμ) and infrared (805 mμ) light were transmitted twenty times per second down a fiber bundle in one lumen of a double-lumen catheter. The diffusely reflected light from the blood at the tip of the catheter was conducted to the external photodetector via a second fiber bundle in the other lumen of the catheter. The photodetecting apparatus consisted of a photomultiplier and oscilloscope, the screen of which showed the red and infrared signals. The ratio of these signals was found to vary linearly with oxygen saturation. The calibration graph presented showed a standard deviation of $\pm$ 1.9% around the regression line.

It is possible to measure the output of the heart per minute by injecting a known amount of indicator into the venous system and measuring its passage in the arterial system with a calibrated detector. With a stable flow for the period of measurement, the prime requisites are that the indicator mixes uniformly with the blood and that it is not lost from the circulation in the time between injection and measurement. A variety of indicators has been employed, the most popular of which are dyes.

The dye-injection method was widely accepted after Hamilton et al. (1948)

[1] The Waters Co., Box 529, Rochester, Minn.

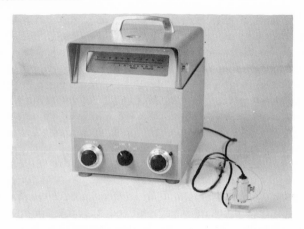

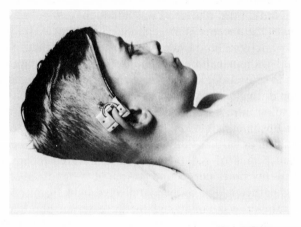

Figure 6–8. Oximeter and earpiece. (Courtesy Waters Co., Rochester, Minn.)

demonstrated that results obtained thereby agreed with those obtained with the Fick technique, and after recording densitometers for arterial blood became available the method was widely accepted. Although many dyes have been employed, the three that appear to be the most popular at present are Evans blue (T1824), indocyanine green (cardio-green), and Coomassie blue. These dyes are nontoxic and nonstimulating. Each has its own characteristics that recommend it for certain purposes. Table 6–2 summarizes the two most important characteristics of each dye, the wavelength for maximum absorption and the retention time in the vascular system.

A few comments will help to identify the relative advantage of each dye. Those that are retained in circulation for a long time yield the highest accuracy. Because of the long retention time, however, the circulation soon

Table 6–2   Characteristics of Dyes

Name	Absorption Wavelength (mμ)	50% Retention Time	Reference
Evans Blue (T1824)	640	5 days	Connolly and Wood (1954)
Indocyanine (cardio-green)	800	10 minutes	Fox (1960), Wheeler et al. (1958)
Coomassie blue	585–600	15–20 minutes	Taylor (1959)

becomes loaded with the dye if repeated determinations are made. Such dyes, although they may be harmless, often discolor the skin if large amounts are injected. On the other hand, dyes which disappear rapidly permit more frequent measurements but, because they soon leave the circulation, accuracy is compromised.

The wavelength for measurement of the dye concentration merits special consideration. Oxygenated blood transmits maximally around 640 mμ; blood without oxygen (reduced blood) and fully oxygenated blood transmit equally well around 800 mμ. Measurements with dyes which absorb around 640 mμ are subject to errors with changes in oxygen saturation. Dyes with maximal transmission around 800 mμ are immune to such errors.

The type of dilution curve following the injection of a dye is shown in Fig. 6–9. Cardiac output is calculated by measuring the area under the first time-concentration curve as shown. Because recirculation usually obscures identification of the end of the first pass, the falling phase is extrapolated to the baseline, or, as was proposed by Kinsman et al. (1929), a semilogarithmic plot of this portion of the curve and linear extrapolation to a negligible concentration (ca. 1% of maximum) are carried out to determine the end of the first pass. The area under the first pass is then determined, and the mean concentration for that time is calculated. The mean concentration for 1 minute is then determined, and cardiac output per minute is calculated by dividing this figure into the amount initially injected. Sample calculations are shown on Fig. 6–9.

When the optical transmission of flowing blood is recorded continuously, scattering and reflection from blood cells cause variations. The transmission varies therefore with the velocity of the blood stream. For this reason it is often difficult to obtain a stable baseline in the recording. A method of overcoming some of these difficulties was reported by Sutterer (1960), who described a compensating densitometer for dye dilution studies using indocyanine green. In this instrument he placed two photodetectors, one sensitive to a wavelength of 800 mμ, the other to all wavelengths but

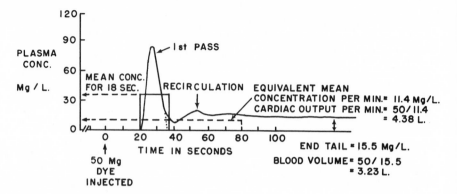

Figure 6–9.   Dye dilution curve.

800 mμ. By combining the outputs of the two photocells, he was able to compensate for changes in flow.

If the dye is retained in the circulation, after several circulations a stable concentration called the "end-tail" is obtained and is often utilized for calibrating the densitometer by withdrawing a sample of blood and analyzing it for the dye concentration existing at this time. This calibration technique is frequently employed when ear oximeters are used to determine cardiac output. It is apparent that calibration by this technique is inaccurate if the dye is cleared rapidly. Because the end-tail calibration point is low on the concentration scale, high accuracy can be attained only if the sample is carefully analyzed.

There is another use for the end-tail concentration, namely, calculation of blood volume. With total mixing of the dye and no loss from the cardiovascular system, blood volume is calculated by dividing the amount injected by the end-tail concentration. The figure obtained in this way assumes that the sample analyzed is representative of all the blood in the body.

Various penetrating mathematical studies of the dilution method have been carried out by Meier and Zierler (1954), Stephenson (1958), Grodins (1962), and Zierler (1962a, 1962b, 1963). These studies are recommended reading for those who wish to investigate current concepts of the dye dilution method. A number of investigators have developed mathematical expressions for the different types of concentration-time curves obtained with normal and abnormal circulatory dynamics. The goal in these studies has been to assign numerical values to the symbols in the equations and by so doing to quantitate the factors underlying the development of the concentration-time curve. An excellent review of the work in this area was presented by Thompson et al. (1964). From their own studies, they developed the following expression for the concentration versus time curve $C(t)$:

$$C(t) = \frac{K(t - T)^\alpha}{e^{(t-T)/\beta}},$$

where t = time after injection,
K = the scale factor constant,
T = appearance time,
α, β = system parameters.

After evaluation of α, β, it was found that this equation very closely fitted the concentration-time curves obtained on a group of normal subjects and patients.

Another *in vivo* colorimetric application of a photodetector is due to Baker (1961), who used the high infrared-sensitivity characteristics of a lead selenide photoresistor to construct a rapidly responding carbon dioxide analyzer to record breath-by-breath changes in the concentration of this gas in expired air. The 4.26-micron absorption band of carbon dioxide was employed to detect the amount of this compound in a gas sample passing between an infrared source and the photoconductive detector. The response time obtained was limited by the speed of admission of the gas sample and the frequency of the chopper amplifier. In practice an overall response time of about 50 ms was obtained.

6-6. NONCOLORIMETRIC APPLICATIONS

There are numerous instances in which photodetectors have been used non-colorimetrically for the transduction of physiological events. One of the earliest was due to Rein et al. (1940), who constructed a blood pressure transducer by affixing a shade to the free end of a Bourdon tube. On one side of the shade was a photovoltaic cell, and on the other was a $\frac{1}{4}$-watt exciter lamp. Pressure applied to the Bourdon tube moved the shade and exposed the photodetector to the light bulb, thereby producing a voltage which was recorded by a rapidly responding galvanometer. The response time reported was 12.5 ms, and the volume displacement was 13.5 mm^3 per 100 mm Hg.

There have been other interesting applications of photodetectors to measure blood pressure; for example, Feitelberg (1942) described an ingenious servosystem with a phototube and light source in an assembly which was mounted on a lead screw and driven by a reversible motor. Between the phototube and light bulb was placed one arm of a mercury manometer which displayed mean blood pressure. In operation the phototube and exciter lamp assembly was made to track the level of mercury.

Mechanically coupled to the photodetector assembly was an ink-writing recorder which displayed changes in mean blood pressure. The advantage of this early servosystem was the elimination of stylus friction, so bothersome in the smoked-drum kymographic recording systems. Feitelberg reported that the system worked well and achieved a tracking rate of 20 mm Hg per second.

Gilson (1943) described the application of the photoelectric principle to detect the movement of the light beam of a Wiggers membrane manometer and the movement of a myograph lever. This method of transduction added sensitivity to an already high-quality photographic recording pressure transducer. His myograph was one of the first to produce an electrical signal from muscle pull. An ingenious method of using the photoelectric principle to develop a catheter-tip blood pressure transducer was described by Clark et al. (1965). In this device a tiny reflecting diaphragm was mounted at the tip of a catheter (0.11 inch diameter) which contained two concentrically mounted bundles of optical fibers. Light was transmitted down one bundle of 3-mil fibers and reflected back to a silicon photocell affixed to the end of the other. Pressure applied to the tiny diaphragm changed the curvature and altered the amount of light reflected to the photocell. With a silvered Mylar diaphragm of appropriate thickness (1 to 3 mils) the change in output was 200 μv for 0 to 50 mm Hg change in pressure. The resonant frequency of the diaphragm was reported by these investigators to be 10kc, indicating that the device had an extremely high frequency response and was capable of recording the briefest of transients in the cardiovascular system.

Figure 6–10 summarizes several applications of the photoelectric principle described by Geddes et al. (1956, 1957). Figure 6–10a illustrates a blood pressure transducer which resembles Rein's except that a high-efficiency miniature photoemissive vacuum tube is employed instead of a photovoltaic cell. With a 15 psi Bourdon tube, a response time of 20 ms is easily attainable when the tube is filled with saline. Below the blood pressure transducer is a pneumograph (Fig. 6–10b) which detects respiration by measuring changes in chest circumference. When the closed rubber bellows is wrapped around the chest, the pressure in it decreases with inspiration. The reduced pressure is sensed by the metal bellows, which causes a shade to alter its position between a photoemissive tube and light bulb. Figure 6–10c shows a photoelectric myograph. The stiff member with the hook carries the shade. When the muscle force is applied to the hook, the elastic member is deflected and the shade is made to move parallel to the face of the phototube by means of a parallelogram arrangement of springs. A series of different elastic members is employed to extend the range of the basic transducing element.

Photodetectors, particularly photovoltaic cells and photoresistors, are extremely practical for detecting pulsatile blood volume changes. For

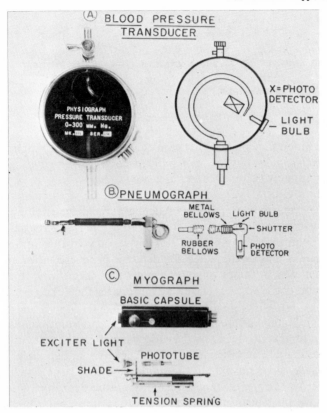

Figure 6–10. Photoelectric transducers: (a) blood pressure transducer; (b) pneumograph; (c) myograph.

detecting the pulse the two techniques diagramed in Fig. 6–11 are employed. Sometimes the vascular bed is placed between the light bulb and photodetector; at other times the exciter lamp is adjacent to the photodetector. In the first technique, the capillary pulse modulates the optical density; in the second, the pulse alters the amount of reflected and scattered light.

The reflectance transducer was introduced by Hertzman (1938). With this device connected to an amplifier and recorder having a time constant longer than 2 seconds, excellent pulse tracings can be recorded for human and small animal subjects. The pulsatile signal recorded reflects the difference in the instantaneous inflow and the outflow of blood. Hertzman standardized the sensitivity of his system with clear glass filters. He computed an approximate relationship between one filter unit and the volume pulse derived from other plethysmographic techniques. It is to be emphasized that the volume pulse when so calibrated yields only information on the temporal

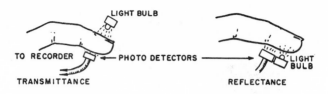

Figure 6–11.   Photoelectric pulse transducers.

changes in blood flow in the skin below the transducer. Although the photo-electric plethysmograph does not indicate total flow, it produces a signal which immediately shows changes in flow.

With photoelectric pulse pickups, detection of stray light sometimes produces artifacts in the recordings. Adequate shielding will eliminate much of this interference. Sensitivity to stray lighting can be decreased consider-ably if a photodetector which is responsive only to the infrared region near 800 mμ is employed. When the detector is covered with an infrared gelatin filter which passes this wavelength, variations in ambient visible light are not detected. An added advantage is that changes in oxygen saturation do not affect the detector.

When employing photoelectric pickups, an important consideration is the amount of heat produced by the exciter lamp. Heat causes dilatation of blood vessels and hence alters the state of the vascular bed under examina-tion. Although the heat aids in the production of a large signal from the pulse detector, in some instances this may not be desirable. One solution to the problem has been the creation of a reflectance pulse pickup which employs cold light.[2] In this interesting device, illustrated in Fig. 6–12, an electroluminescent panel emits light at 640 mμ and illuminates the vascular bed. In the center of this panel is mounted a photoconductive cell which detects the variations in reflected and scattered light caused by changes in blood flow under the transducer. Because it weighs little, is easily attachable, and measures only 0.5 × 0.5 × 0.1 inch, this device should see considerable service in monitoring the pulse.

A photoelectric pulse pickup can be employed in systems that measure blood pressure, heart rate, and blood flow in the region examined by the photodetector. Capacitance coupling with a relatively short time constant (1 second for human beings) can be used in the former cases; direct coupling or condenser coupling with a long time constant is necessary in the latter. If an artery central to a photoelectric pulse pickup is occluded by a pres-surized cuff[3] the pulse disappears. As the pressure is reduced, the pulse appears when the pressure in the cuff is slightly below systolic. If the pressure

[2] Statham Medical Instruments, Los Angeles, Calif.
[3] The width of the cuff merits special consideration (see Geddes et al., 1966).

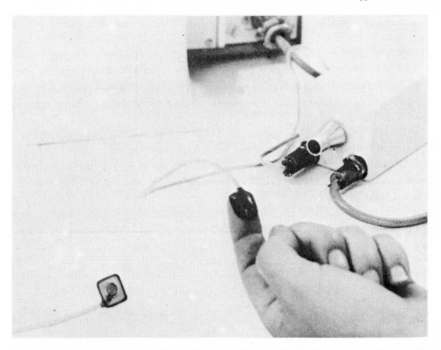

Figure 6–12. Cold light pulse pickup. (Courtesy Statham Medical Instruments, Los Angeles, Calif.)

is read at the first appearance of the pulse, the value obtained is very close to the systolic blood pressure in the artery under the cuff. As the pressure in the cuff is further decreased, the pulse increases in amplitude and reaches a stable level. There is no consistently identifiable transitional point as the cuff pressure passes through diastolic pressure.

An ingenious use of the photoelectric method to obtain a good approximation of systolic and diastolic pressures was described by Wood et al. (1950). With their method an oximeter earpiece with a pressure capsule was employed. A continuous record of the capsule pressure and the optical pulse was made. With a capsule pressure above systolic pressure, the optical pulse record showed no oscillations. As the capsule pressure was reduced, the pulse appeared at pressure just below the systolic value. As the pressure was further reduced, the amplitude of the photoelectric pulse increased, passed through a maximum, and then stabilized at a reduced amplitude. When the pulses were maximal the capsule pressure was taken as diastolic pressure, this point being the diastolic criterion in the oscillometric method. A simultaneous recording of direct blood pressure in the radial artery revealed a good degree of correspondence for systolic and diastolic pressures.

Geddes et al. (1961) employed the photoelectric transduction principle to obtain an electrical signal related to the partial pressure of oxygen in a gas sample by the method shown in Fig. 6–13. In this illustration the detector is the Pauling (1946) paramagnetic oxygen analyzer, which is now available commercially.[4] By replacing the scale with a photodetector having a triangular aperture and replacing the light source with an illuminated slit, the position of the mirror-carrying sensor in the analyzer was converted to an electrical signal.

When fluids flow at low rates, it is advantageous to count drops. Although the size of a drop depends on many factors, in most situations 15 to 30 drops constitute 1 cc of fluid. With a given orifice, drop size is fairly constant. Drop counters in which the fluid strikes a pair of contacts have never been dependable. To eliminate direct contact with the drops of fluid, the photoelectric principle has been employed with considerable success. In some instances the drop interrupts the beam of light to the photodetector; in others the drop reflects and scatters the light sensed by the photodetector. Among the investigators who have described such drop counters are Goetz (1948), Clementz and Ryberg (1949), Hilton and Lywood (1954), Lindgren and Unvas (1954), and Peiss and McCoole (1958).

Another interesting use of the photoelectric principle is in recording

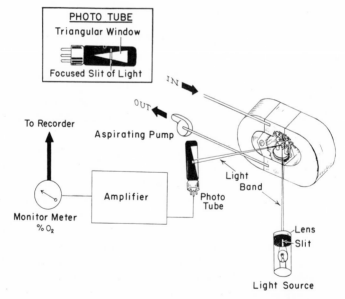

Figure 6–13. Photoelectric transducer applied to paramagnetic Beckman oxygen analyzer. Model C (modified). [From Geddes et al., IRE Trans. *Bio-Med. Electron.* **8**:38 (1961). By permission.]

[4] Beckman Instruments, Scientific and Process Instruments Division, Fullerton, Calif.

the movements imparted to the body when the heart beats. Such a recording is called a ballistocardiogram, and from it may be derived body displacement, velocity, and acceleration. In order to record body movements directly rather than those of a table on which a subject was placed, Dock and Taubman (1949) developed a photoelectric transducer which was coupled to the shins or head of a supine subject. Body movements altered the position of a shade placed between a photodetector and a light source. For a time it was hoped that this signal could be calibrated directly in terms of the systolic discharge from the heart, but this has not been possible to date. In a given subject however, ballistocardiograms do indicate changes in stroke volume.

As a practical and efficient transducer for large or small mechanical movements the photodetector is difficult to surpass. A wide range of photodetectors is available with small or large photosensitive surfaces. By suitable masking, a variety of output versus shade motion relationships is available. Figure 6–14 illustrates a few of the types of transfer characteristic attain-

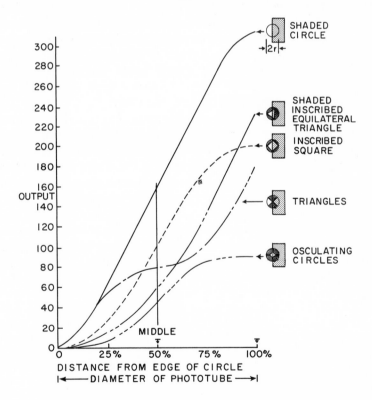

Figure 6–14.   Phototube mask curves.

able by masking a circular photodetector with simple geometric shapes. When a light source is chopped by rotating a disk with a hole in it, various useful waveforms can be generated. For example, a curve closely approximating a sinusoid can be obtained when a square aperture passes over a circular photosensitive area having its diameter equal to the diagonal of the square. The same waveform can be obtained if the photosensitive surface is circular and the aperture is square. The direction of motion is such that the diagonal of the square moves coincidently with and along the diameter of the circle. A sinusoidal variation in light can also be obtained by rotating an eccentrically mounted circular mask made to vary the length of a slit exposed to light. This technique was used by Geddes (1951) to generate a variable-frequency sine wave with a notch fixed at its positive peak. This complex waveform was employed for testing phase distortion in amplifiers.

Suitable choice of the type of photodetector will produce an appreciable voltage or current for a small change in light level. Thus, a high conversion efficiency is easy to obtain. Because the shade mounted on a moving member can usually be made small and lightweight, it adds little inertia to the system. Freedom from contact also eliminates frictional and hysteresis errors. With a proper choice of photodetector, the response time is determined by the mechanical characteristics of the moving element. Alternating and direct current can energize exciter lamps. If alternating current is employed, the photodetector output contains a ripple signal with twice the frequency of the current used to excite the lamp.

There are disadvantages in using phototransducers. In most applications it is necessary to provide shielding to prevent stray light from entering the transducer; in nearly all, a constant-intensity light source is required. With many lamps the light output varies nearly as the square of the applied voltage; hence the lamp voltage must be well regulated. One way of reducing the need for regulation is to use two identical photodetectors in a differential configuration. In such a circuit arrangement one photodetector monitors the light intensity and the other senses the changes in light produced by the event being transduced. In practice, a signal derived from the difference in the ouputs of the two photodetectors is immune to changes in light intensity over a considerable range.

REFERENCES

Acker, R. M., R. P. Lipkis, R. S. Miller, and P. C. Robinson. 1960. Solar cell power supplies for satellites. *Electronics* **33**:167–172.

Baker, L. E. 1961. A rapidly responding narrow-band infrared gaseous CO_2 analyzer for physiological studies. *IRE Trans. Bio-Med. Electron.* BME-8:16–24.

Clark, F. J., E. M. Schmidt, and R. F. De La Croix. 1965. Fiber optic blood pressure catheter with frequency response from DC into the audio range. *Proc. Natl. Electron. Conf.* **21**: 213–216.

Clementz, B., and C. E. Ryberg. 1949. An ordinate recorder for measuring drop flow. *Acta Physiol. Scand.* **17**:339–344.

Connolly, D. C., and E. H. Wood. 1954. Simultaneous measurement of the appearance and disappearance of T1824 (Evans Blue) in blood and tissue after intravenous injection in man. *J. Appl. Physiol.* **7**:73–83.

Dock, W., and F. Taubman. 1949. Some techniques for recording the ballistocardiograph directly from the body. *Am. J. Med.* **7**:751–755.

Elam, J. O., J. F. Neville, W. Sleator, and W. N. Elam. 1949. Sources of error in oximetry. *Ann. Surg.* **130**:755–773.

Enson, Y., W. A. Briscoe, M. L. Polanyi, and A. Cournand. 1962. *In vivo* studies with an intravascular and intracardiac reflection oximeter. *J. Appl. Physiol.* **17**:552–558.

Feitelberg, S. 1942. A photoelectrical recorder for biological purposes. *Proc. Soc. Exptl. Biol. Med.* **49**:177–178.

Fox, I. J., and E. H. Wood. 1960. Indocyanine green: physical and physiologic properties. *Proc. Staff Meetings Mayo Clinic* **35**:732–744.

Geddes, L. A. 1951. A note on phase distortion. *EEG Clin. Neurophysiol.* **3**:517–518.

Geddes, L. A., H. E. Hoff, and A. S. Badger. 1966. Introduction of the auscultatory method of measuring blood pressure. *Cardiovascular Res. Center Bull.* **5**:57–74.

Geddes, L. A., H. E. Hoff, and W. A. Spencer. 1957. The Physiograph—an instrument in teaching physiology, *J. Med. Educ.* **32**:181–198; also: 1956. *IRE Conv. Record* **9**:29–37.

Geddes, L. A., H. E. Hoff, and W. A. Spencer. 1961. The center for vital studies—a new laboratory for the study of bodily functions in man. *IRE Trans. Bio.-Med. Electron*, BME-**8**:33–45.

Gilson, W. E. 1943. Applications of electronics to physiology. *Electronics* **16**:86–89.

Goetz, R. H. 1948. A photoelectric drop recorder. *Lancet* **1**:830–831.

Grodins, F. 1962. Basic concepts in the determination of vascular volumes by indicator dilution methods. *Circulation. Res.* **10**:429–446.

Hamilton, W., R. L. Riley, A. M. Attyah, A. Cournand, D. M. Powell, A. Himmelstein, R. P. Noble, J. W. Remington, D. W. Richards, N. C. Wheeler, and A. C. Witham. 1948. Comparison of the Fick and dye injection methods of measuring the cardiac output in man. *Am. J. Physiol.* **153**:309–321.

Hertzman, A. 1938. The blood supply of various skin areas as estimated by the photoelectric plethysmograph. *Am. J. Physiol.* **124**:328–340.

Hilton, S. M., and D. W. Lywood, 1954. Photoelectric drop counter. *J. Physiol.* **123**:64.

Jacobs, S. F. 1960. Characteristics of infra-red detectors. *Electronics* **33**:72–73.

Kinsman, J. M., J. W. Moore, and W. F. Hamilton. 1929. Studies on the circulation. *Am. J. Physiol* **89**:322–330.

Lindgren, P., and B. Unvas. 1954. Photoelectric recording of the venous and arterial blood flow. *Acta Physiol. Scand.* **32**:259–263.

Meier, P., and K. L. Zierler. 1954. On the theory of the indicator-dilution method for measurement of blood flow and volume. *J. Appl. Physiol.* **6**:732–744.

Millikan, C. A. 1942. The oximeter, an instrument for measuring continuously the oxygen saturation of arterial blood in man. *Rev. Sci. Instrs.* **13**:434–444.

Moss, T. S. 1949. The temperature variation of the long wave limit of infra-red conductivity in lead sulphide and similar substances. *Proc. Phys. Soc.* (London) **B62**:741–748.

Pauling, L., R. E. Wood, and J. H. Strudivant. 1946. An instrument for determining the partial pressure of oxygen in a gas. *Science* **103**:338.

Peiss, C., and R. D. McCoole. 1958. Simple optically recording flowmeter for drop or integrated flow measurement. *J. Appl. Physiol.* **12**:137–139.

RCA Phototubes-Photocells. *Bulletin* 1G1018. Radio Corporation of America, Electron Tube Div., Harrison, Pa.

Rein, H., A. A. Hampel, and W. A. Heinemann. 1940. Photoelectrische Transmission-manometer zur Blutdruckschreibung. *Arch. ges. Physiol.* **243**:329–335.

Stephenson, J. L. 1958. Theory of measurement of blood flow by dye dilution technique. *IRE Trans. Med. Electron.* PGME-**12**:82–88.

Sutterer, W. F. 1960. A compensated densitometer for indocyanine green. *Physiologist*, **3**:159.

Taylor, S. H., and J. P. Shillingford. 1959. Clinical applications of coomassie blue. *Brit. Heart J.* **21**:497–504.

Taylor, S. H., and J. M. Thorp. 1959. Properties and biological behavior of coomassie blue. *Brit. Heart J.* **21**:492–496.

Thompson, H. K., C. F. Starmer, R. E. Whalen, and H. D. McIntosh. 1964. Indicator transit time considered as a gamma variate. *Circulation Res.* **14**:502–515.

Wheeler, H. O., W. I. Cranston, and J. I. Meltzer. 1958. Hepatic uptake and biliary excretion of indocyanine green in the dog. *Proc. Soc. Exptl. Biol. Med.* **99**:11–14.

Wood, E. H., and J. E. Geraci. 1949. Photoelectric determination of arterial oxygen saturation in man. *J. Lab. Clin. Med.* **34**:387–401.

Wood, E. H., J. R. B. Knutson, and B. E. Taylor. 1950. Measurement of blood content and blood pressure in the human ear. *Proc. Staff Meetings Mayo Clinic* **25**:398–405.

Zierler, K. L. 1962a. Circulation times and the theory of indicator-dilution methods for determining blood flow and volume. *Handbook of Physiology*, Vol. 1, Sec. 18. Washington, D.C.: American Physiological Society.

Zierler, K. L. 1962b. Theoretical basis of indicator-dilution methods for measuring flow and volume. *Circulation Res.* **10** (Part 2): 393–407.

Zierler. K. L. 1963. Theory of use of indicators to measure blood flow and extracellular volume and calculation of transcapillary movement of tracers. *Circulation Res.* **12** (Part 1): 464–471.

Zijlstra, W. G. 1951. *Fundamentals and Applications of Clinical Oximetry.* Assen, The Netherlands: Van Gorcum and Co.

7

Piezoelectric Transducers

The piezo- (pressure)- electric effect, discovered in 1880 by Pierre and Jacques Curie, is a property of some natural crystalline substances to develop electrical potential along certain crystallographic axes in response to the movement of charge as a result of mechanical deformation. Figure 7–1 diagrams the method of designating crystallographic axes is some of the more familiar crystals. A necessary condition for the presence of the effect is the absence of a center of symmetry of charge distribution. Twenty-one of the thirty-two crystal classes lack this symmetry, and crystals in all but one of these classes can exhibit the piezoelectric phenomenon. Although about one thousand crystalline substances have been observed to have the property, for only about one hundred are quantitative data available. The magnitude of the effect is of practical value in about ten substances.

It is to be noted that the application of an electric field to a piezoelectric crystal distorts it. Thus the phenomenon is reversible. These two features

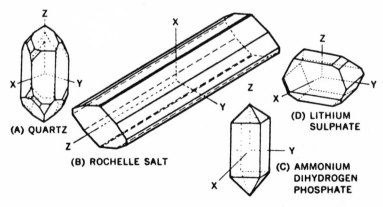

Figure 7–1. Crystals and axes. Clevite Corp., Bedford, Ohio. By permission.

of piezo crystals are responsible for their widespread application in industry and in biomedical studies.

To observe the piezoelectric effect, electrodes must be placed on specific faces of the crystal and the deforming force applied in the appropriate direction (Fig. 7–2). The voltage appearing between the electrodes is linearly related to the deformation. In practice, piezo elements are slabs removed from the parent crystal by cutting along certain crystallographic axes. The magnitude of the piezoelectric effect is dependent on the axis of the cut. The unit employed to designate the magnitude of the effect is the micromicrocoulomb per square meter per newton per square meter. Table 7–1 lists the constants for some of the more common piezoelectric materials.

The slabs cut from the parent crystal can be mounted to permit the development of a piezoelectric voltage in response to bending, twisting, or shearing forces. Frequently the slabs are assembled in pairs or in stacks. One configuration, the bimorph,[1] is particularly useful since it permits a

Table 7–1   Characteristics of Piezoelectric Materials*

	Piezoelectric Constant ($\mu\mu c/m^2/$ newton/m²)	Maximum Humidity Range (%)	Dielectric Constant†	Temperature (°C)
Rochelle salt (30°C)	$d14 + 550$		350	-18 to $+24$
Rochelle salt (30°C)	$d25 - 54$	40–70	9.2	45
Rochelle salt (30°C)	$d36 + 12$		9.5	45
Quartz	$d11 + 2.3$		4.5	550
Quartz	$d14 - 0.7$		4.5	550
Ammonium dihydrogen phosphate (ADP)	$d14 - 1.5$	0–94	56	120 to 125
Ammonium dihydrogen phosphate (ADP)	$d36 + 48$		15.5	120 to 125
Barium titanate (XTAL)	$d31 - 34$		170	125
Barium titanate (XTAL)	$d33 + 86$		170	125
Barium titanate (XTAL)	$d15 + 392$		2900	125
Barium titanate (ceramic)	$d31 - 7.8$		1700	70 to 100
Barium titanate (ceramic)	$d33 + 190$		1700	
Barium titanate (ceramic)	$d15 + 260$		1450	

Encyclopaedia Britannica, 1963, Encyclopaedia Britannica, Inc., Chicago, London, Toronto, Geneva. 24 vols.
† Relative to air.

[1] Clevite Corp., Bedford, Ohio.

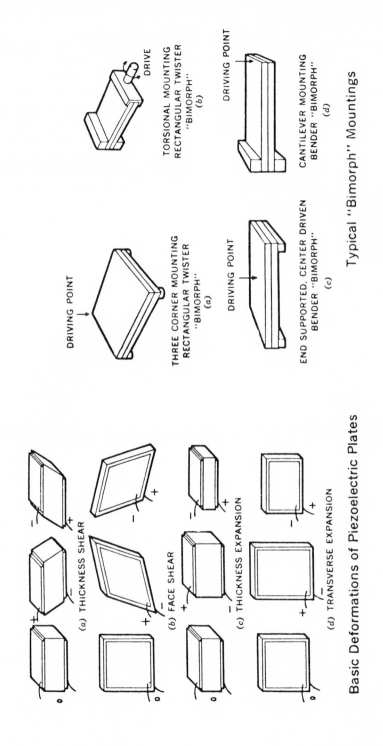

DRIVE

TORSIONAL MOUNTING
RECTANGULAR TWISTER
"BIMORPH"
(b)

DRIVING POINT

CANTILEVER MOUNTING
BENDER "BIMORPH"
(d)

DRIVING POINT

THREE CORNER MOUNTING
RECTANGULAR TWISTER
"BIMORPH"
(a)

DRIVING POINT

END SUPPORTED, CENTER DRIVEN
BENDER "BIMORPH"
(c)

Typical "Bimorph" Mountings

(a) THICKNESS SHEAR

(b) FACE SHEAR

(c) THICKNESS EXPANSION

(d) TRANSVERSE EXPANSION

Basic Deformations of Piezoelectric Plates

Figure 7-2. Piezoelectric crystal elements. Clevite Corp., Bedford, Ohio. By permission.

greater range of motion than is attainable with a single plate. Some of the typical mounting arrangements are illustrated in Fig. 7–2.

In addition to the naturally occurring crystals it is possible to induce the piezoelectric property in certain ceramics, notably barium titanate. With the application of a high voltage to electrodes on the material, there is a reorientation of the crystalline structure which persists after removal of the polarizing voltage. Often this induction process is carried out at an elevated temperature. This technique, in addition to producing a material with a high piezoelectric constant, removes the geometrical constraints of crystallographic axes and makes it possible to cast piezo crystals having any desired form.

A piezo crystal need be distorted only a tiny amount to obtain a voltage in the fractional volt range. For this reason it may be called an efficient isometric transducer. The stiffness of piezo crystals is high, and the permissible deformations are small. Donaldson (1958) stated that the deformation of crystals used in phonograph pickups is 10 microns per gram of weight and that crystals used in accelerometers are distorted only 1 micron per kilogram weight.

A close electrical analog to the piezo crystal is a condenser which is charged by the application of mechanical force. Figure 7–3 illustrates the simplest equivalent circuit. Typical phonograph crystals develop signals in the fractional volt range. With very large crystals and high forces, it is possible to develop many hundreds of volts. Materials lose their piezoelectric property if heated. The temperature at which this occurs is called the Curie point. With most piezoelectric materials there is an upper and a lower temperature limit for retention of the property. The safe operating range is usually much smaller than these two temperature extremes indicate. The upper temperature limits for many piezo crystals are shown in Table 7–1. With an increase in temperature, a slight deterioration of the piezoelectric effect occurs in the piezoelectric ceramics. Although the effect is small, it is nonetheless present and must be considered if techniques involving high accuracy are employed. Some natural crystals are deliquescent, and therefore their performance is adversely affected by a high relative humidity.

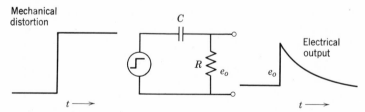

Figure 7–3. Piezoelectric crystal equivalent circuit.

Piezo crystals, being high-impedance devices, can deliver only very small currents. Connecting a resistive load across them reduces the output voltage markedly. A more serious drawback is that, because of leakage resistance, the voltage cannot be maintained when a sustained force is applied. Therefore piezo crystals are only suited to the measurement of changing mechanical forces. They can develop a voltage for changes in mechanical deformation having a frequency of a few cycles per second to many megacycles per second. The upper limit is determined by the total mass and stiffness of the moving system. Because of the high stiffness and low mass of such crystals, they see service as the transducing unit in phonograph pickups, microphones, and vibration detectors. A survey of these industrial uses was presented by Siegel (1959).

In biomedical studies there have been numerous applications of the piezoelectric crystal. Because of its low cost, small size, isometric nature, and large electrical output, it is most useful for the transduction of a variety of time-varying events. A survey of some of the typical uses in physiology was presented by Malcolm (1946), who described a piezo crystal, in a holder of unique design, which served as a general-purpose transducer for ballistocardiography, heart sounds, pulse wave recording, drop counting, muscle pull, and respiration.

The piezoelectric transducer is particularly well suited to the detection of the pressure pulse and of low-energy acoustic phenomena such as heart and Korotkoff sounds. Just after the piezo crystal appeared in industry, Gomez and Langevin (1937) recognized its value for pulse wave recording in the human subject and discussed this application extensively. Miller and White (1941) employed a crystal microphone air-coupled to a chamber placed on the skin to measure arterial and venous pulses. The small pulsation seen in blood pressure cuffs were recorded with good fidelity by Rappaport and Luisada (1944) and Lax et al. (1956). Both teams rebuilt crystal microphones to operate as differential pressure transducers, in which the mean cuff pressure was applied to one side of the diaphragm and the total pressure (mean plus oscillations) to the other.

In many respects the crystal element is ideal for heart sound transduction; almost as soon as the crystal microphone was available commercially, it was called into service for this purpose. Sachs et al. (1935) and Bjerring et al. (1935) used the crystal microphone and described an amplifying device for heart sounds. This instrument, one of the first of its kind to become available commercially, was described in more detail by Lockhart three years later (1938). Narat (1936) eliminated the air coupling from the surface of the body to the microphone diaphragm by developing a contact crystal microphone for the transduction of all vibrations produced by the heart; however, this technique did not attract much attention. Nearly all subsequent workers have used the air-coupling method, probably to attenuate the large amount of low-frequency vibrational energy generated by the beating heart. Boone (1939) employed a crystal microphone with a cathode ray oscilloscope to guarantee maximum fidelity in reproduction of all the cardiac vibrations. Mannheimer (1941) used the high-efficiency and high-fidelity qualities of the crystal microphone in an attempt to calibrate phonocardiography by separating the sounds into four frequency bands. Rappaport and Sprague (1941, 1942) also selected the crystal microphone for their extensive studies on the nature of heart sounds and the frequency response of stethoscopes. The high-efficiency feature of the crystal microphone showed itself again in the transduction of fetal heart sounds. Wood and Gunn (1953) recorded, counted, and monitored these feeble sounds with the aid of an amplifying system with variable frequency tuning.

Contact crystal transducers are beginning to be used more frequently in biomedical investigations. One interesting application is due to Wallace et al. (1957) and Lewis et al. (1957), who constructed miniature phonocatheters by mounting hollow tubular barium titanate crystals on the ends of catheters to detect the intracardiac sounds during heart catheterization studies.

Among the feeblest of auscultatory phenomena are the Korotkoff sounds, and the high-efficiency feature of the piezo crystal has been put to use in their detection. Omberg (1936) used a crystal microphone to control the cycling of a pump connected to a blood pressure cuff. As the cuff pressure decayed, the systolic sounds detected by the microphone restarted the pump; when they disappeared the pump stopped, thereby maintaining the cuff pressure very nearly equal to systolic blood pressure. Gilson et al. (1941, 1942) recorded human blood pressure indirectly by presenting two channel records of cuff pressure and Korotkoff sounds detected by a crystal microphone. These sounds, as they appeared in a smaller cuff located below the blood pressure cuff on the subject's arm, were detected by Rappaport and Luisada (1944). Like Omberg, Gilford and Broida (1954) used a crystal microphone as the primary detector in their fully automatic recording machine which plotted and indicated both systolic and diastolic human blood pressures. Detection of the Korotkoff sounds by crystal elements and their superimposition on the occluding cuff pressure was described by Currens et al. (1957) and Geddes et al. (1959).

Both properties of piezoelectric crystals are employed in ultrasonic blood flowmeters. In such devices two piezo crystals are mounted on a blood vessel. A pulse of high-frequency voltage is applied to one, and the sound created travels to the second piezo element with a velocity which is the algebraic sum of the velocity of the sound in blood and the velocity of the blood. Measurement of the time of arrival of the sound permits continuous determination of the mean velocity of the blood flowing in the vessel. The first instruments operating on this principle were described by Kalmus (1954), Herrick (1959), and Farrall (1959). Because of the small time differences resulting from the flow velocities encountered and the close spacing between crystals, the phase shift is usually measured and is the quantity which is related to velocity. In a slightly different approach taken by Franklin et al. (1959), the transmitting and receiving crystals were alternately switched; the difference between the upstream and downstream times was written out as the signal proportional to the mean velocity of blood flow.

Another system described by Franklin et al. (1961) employed the Doppler effect to measure blood velocity. In this device an ultrasound beam was reflected from the blood cells, and the difference in frequency between the incident and the back-scattered beam was proportional to the velocity of blood in the vessel.

With ultrasonic and other velocity flowmeters, in order to determine the volume rate of flow it is necessary to know the velocity profile and the vessel diameter, both of which are difficult to determine. Often the mean velocity is determined and multiplied by the cross-sectional area to give a figure which approximates flow. It is interesting to observe that Herrick (1959) suggested that the vessel diameter could be determined by ultrasound. This suggestion has not yet been adopted in ultrasonic flowmeter technology.

Piezo crystals are employed also in sonar-like devices in biomedicine. There are many echo-sounding instruments in which the time of return of an echo from a structure within the body is displayed on a cathode ray tube. The position of the echo signal indicates the distance between the target and the piezoelectric transducer. Both Wagai (1965) and Jacobs (1966) have reviewed these techniques.

An ingenious application of the ability of the piezo crystal to produce movement was described by Pascoe (1955). He faced the problem of advancing a microelectrode into a nerve cell which was enveloped in a tough membrane. By mounting the microelectrode on a piezo crystal and applying a pulse of voltage, the electrode was suddenly advanced 20 microns and the tip of the electrode penetrated the cell without damage.

For experimental purposes piezo crystals are readily obtained in a variety of inexpensive commercially available devices such as crystal microphones, phonograph cartridges, earphones, and loudspeakers. The crystal elements are easily removed and are readily adaptable to a wide variety of tasks. Figures 7–4, 7–5, and 7–6 illustrate some of the uses for such piezoelectric elements. Figure 7–4 shows a piezoelectric pulse pickup constructed by Geddes and Hoff (1960), which uses a piezo crystal

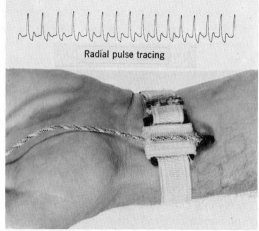

Radial pulse tracing

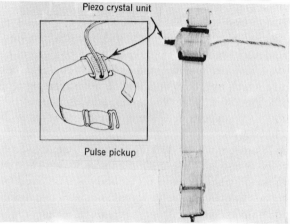

Piezo crystal unit

Pulse pickup

Figure 7–4.   Piezoelectric pulse pickup.

removed from a phonograph cartridge. The element was first coated with an insulating spray and then wrapped with aluminum foil for electrical shielding. A coating of flexible insulation (Insul − X)[2] was then applied, and the element assembled in the bracelet.

Figure 7–5 illustrates a piezoelectric drop counter. This device is merely a phonograph pickup mounted in a metal case; in place of the needle is a mesh pan. Drops striking the pan twist the piezo element and give rise to a voltage pulse of approximately 100 mv.

Figure 7–6 shows a phonograph cartridge piezo element mounted in the lower third of a blood pressure cuff (Geddes, 1959) to detect the Korotkoff sounds in the measurement of blood pressure. If the method

[2] Insul-X Products Corp., Yonkers, N.Y.

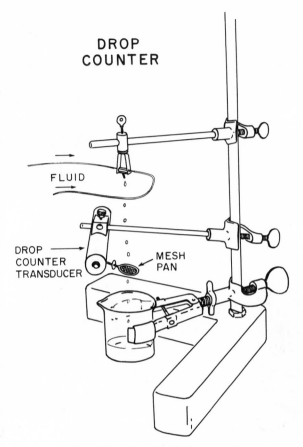

Figure 7–5. Piezoelectric drop counter.

is to be used on subjects with low blood pressure, a larger signal can be obtained by taping the crystal element directly to the skin distal to the cuff and over the brachial artery.

In summary, the piezoelectric crystal is characterized by a high conversion ratio and stiffness, being almost isometric. Electrically it resembles a condenser which becomes charged when distorted. It is thus a voltage generator having a high internal impedance. The piezo crystal cannot be used for the measurement of static forces because of its own leakage resistance, but it is ideally suited to the detection of transient forces which change at rates from a few cycles per second to many megacycles per second, the upper limit being determined by the mechanical resonant frequency of the system.

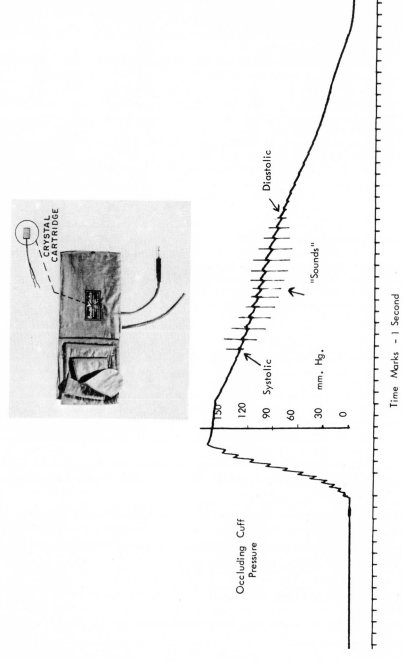

CRYSTAL
CARTRIDGE

Occluding Cuff
Pressure

Systolic

Diastolic

"Sounds"

150
120
90
60
30
0

mm. Hg.

Time Marks – 1 Second

Figure 7-6. Korotkoff sound detector.

REFERENCES

Bjerring, W. L., H. C. Boone, and M. L. Lockhart, 1935. Use of electrostethophone for recording heart sounds. *J. Am. Med. Assoc.* **104**:628–637.

Boone, B. R. 1939. An amplifier for recording heart sounds through use of the cathode ray tube. *J. Lab. Clin. Med.* **25**:188–193.

Currens, J. H., G. L. Branwell, and S. Aronow. 1957. An automatic blood pressure recording machine. *New Engl. J. Med.* **17**:780–784.

Donaldson, P. E. K. 1958. *Electronic Apparatus for Biological Research*. London: Butterworth's Scientific Publications.

Farrall, W. R. 1959. Design considerations for ultrasonic flowmeters. *IRE Trans. Med. Electron.* Me-**6**:198–201.

Franklin, D. L., D. W. Baker, R. M. Ellis, and R. F. Rushmer, 1959. A pulsed ultrasonic flowmeter. *IRE Trans. Med. Electron.* ME-**6**:204–206.

Franklin, D. L., W. Schlegel, and R. F. Rushmer, 1961. Blood flow measurement by doppler frequency shift. *Science* **34**:564–565.

Geddes, L. A., and H. E. Hoff 1960. Graphic recording of the pressure pulse wave *J. Appl. Physiol.* **15**:959–960.

Geddes, L. A., W. A. Spencer, and H. E. Hoff. 1959. Graphic recording of the Korotkoff sounds. *Am. Heart J.* **57**:361–370.

Gilford, S. R., and H. P. Broida. 1954. Physiological monitoring equipment for anesthesia and other uses. *Natl. Bur. Std. (U.S.) Ann. Rept.* 3301, Project 1204–20–5512.

Gilson, W. E. 1942. Automatic blood pressure recorder. *Electronics* **15**:54–56.

Gilson, W. E., H. Goldberg, and H. Slocum. 1941. Automatic device for periodically determining and recording both systolic and diastolic blood pressure in man. *Science* **94**:194.

Gomez, D. M., and A. Langevin. 1937. *La piézographe directe et instantanée*. Paris; Hermann & Cie.

Herrick, J. F. 1959. An ultrasonic flowmeter. *IRE Trans. Med. Electron.* ME-**6**:195–197.

Jacobs, J. E. 1966. *Advances in Bioengineering and Bioinstrumentation* (F. Alt, Ed.) New York: Plenum Press.

Kalmus, H. P. 1954. An electric flowmeter. *Rev. Sci. Instrs.* **25**:201–206.

Lax, H., A. W. Feinberg, and B. M. Cohen. 1956. Studies of the arterial pulse wave. J. Chronic Diseases 3:618–631.

Lewis, D. H., G. W. Dietz, J. D. Wallace and J. R. Brown. 1957. Intracardiac phonocardiography in man. *Circulation* **16**:764–775.

Lockhart, M. L. 1938. The stethograph. *Am. Heart J.* **10**:72–78.

Malcolm, J. L. 1946. A piezoelectric unit for general purpose physiological recording. *J. Sci. Instrs.* **23**:146–148.

Mannheimer, E. 1941. Calibrated phonocardiography. *Am. Heart J.* **21**:151–162.

Miller, A., and P. D. White. 1941. Crystal microphone for pulse wave recording. *Am. Heart J.* **21**:504–510.

Narat, J. K. 1936. New electronic stethoscope and stethograph. Preliminary Report. *Illinois Med. J.* **70**:131–134.

Omberg, A. C. 1936. Apparatus for recording systolic blood pressure. *Rev. Sci. Instrs.* **7**:33–34.

Pascoe, J. E. 1955. A technique for introduction of intracellular electrodes. *J. Physiol.* **128**:26P-27P.

Rappaport, M. B., and A. Luisada, 1944. Indirect sphygmomanometry. *J. Lab. Clin. Med.* **29**:638–565.

Rappaport, M. B., and H. B. Sprague. 1941. Physiologic and physical laws that govern auscultation and their application. *Am. Heart J.* **21**:257–318.

Rappaport, M. B., and H. B. Sprague. 1942. Graphic registration of normal heart sounds. *Am. Heart J.* **23**:591–623.

Sachs, H. A., H. Marquis, and B. Blumenthal. 1935. A modification of the Wiggers-Dean system measuring heart sounds using audio amplification. *Am. Heart J.* **10**:965–8.

Siegel, J. J. 1959. Piezoelectric transducers measure fluctuating forces, pressures, accelerations. *Prod. Eng.* **30**:61–63.

Wagai, T. 1965. Diagnostic application of ultrasound. *Japan Electron. Eng.* **2**:25–30.

Wallace, J. D., J. R. Brown, D. H. Lewis, and G. W. Dietz. 1957. Phonocatheters: Their design and application. Part 1. *IRE Trans. Med. Electron.* PGME-**9**:25–30.

Wood, M. C., and A. C. Gunn. 1953. The amplification and recording of foetal heart sounds. *Electron. Eng.* **25**:90–93.

8

Thermoelectric Transducers

When two metals are joined, a temperature-dependent potential, called the contact potential, develops. First demonstrated in 1821 by Seebeck, the phenomenon has been used extensively for the measurement of temperature for over a century. The contact potential is related to the differences in work function of the two metals. Although a single junction of two metals can be employed to develop the potential, such a simple arrangement is often impractical; the usual configuration for utilization of the thermoelectric effect is illustrated in Fig. 8–1a. The two metals (1, 2) constitute the thermocouple, and the potential developed is then dependent on the temperature difference between the two bimetal junctions $J_{1\text{-}2}$ and $J_{2\text{-}1}$. In practice, it is customary to keep one junction at a reference temperature and employ the other to measure the unknown temperature. Usually the reference point chosen is 0 or 100°C, although room temperature is sometimes employed.

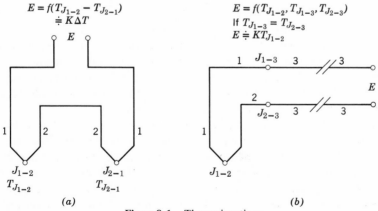

$$E = f(T_{J_{1-2}} - T_{J_{2-1}})$$
$$\doteq K\Delta T$$

$$E = f(T_{J_{1-2}}, T_{J_{1-3}}, T_{J_{2-3}})$$
$$\text{If } T_{J_{1-3}} = T_{J_{2-3}}$$
$$E \doteq KT_{J_{1-2}}$$

(a)

(b)

Figure 8–1. Thermojunctions.

Because the measuring junction must often be located some distance from the reference junction and the indicating instrument, it is usually impractical to choose the same metal for both the interconnecting cable conductors and the thermojunctions. For this reason conducting wires of a different material are introduced into the circuit. Under these conditions the thermodetector takes the form shown in Fig. 8–1b. Thus there are really three important thermal junctions: J_{1-2}, J_{1-3}, and J_{2-3}. The temperature $T_{J_{1-2}}$ can be measured only if the temperatures of the two remaining junctions are kept constant. Usually the connecting wires are made of materials chosen so that the thermal voltages between junctions J_{1-3} and J_{2-3} are small. Thus minor variations in the temperature of J_{1-3} and J_{2-3} will contribute only insignificant error voltages, and the voltage presented to the indicator is largely a function of $T_{J_{1-2}}$.

It is to be noted that the potential developed by thermojunctions depends on the temperature of the metals and not on the size of their junctions. However, it is important to note that the resistance of the circuit does depend on the size of the metallic conductors; if the thermoelectric voltage is to be employed to drive a current-drawing indicator, total circuit resistance must be considered. Another factor, the Peltier effect, is also involved and is discussed later.

The ability of a particular thermojunction to develop a voltage is specified by its thermoelectric power, an old term now of dubious merit. The voltages developed by couples of various metals are usually small. Certain special alloys that produce a large voltage per degree of temperature difference between the reference and exploring junctions have been developed. Typical values for some familiar thermocouples are given in Table 8–1. Over a limited range the voltage is linear with temperature difference.

From these data it is apparent that the thermocouples produce a small voltage per degree of temperature difference between the junctions. For precise determination of temperature, the voltage must be measured with a potentiometer. If current is passed through the junctions, one is warmed and the other cooled. This phenomenon is known as the Peltier effect, and, although its magnitude is small, it must be considered in terms of both changing the resistance of the circuit and adding heat to or abstracting heat from what is being measured.

Although the thermocouple has been somewhat overshadowed by the thermistor as a temperature sensor, new techniques of fabrication indicate that it may see wider application in biomedicine. For example, Reed and Kampwirth (1964) described thermocouples of micron dimensions which could easily be inserted into single living cells to measure the temperature of the cytoplasm. The fabrication technique employed by

Table 8–1   Thermoelectric Sensitivities*'†

Thermojunctions	Thermoelectric Sensitivity (μv/°C)
Nickel-platinum	– 15
Lead-platinum	4
Silver-platinum	6.5
Copper-platinum	6.5
Iron-platinum	18.5
Nichrome-platinum	25
Platinum/rhodium-platinum	6
Chromel-Alumel	40–55
Copper-constantan	40
Iron-constantan	53
Germanium-platinum	300
Silicon-platinum	440
Selenium-platinum	900

*From K. S. Lion, *Instrumentation in Scientific Research*, McGraw-Hill, Book Co., New York, 1959.
†Reference junction, 0°C.

these investigators consisted of vapor deposition of thermoelectric materials on quartz fibers. The thermoelectric voltages developed were those of the metals employed. The resistance of the fibers carrying the thermojunctions approximated 20 kilohms per 5 cm of length. A response time resolvable in microseconds was reported. The response time for slightly larger thermocouples (25 microns) was given by Gelb et al. (1964) as 115 ms for 95% response. Thermocouples made from 40-gauge wire by a commercial firm[1] are advertised as having a time constant of 0.1 second, and the time constant of its ultraminiature couples is given as 0.05 second. Another supplier[2] has advertised fine wire (0.002 to 0.005 inch) iron-constantan thermocouples having time constants in the range of 0.002 to 1 second. Such devices merely await application.

In biomedical studies thermocouples find a variety of uses as detectors of temperature which reflect circulation in the regions measured. Scott (1930) described the use of four couples in series (a thermopile) for measuring skin temperature. Hardy (1934) measured radiant heat from the body with such a device. Miniature thermocouples for determining the temperatures of deep tissues and blood have been constructed and placed in hypodermic needles by Clark (1922), Bazzett and McGlone (1927), Sheard (1931), and Foster (1936). Bazzett and McGlone have

[1] High Temperature Instruments Corp., Philadelphia 33, Pa.

[2] Omega Engineering Inc., Springdale, Conn.

called attention to the fact that thermocouples were used to measure the temperature in human muscle as long ago as 1835. In all probability the thermocouple was the first electrical transducer in physiology. In the hands of Hill (1932) the thermocouple showed that the temperature rise in nerve during the passage of an impulse was 7×10^{-8} °C.

Rein (1928) described his blood flow transducer, the thermostromuhr, which employed a pair of small thermocouples and a heating element to measure blood flow. The apparatus consisted of a tube with the heating element located in the axial stream; proximal and distal to the heating element were mounted the thermocouples. Blood flowing past the heating element was warmed. The upstream couple detected the temperature of the blood before heating, and the downstream unit monitored the temperature of the warmed blood. The temperature difference was thus dependent on blood flow. By improving Rein's instrument, Baldes et al. (1933) were able to measure very tiny blood flows. Their contribution consisted of warming the blood with dielectric heating instead of using a heating element in the blood stream.

For a considerable time the thermostromuhr was a standard blood flow transducer. Burton (1938) analyzed the theoretical considerations underlying the functioning of the device. Applications, advantages, and limitations were set forth by Gregg (1948) and Linzell (1953).

Thermocouples can be small or large in size; the smaller they are the more rapidly they respond to temperature changes. Furthermore, because small units have a low thermal mass, they will not appreciably alter the temperature of whatever is being measured. It is well to remember that with any temperature sensor there is always the problem of heat transfer by conduction along the wires connecting the device to the indicating apparatus.

In the construction of thermocouples certain precautions must be observed. The material from which the junctions are made must be homogeneous, and considerable attention is needed to the fusing of the elements to form the active junction. *Bulletin* 15A-RP 1.4 of the Leeds and Northrup Co. covers the important details of construction and describes gas, electric arc, and resistance welding of the thermojunctions.

An ingenious laboratory method of arc-welding thermocouple junctions electrically, described by Riley (1949), employs a metal cup in which is placed a small quantity of mercury covered with mineral or motor oil to a depth of 2 to 3 cm. The metal cup and the mercury within it constitute one electrode connected to the 115-volt power line. The ends of the thermocouple wires are cleaned and twisted tightly together for a distance of several millimeters. The distal end, which is to become the thermojunction, is then cut, leaving only a little more than a single turn of the twisted wires. The other ends of the wires are then joined and connected via a variable resistor to the other side of the power line. The resistor that Riley used consisted of a 400-watt heating element to fabricate a 0.3-mm thermocouple. Welding is accomplished by lowering the twisted ends of the thermocouple wires into the oil to make contact with the surface of the mercury. The assembly is then withdrawn; as contact is broken, the high-temperature arc formed between the wires and the pool of mercury fuses the ends to form the thermojunction. Iron-constantan, platinum, platinum-rhodium, chromel-alumel, and copper-constantan wires have been welded by using this easily mastered technique. Riley reported that the magnitude of the resistor is dictated by the diameter of the wires chosen for the thermocouple. In his experience wires ranging from 0.1 to 4 mm were successfully welded.

By virtue of its ability to generate an electrical potential which can drive a current through a load and so produce power, the thermocouple is a thermoelectric converter. Although the efficiency is low, it may permit the heat of metabolism to be employed as a source of electrical energy.

Thermojunctions are beginning to be used in biomedical research as heat pumps. Yamazaki (1965) and Hayward (1965) have reviewed many of the applications in which the Peltier effect has been used to cool tissues and fluids. Because the cold produced by thermojunctions is easily controlled, precise temperatures can be maintained. Smallness of size, quietness of operation, freedom from moving parts, and ability to switch over instantly from cooling to heating make these devices attractive for biothermal studies.

REFERENCES

Baldes, E. J., J. F. Herrick, and H. E. Essex. 1933. Modification in thermostromuhr method of measuring flow of blood. *Proc. Soc. Exptl. Biol. Med.* **30**:1109–1111.

Bazzett, H. C., and B. McGlone. 1927. Temperature gradients in tissues in man. *Am. J. Physiol.* **82**:415–451.

Burton, A. C. 1938. Theory and design of the thermostromuhr. *J. Appl. Physics.* **9**:127–131.

Clark, H. 1922. The measurement of intravenous temperatures. *J. Exptl. Med.* **35**:385–389.

Foster, P. C. 1936. Thermocouples for the medical laboratory. *J. Lab. Clin. Med.* **22**:68–81.

Gelb, G. H., B. D. Marcus, and D. Dropkin. 1964. Manufacture of fine wire thermocouple probes. *Rev. Sci. Instrs.* **35**:80–81.

Gregg, D. E. 1948. *Thermostromuhr: Methods in Medical Research,* Vol. I. Chicago: Year Book Publishers.

Hardy, J. D. 1934. The radiation of heat from the human body. *J. Clin. Invest.* **13**:593–620.

Hayward, J. N., L. H. Ott, D. G. Stuart, and F. C. Cheshire. 1965. Peltier biothermodes. *Am. J. Med. Electron.* **4**:11–19.

Hill, A. V. 1932. A closer analysis of the heat production of nerve. *Proc. Roy. Soc.* (*London*) **BIII**:106–164.

Leeds and Northrup Co. *Bulletin* 15A-RP 1.4. Pittsburgh: The Instrument Society of America.

Linzell, J. L. 1953. Internal calorimetry in the measurement of blood flow with heated thermocouples. *J. Physiol.* **121**:390–402.

Reed, R. P., and R. T. Kampwirth. 1964. Thermocouples of micron size by vapor deposition. *Direction*, **10**:8.

Rein, H. 1928. Die Thermo-Stromuhr. *Z. Biol.* **87**:394–418.

Riley, J. A. 1949. A simple method for welding thermocouples. *Science* **109**:281.

Scott, W. J. M. 1930. An improved electrodermal instrument for measuring the surface temperature. *J. Am. Med. Assoc.* **94**:1987–1988.

Sheard, C. 1931. The electromotive thermometer, an instrument for measuring intramural, intravenous, superficial and cavity temperatures. *Am. J. Clin. Path.* **1**:209–226.

Yamazaki, Z. 1965. Medical application of thermoelectric cooling. *Japan. Elect. Eng.* **2**:32–35.

9

Chemical Transducers

9-1. INTRODUCTION

The survival of a living cell and of a whole organism depends entirely on the existence of chemical reactions which are precisely ordered and controlled by biological catalysts called enzymes. To understand the processes which characterize life, there is a need to measure the molecular and ionic concentrations of the materials which participate in these reactions. Accordingly, the measurements of pH, pCO_2, and pO_2 are of prime importance in understanding the chemical energy exchanges which are called metabolism. This chapter is devoted to a study of the methods of transduction of these quantities, as they appear in solution, into an electrical signal. Attention will be devoted also to the detection of other important ions, such as sodium, calcium, and potassium.

9-2. ELECTRODE POTENTIAL

The concept of electrode potential is fundamental to an understanding of the measurement of the concentration of ions in solution. Electrode potential is the potential produced at the interface between two material phases. For example, in the case of a metal-solution interface, an electrode potential results from the difference in rates between two opposing processes: (a) the passage of ions from the metal into the solution, and (b) the combination of metallic ions in solution with electrons in the metal to form atoms of the metal. When equilibrium is reached, a layer of charge is formed in proximity to the electrode; that next to the electrode is of one sign, that in the solution is of the opposite. The charge distribution is called the electrical double layer. Although diffuse, the layer in its simplest form was considered by Helmholtz to be a uniform layer of charge. This double layer of charge constitutes a capacitance which is of importance in determining the electrical impedance of the interface as discussed in Chapter 11. The

119

potential appearing across the metal-electrolyte interface at equilibrium is the electrode potential. Table 9–1 lists various ion-to-metal potentials.

Table 9–1   Half-Cell Potentials*

	Potential (volts)
Aluminum^{+++} / aluminum	−1.66
Iron^{++} / iron	−0.44
Nickel^{++} / nickel	−0.250
Lead^{++} / lead	−0.126
Hydrogen^{+} / hydrogen	0.0 (Reference)
Copper^{++} / copper	+0.337
Copper^{+} / copper	+0.521
Silver^{+} / silver	+0.799
Platinum^{++} / platinum	+1.2
Gold^{+} / gold	+1.68
Gold^{+++} / gold	+1.50

Handbook of Chemistry and Physics, 45th Ed., Chemical Rubber Publishing Co., Cleveland, Ohio, 1958.

NOTE: These potentials are listed in the reference as oxidation potentials and accordingly carry a sign opposite to that shown here.

An electrode potential is also developed if an interface is created by imposing a semipermeable barrier (membrane) between two liquid phases so that the membrane allows reversible transfer of a particular ion. After equilibrium has been established, the potential created is proportional to the logarithm of the ratio of the concentrations of the ion to which the membrane is selectively permeable. For a membrane which is ideally selective the potential developed is given by the Nernst equation:

$$E = -\frac{RT}{nF} \ln \frac{C_1}{C_2} = -2.303 \frac{RT}{nF} \log_{10} \frac{C_1}{C_2},$$

where n = valence of the ion,
  R = gas constant (8.315×10^7 ergs per degree per mole),
  T = absolute temperature (degrees Kelvin),
  F = number of coulombs transferred (96,500 coulombs, i.e., 1 faraday, is required to convert one equivalent of an element to an equivalent of ions)
C_1 and C_2 = concentration of the selected ion on the two sides of the membrane.

This form of the Nernst equation is based upon ideal thermodynamic considerations and is valid only for very dilute solutions. It has been found to be in error as the ionic concentrations are increased. This departure from ideal thermodynamic behavior is expressed in terms of the ionic activity, which is related to the ionic concentration in accordance with the expression

$$a = C \times \gamma,$$

where a = the activity of a specific ion,
C = the concentration of the ion,
γ = the activity coefficient.

The Nernst equation is usually written in terms of ion activity as follows:

$$E = -\frac{RT}{nF} \ln \frac{a_1}{a_2} = -2.303 \frac{RT}{nF} \log_{10} \frac{a_1}{a_2}.$$

The activity of an ion species is a measure of the effective concentration rather than the actual concentration. For very dilute solutions γ approaches unity, and the ideal situation in which the potential developed is proportional to the logarithm of the ratio of concentrations more nearly holds. Activity coefficients must be known if the ion concentration is to be determined in terms of the electrical potential developed. The Debye-Hückel equations have been found to yield accurate values for the activity coefficients of dilute solutions such as those encountered in living matter. For a discussion of the application of the Debye-Hückel theory of electrolytes to biological systems a textbook such as that of Bull (1964) is recommended.

The availability of a membrane which exhibits a selective permeability for a particular ion provides, therefore, a means of creating a transducer for that species of ion.

9-3. THE HYDROGEN ELECTRODE

Knowledge of the behavior of the hydrogen electrode is fundamental to an understanding of the determination of pH and pCO_2 by electrometric methods. It is impossible to measure the potential of a single interphase boundary because in the measuring process an additional interface is introduced. It is necessary, therefore, to specify one electrode or interface as the standard to which others may be compared. The hydrogen electrode has been chosen as the standard and its potential specified as zero, as shown in Table 9-1; the potentials of other metal-to-ion interfaces are measured with reference to it.

Of the interfaces listed in Table 9–1, hydrogen⁺/hydrogen is the only one that does not consist of a solid metal in equilibrium with its ion. It is appropriate to inquire how electrical connection can be made to a gas. Because platinum adsorbs hydrogen readily and is itself a good conductor, electrical connection to the hydrogen is accomplished by electrolytically coating a platinum wire or plate with finely divided platinum (platinum black) to increase its surface area. The wire or plate is then said to be platinized. When such an electrode with its adsorbed hydrogen is placed in a solution containing hydrogen ions, a difference of potential, depending on the tendency of the gas to go into solution and on the concentration of hydrogen ions in solution, will develop. The platinum black must remain in external contact with hydrogen gas to ensure that the supply of gas will not be depleted. Hydrogen electrodes have been made in many forms, one of which is the Hildebrand type shown in Fig. 9–1. In using this electrode, the platinized plate is submerged to one half its height in the solution. Hydrogen gas is admitted through the tube as shown and completely surrounds the upper half of the plate. The gas escapes through the holes at the level of the middle of the plate.

Because the potential of the hydrogen electrode is dependent on the concentration of hydrogen ions in solution, it has been possible to design intracardiac catheters with single and double platinum electrodes for detecting and localizing left-to-right heart shunts (Vogel et al., 1962). In this method the catheter containing the hydrogen electrode is placed in the main pulmonary artery. A single breath of hydrogen gas is then administered to the patient, which results in the almost immediate

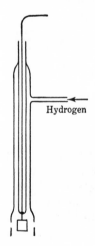

Figure 9–1.   The Hildebrand hydrogen electrode. (From Glasstone, *The Elements of Physical Chemistry*, D. Van Nostrand Co., Princeton, N.J., 1946.)

appearance of hydrogenated blood in the left side of the heart. If a left-to-right shunt is present, it is detected by the development of an electrode potential. The shunt is then localized by repeating the single breath inhalation of hydrogen and searching for the maximum developed potential as the catheter is moved about the right heart while monitoring the position of the catheter with a fluoroscope.

The hydrogen electrode could be used (in theory at least) to measure the pH of solutions. It does, however, possess certain practical inconveniences that are obvious from the foregoing description, and which limit its everyday use both as a pH-determining electrode and as a practical standard electrode in the laboratory. Accordingly, electrodes of high stability and convenience (called standard or reference electrodes) are normally used to measure and compare potentials. Perhaps the two most practical reference electrodes are the calomel and the silver-silver chloride electrodes.

9–4. THE CALOMEL ELECTRODE

The calomel electrode (Fig. 9–2) is one of the most stable of the practical reference electrodes. The potential is developed across a junction

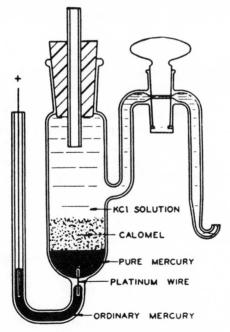

Figure 9–2. The calomel electrode. (From Wellard, Merritt, and Dean, *Instrumental Methods Analysis*, D. Van Nostrand Co., Princeton, N.J., 1951.)

of pure mercury and potassium chloride solution which is saturated with calomel (mercurous chloride). The potential of the calomel electrode is dependent upon the concentration of potassium chloride solution used. Measurement of potential by means of the calomel electrode (or calomel half cell, as it is often called) and other half cells, which may likewise possess a fluid boundary, gives rise to a potential between the two liquid junctions. Such liquid-to-liquid junction potentials are minimized by the use of a "salt bridge," which usually consists of a saturated solution of potassium chloride held in an agar gel in a glass tube and serves as a liquid conductor to connect one liquid with the other. Potassium chloride is especially useful for this purpose because the potassium and chloride ions possess approximately the same mobilities and hence minimize the formation of concentration gradients and resulting electrical potentials. If potassium chloride cannot be used because the presence of certain ions (such as silver) in one or both solutions may produce undesirable chemical reactions, ammonium nitrate may be substituted.

Apart from the practicality of the calomel cell, its chief advantage lies in the stability of its potential over long periods. Because it is a chemical cell, temperature influences the mobility of the ions and hence a small temperature correction is necessary. The emf's of typical calomel cells are shown in Table 9–2.

9–5. THE SILVER-SILVER CHLORIDE ELECTRODE

Silver-silver chloride (Ag-AgCl) is widely used as a reference electrode because it is easy to prepare, reproducible, and small in size. A most complete summary of the preparation, characteristics, and application of this type of electrode was presented by Janz and Taniguchi (1953). Although there are many techniques for preparing these electrodes, one of the easiest methods consists of placing the cleaned silver specimen which is to be chlorided in a solution of sodium chloride. The specimen is then made positive with respect to a silver plate or wire also in the solution. The silver ions combine with the chloride ions to produce neutral silver chloride molecules which coat the silver anode. For general-purpose Ag-AgCl electrodes, Cooper (1963) recommended chloriding at the rate of about 2.5 ma/cm² for several minutes in bromide-free sodium chloride solution. The strength of this solution is not critical but should be at least that of physiological saline (0.9%). Cooper pointed out further that, contrary to general belief, the properties of the chloride layer are not materially changed by continued exposure to light, although Ag-AgCl is photosensitive and produces photovoltaic potentials that can be trouble-

Table 9–2   The EMF's of Reference Cells*

Cell Type	EMF† (volts)	Correction (volts/°C)
Mercury-calomel		
Hg/HgCl$_2$/0.01 MKCl	+0.388	+0.00094
Hg/HgCl$_2$/0.1 MKCl	+0.333	+0.00079
Hg/HgCl$_2$/1.0 MKCL	+0.280	+0.00059 avg.
Hg/HgCl$_2$/3.5 MKCl	+0.247	+0.00047
Silver-silver Chloride		
Ag/AgCl/ 0.01 MKCl	+0.343	+0.000617
Ag/AgCl/ 0.1 MKCl	+0.288	+0.000431
Ag/AgCl/ 1.0 MKCl	+0.235	+0.000250

*From *Encyclopedia of Electrochemistry* (C. A. Hampel, Ed.), Reinhold Publishing Corp., New York, 1964.
† Referred to standard hydrogen electrode at 25°C.

some in some cases, such as recording the EEG while employing photic stimulation. The potential of the Ag-AgCl electrode is dependent on the solution which it contacts and the temperature. Typical values are presented in Table 9–2. Additional information regarding use of the Ag-AgCl electrode for recording bioelectric events is found in Chapter 11.

9–6.   THE pH ELECTRODE

Because it is impractical to use the standard hydrogen electrode to determine pH, the glass electrode is ordinarily employed. A typical glass electrode is illustrated in Fig. 9–3. According to Bull (1943), the glass electrode was discovered by Cremer and was developed by Haber and Klemensiewicz. It consists of a thin glass membrane which permits the passage of only hydrogen ions (in the form H_3O^+). The usual configuration consists of a spherical bulb $\frac{1}{4}$ inch in diameter. On the inside of the pH-responsive glass bulb is placed a buffer solution usually of pH = 1 in which is immersed an Ag-AgCl nonpolarizable electrode. The other side of the glass bulb is exposed to the solution of unknown pH. The connection to the potential-measuring circuit and the solution being tested is completed through a potassium chloride salt bridge and a calomel cell.

The mechanism underlying the operation of the glass electrode is far from simple, and several theories have been proposed to explain the origin of the pH-dependent potential. According to Eisenman (1967), opinion regarding the origin of the glass electrode potential was for many years divided into essentially two schools of thought. One view

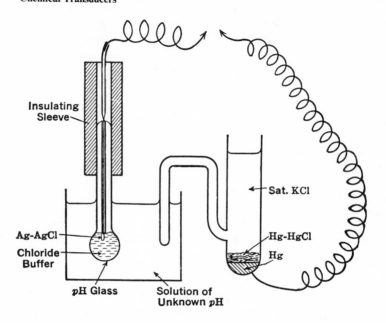

Figure 9–3. The glass electrode used with the calomel half cell to measure pH. (From H. B. Bull, *Physical Biochemistry*, John Wiley & Sons, New York, 1943. By permission.)

held that the potential was exclusively a phase-boundary potential produced at the membrane-solution interfaces. The other view attributed it to a diffusion potential arising within the membrane. These views have been reconciled, and Eisenman states, "It now seems virtually certain that the glass electrode is nothing more or less than a perfect cation-exchange membrane, whose electrode potential represents a sum of contributions from both diffusion and phase-boundary processes." The total glass electrode potential is therefore expressed as the sum of the two boundary potentials produced at the membrane-solution interfaces and the diffusion potential arising within the glass. The interested reader is referred to Eisenman (1967) for detailed theoretical and practical information pertaining to glass electrodes.

The potential developed across the glass membrane is about 60 mv per unit of pH at 30°C. Operation at a different temperature requires the application of a small correction.

The glass electrode made the determination of pH in the laboratory a simple and routine procedure. Bull (1943) listed the following advantages of the glass electrode as compiled by Dole et al. (1941):

1. The glass electrode is independent of oxidation-reduction potentials.

2. It is not necessary to pass a gas through the solution or to add any material to it.
3. It is possible to use very small quantities of solution.
4. The electrode can be used in colored or turbid solutions.
5. The electrode gives accurate values in unbuffered solutions.
6. Equilibrium is reached rapidly.

The glass electrode does, however, possess some limitations. The range of pH over which accurate response is obtained may be restricted unless special glasses are used. For example, some error often exists in both highly acidic solutions (near pH = 0) and alkaline solutions (above pH = 9). Figure 9–4 shows the error in pH for both acid and alkaline solutions for electrodes constructed from the classical Corning 015 glass. This figure shows the amount of error encountered because of sodium and potassium ion concentration. Errors in pH measurement in the range above pH = 9 are known as "salt" or "alkaline" errors. It is now possible to purchase pH electrodes constructed from special glass which may be used over the range pH = 0 to 14 with only a slight correction required above pH = 13.

Because the pH is determined in terms of the potential developed by the pH electrode, it is important that the magnitude of the potential be accurately measured. The fact that the potential is developed by the diffusion of relatively few ions across a glass surface, which in itself is a good insulator, means that the pH electrode has the characteristics of a potential source with a very high internal impedance. Typical

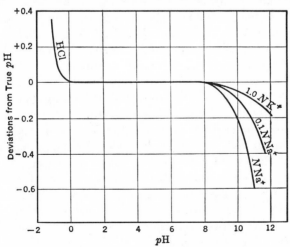

Figure 9–4.   Glass electrode error as a function of solution pH. (From M. Dole, *Theoretical and Experimental Electrochemistry*, McGraw Hill Book Co., New York, 1935. By permission.)

values are in excess of 200 megohms. To prevent the device used to measure this potential from drawing current from the electrode it must possess an input impedance much higher than that of the pH electrode. (The problem of loading is discussed in Chapters 11 and 13.) This requirement is met by use of a potentiometer or a voltage-measuring instrument which employs an electrometer tube or a field-effect transistor in the input stage.

While *in vitro* measurements of pH abound in the life sciences, the continuous recording of pH changes *in vivo* has been carried out less frequently, although the number of investigations has increased with the improvement of pH-monitoring equipment. The stability and sensitivity requirements of pH-measuring devices for *in vivo* work can be appreciated by recalling that the range of hydrogen ion concentration compatible with normal cellular function is about one pH unit; therefore, to record continuously pH *in vivo* means that the recording system is never presented with a signal greater than 60 mv. When measuring mammalian arterial blood, the permissible pH range is about 7.35 to 7.45 and the signal obtainable is only 6 mv. Accordingly, this amplitude must be adequately displayed by the recording stylus or indicator. If smaller changes within the normal range are to be registered, the recording system must possess a sensitivity in the microvolt range.

One of the earliest to measure pH *in vivo* electrically was McClendon (1915), who passed a platinum gaseous-hydrogen calomel-electrode assembly into the stomachs and duodenums of adults and infants to make readings of the pH. Continuous recording of pH was introduced by Gesell and Hertzman (1926). Using a cuvette equipped with a MnO_2 electrode paired with a calomel cell affixed to a continuous aspirating device, they recorded pH changes of arterial and venous blood under a variety of circumstances in order to investigate the effect of pH on the respiratory center. Voegtlin et al. (1930) introduced the application of the glass electrode for continuously measuring blood pH, using electrodes mounted in a flow-through cuvette. They referred to graphic recording and proved that such an electrode system is insensitive to changes in blood flow. A similar electrode system described by Fruhling and Winterstein (1934) was used to make recordings of the pH of carotid artery blood of dogs. Dubuisson (1937) recorded a pH change of a few tenths of a pH unit within a second after the beginning of contraction of skeletal muscle. Continuous records of pH changes on the surface of the cortices of monkeys were made by Dusser de Barenne et al. (1937). They employed a glass electrode paired with a Ag-AgCl electrode filled with physiological saline to avoid the injurious action of the potassium ion in the calomel electrode.

The technique of prolonged recording of pH in the blood of experimental animals was investigated thoroughly by Nims and his co-workers. In a series of papers (1937) they discussed the construction of electrodes suitable for recording pH in flowing blood and described experiments in which continuous records of pH changes were made for periods up to 8 hours. Elegant records of rhythmic changes of approximately 0.1 pH unit in the anesthetized dog were presented. Marshall and Nims (1937) recorded the blood pH response to a variety of injected substances, while Nims et al. (1938) showed that by careful adjustment of the respirator, the pH could be maintained at a chosen level in the curarized dog.

Band and Semple (1967) developed a rapidly responding, indwelling arterial glass electrode for the continuous measurement of blood pH. The pH-sensitive cell consisted of a glass electrode and a Ag-AgCl reference electrode, both lying in the lumen of an intra-arterial needle. The outside diameter of the pH-sensitive glass portion of the electrode measured 0.5 to 0.8 mm, the wall thickness 0.0025 to 0.50 mm, and the length 1.5 to 2.0 cm. The 90% response to a change in pH of blood flowing past the electrode at 2 ml per minute was 0.5 second. The two samples of blood used to measure the response time had been equilibrated previously with 4 and 6% CO_2. In a test performed by driving buffers past the electrode *in situ* at high flow rates (10 ml per minute), 90% of the response occurred in about 40 ms.

For the most part, the glass electrode is an excellent device for monitoring pH and changes in pH. Some limitations and precautions, however, should be mentioned in connection with its use. The glass electrode exhibits a loss of sensitivity and decreased speed of response after a period of service (i.e., a couple of months). This deterioration may be accelerated and become more severe when the electrode is employed in solutions containing proteins. The electrode may be restored repeatedly by etching the glass surface to remove the inactive outer layer. According to Brems (1962), the sensitivity of the glass electrode increases by 0.34% per °C with rising temperature, and the electrical resistance of the glass increases with falling temperature, increasing accordingly the required input impedance of the recording device. Because the active portion of the electrode consists of a thin glass bulb, obvious precautions are required to prevent breakage.

Mattock and Band (1967) have called attention to the limitations of glass electrodes for both pH and cation determinations. In regard to accuracy of measurement, these investigators state:

"It is probably true to say that the accuracy of most pH measurements in terms of interpretative values is relatively poor, and insufficient work has been done to establish how accurate are most of the measurements of cations by electrochemical methods. A good reproducibility or even a good discrimination does not imply good accuracy, since this, if related (as is usual) to an individual ion activity, depends mainly on the validity of the extrathermodynamic assumptions which have to be made in the interpretation of the Nernst equation."

These investigators give the following example showing the degree of difference between accuracy and discrimination which can arise:

"In blood pH measurements it is probably fair to say that a discrimination between samples to within ± 0.004 pH unit ($\equiv \pm 1\%$) is possible, but that accuracy in terms of translation to hydrogen ion activity cannot be any better than ± 0.02 pH unit ($\equiv 4.5\%$). This implies that an operational pH scale for blood can be defined quite closely, without involving interpretation of the pH numbers to beyond a 'notional' activity, but that an absolute activity determination from these numbers can only be uncertain."

9–7. THE pCO_2 ELECTRODE

The pCO_2 electrode was first described by Stow et al. (1957). It consisted of a standard glass pH electrode covered with a rubber membrane permeable to CO_2. Between the glass surface and the membrane was a thin film of water. The solution under test, which contained dissolved CO_2, was presented to the outer surface of the rubber membrane. The film of water equilibrated with the CO_2 in the solution under test by diffusion of CO_2 across the membrane. After equilibration, the pH of the aqueous film was measured by the glass electrode and interpreted in terms of pCO_2 on the basis of the linear relationship between log pCO_2 and pH as described by the Henderson-Hasselbalch equation.

The Stow pCO_2 electrode was improved by Severinghaus and Bradley (1958), who showed both analytically and experimentally that the sensitivity of the electrode could be doubled by including bicarbonate ion in the aqueous medium between the rubber membrane and the glass electrode. These investigators also found that wet Teflon backed with a layer of cellophane 0.002 inch thick was a superior membrane. The optimum aqueous solution consisted of $0.01 M$ $NaHCO_3$ and $0.1 M$ NaCl in which the cellophane had been soaked for several hours. In addition to these modifications of Stow's electrode, Severinghaus and Bradley added NaCl to the solution surrounding the silver reference electrode, thus increasing the conductivity of this solution and stabilizing the reference electrode. The resulting modified CO_2 electrode was twice as sensitive and drifted much less than before. The response time was such that equilibrium was reached in about 2 minutes after a fourfold rise in CO_2 and in about 4 minutes after a fourfold fall in CO_2.

Further improvements in stability and response time, achieved by utilization of a flat-plane membrane glass electrode for tissue measurements, were reported by Hertz and Siesjö (1959). The increase in overall stability was also due to the use of a calomel cell (made an integral part of the electrode) instead of the Ag-AgCl reference cell. The response time was reduced to 25 to 30 seconds for 90% response by employing a more dilute $NaHCO_3$ solution ($0.0001 N$). The use of this dilute solution, however, reduced the sensitivity slightly and introduced an initial rapid drift toward alkalinity, followed later by a slower drift. The use of a $0.001 N$ solution of $NaHCO_3$ appeared to provide a good compromise between drift and response time, although more dilute solutions (even distilled water) were required when rapid response time was the primary consideration. The response times for the electrode at 36°C in saline, equilibrated with different gas mixtures of known CO_2 concentrations, are shown in Fig. 9–5. Because of its unique construction, this electrode could not be used in the horizontal or inverted position.

Severinghaus (1962) reported improvement in both response time and linearity of the Severinghaus-Bradley electrode in the low pCO_2 range by replacing the cellophane spacer used to hold the water film on the surface of the glass electrode with very thin nylon mesh from a stocking. Fibers of glass wool or powdered glass wool were also found to constitute good separators. By using a membrane of 3/8-mil Teflon and glass wool for the separator, electrodes with 95% response in 20 seconds were constructed. It was discovered that glass wool catalyzed the reaction of CO_2 with water. The response time was found to be almost entirely due to the diffusion rate, which was governed by the membrane thickness and temperature. According to Severinghaus, the response time was reduced further by the addition of hemolyzed blood to the electrolyte. The blood provides carbonic anhydrase activity for 1 or 2 days.

In an effort to reduce the response time further, Reyes and Neville (1967) used 0.5-mil polyethylene as a pCO_2 electrode membrane. No separator or spacing material was placed between the glass surface and the membrane. A commercial preparation of carbonic anhydrase was added to the electrolyte. The response time of this electrode was 6 seconds for 90% of a step change from 2% to 5% CO_2.

In commercially available equipment that uses the Astrup method for the determination of blood pCO_2, the same electrode employed for measuring pH directly serves also to determine pCO_2.[1] The procedure makes use of a nomogram shown in Fig. 9–6, the ordinate of which is pCO_2 in

[1] Radiometer Co., Copenhagen, Denmark.

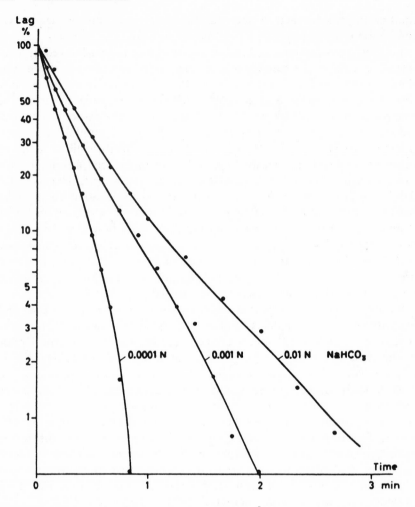

Figure 9–5. The response time of the pCo$_2$ electrode. [From C. H. Hertz and B. Siesjo, *Acta Physiol. Scand.* **47**:115–123 (1959). By permission.]

mm Hg plotted on a log scale, and the abscissa is pH plotted on a linear scale. Briefly, the method employed is as follows. First, the pH of a small sample of heparinized blood (drawn from a capillary bed such as the lobe of the ear) is measured directly. This is the actual pH value, and it determines a vertical line passing through this point on the pH axis. Next, two other small samples taken at the same time as the first are equilibrated under temperature control with two different standard gas mixtures of known pCO$_2$ (60 and 30 mm Hg, for example). The pH of the equilibrated blood

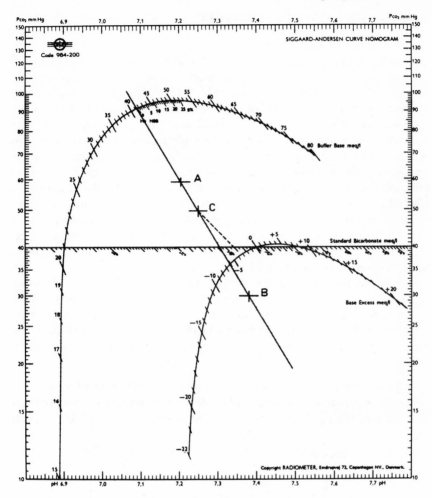

Figure 9–6. Acid-Base nomogram according to Siggaard–Andersen and Engel. (From Radiometer Bulletin 21917E, Copenhagen. By permission.)

samples is then measured directly with the pH electrode. These two values are then plotted on the nomogram (points A and B, respectively), and a straight line is drawn between them. The intersection of line A–B with the vertical line through the actual pH value (point C) is projected to the pCO_2 axis, from which the actual pCO_2 is read. This construction also permits reading values of standard bicarbonate, base excess, and buffer base (all in milliequivalents per liter). The basis of this method was reported by Siggaard-Andersen and Engel (1960), and Siggaard-Andersen (1962).

9–8.   THE pO₂ (OXYGEN) ELECTRODE

In the study of oxygen concentration levels in biological systems, the oxygen electrode provides a means of measuring the partial pressure of oxygen directly at the point of insertion into the tissue. Localization is limited only by the size of the electrode. This is in contrast to manometric methods, which measure the total oxygen concentration in that portion of a biological system that can be isolated and brought to equilibrium with the oxygen in a manometer. An excellent discussion of the principles and techniques pertaining to the use of the oxygen electrode has been presented by Davies (1962). Davies prefers to call this electrode, which is used to measure dissolved oxygen, an oxygen cathode to avoid possible confusion with the oxygen electrode as understood in physical chemistry, which operates under equilibrium conditions and possesses a standard potential of $+1.229$ volts relative to the hydrogen electrode. The term oxygen electrode will be employed in this book since it is the designation most often used by workers in the life sciences.

A method for applying the oxygen electrode to measure the partial pressure of dissolved oxygen is diagramed in Fig. 9–7. The oxygen electrode itself is a piece of platinum wire embedded in an insulating glass holder with the end of the wire exposed to the solution under measurement. According to Davies (1962), the principle of operation of the electrode is as follows:

1. When the platinum electrode is made slightly negative (about -0.2 volt) with respect to the reference electrode, oxygen reaching the surface of the platinum is reduced electrolytically (i.e., the O_2 accepts

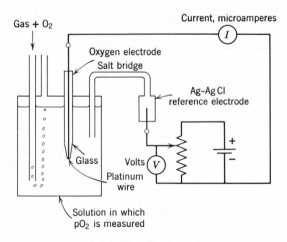

Figure 9–7. The pO₂ electrode.

electrons). The reaction at the cathode is, however, not fully understood.

2. When the platinum is made more negative (-0.6 to -0.9 volt), the velocity of the electrolytic reduction is limited by the maximum rate at which O$_2$ can diffuse to the electrode surface and is not affected greatly by the magnitude of the potential difference. In this voltage range it is found that the current flowing is proportional to the oxygen concentration in the body of the solution.

The shape of the electrode current versus potential relationship is shown in Fig. 9–8a. The electrode is operated in the "plateau" region over which the current shows very little dependence upon the applied voltage. If the potential is held constant (at -0.7 volt, for example), the current is a linear function of the partial pressure of dissolved oxygen, which is expressed as percent O$_2$ in Fig. 9–8b.

Although most of the commercially available pO$_2$ electrodes exhibit a response time of 30 to 60 seconds, it is possible to construct electrodes with a very short response time. Figure 9–9 shows the response time of an open-type oxygen electrode to a sudden change in pO$_2$ as reported by Davies (1962). The 0 to 90% response time of the recording system, including the capacitance of the O$_2$ electrode and wiring, was determined to be about 25 μs. The rise time of this particular electrode is seen to be approximately 0.3 ms (300 μs), which is certainly adequate to monitor continuously localized varying changes in tissue oxygen content.

The oxygen electrode is not free of practical difficulties. The problem known as electrode aging presents itself as a slow reduction in current over a period of time (minutes or hours), even though the O$_2$ tension of the test medium is maintained at a constant level. Aging requires frequent recalibration of the electrode. The exact cause of aging is not known, but it is associated with material attaching itself to the electrode surface. Two measures are often used to combat this problem. First, the electrode is covered with a protective film such as polyethylene, which has the undesirable effect of shielding the electrode from the dissolved O$_2$ and consequently increases the response time (0 to 90%) to as much as 2.5 minutes. The second procedure employed to minimize aging is to reverse the flow of current frequently to lower or reverse the accumulation of surface contaminants.

Another problem encountered with the oxygen electrode is created by the presence of the electrode itself. The O$_2$ diffusion field is maximal in the vicinity of the electrode, causing the concentration of O$_2$ there to be different from what would exist in the absence of the electrode. This source of error is reduced by constantly rotating or vibrating the electrode or by giving it a special geometrical shape.

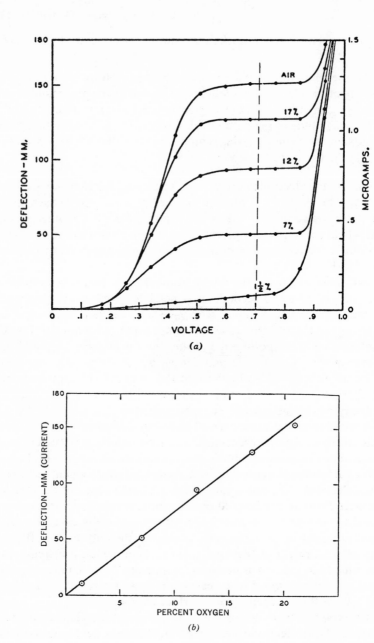

Figure 9–8. (a) The current-voltage characteristics of the pO₂ electrode; (b) the response of pO₂ electrode versus percent oxygen. These values were obtained from Figure 9–8a for polarization voltage of 0.7 volt. [Both (a) and (b) from R. A. Olsen, F. S. Brackett, and R. G. Crickard, *J. Gen. Physiol.* **32**:687–703 (1949). By permission.]

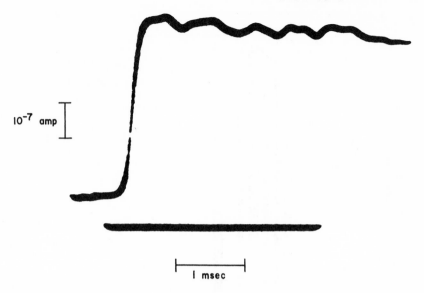

10^{-7} amp

I msec

Figure 9–9.   Response time of open-type pO$_2$ electrode. [From P. W. Davies in Physical Techniques in Biological Research (W. L. Nastuk, ed.), Vol. IV, Academic Press, New York, 1962. By permission.]

Olson et al. (1949) reported an investigation which explored the application of alternating potential techniques to overcome the difficulties attendant on the use of open, static platinum electrodes. This method employed switching the potential pattern imposed on an electrolytic cell consisting of a platinum electrode of 20-gauge wire about 3mm long versus a 0.1M calomel half cell, both immersed in a 0.1M KCl solution. Dual cells were used as a means of comparing electrode performance in oxygen and nitrogen-saturated KCl solutions. The applied potential pattern consisted of a square positive pulse followed by an interval during which the applied potential was suddenly reduced to zero by shorting the cell through a resistance. The short was then removed and a square negative pulse applied, after which the short was again induced before application of the positive pulse to begin the next cycle. Observations were made over the range of 30 cps down to 6 to 12 cpm. Because of the time required for stabilization of the oxygen plateau, the maximum rate at which the potential could be switched and stable values of current output obtained was between 5 and 10 cpm.

The Clark (1956) type of oxygen electrode, which has been employed widely by many biological investigators, is shown in Fig. 9–10. It is of

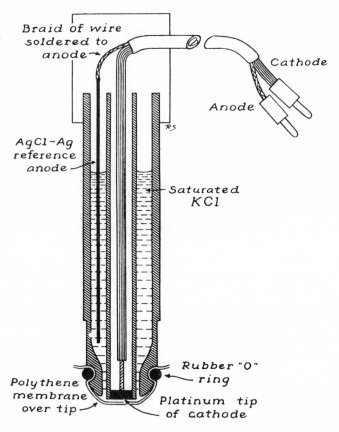

Figure 9–10. The Clark-type pO$_2$ electrode. [From B. J. Sproule et al., *J. Appl. Physiol.* 11:365–370 (1957). By permission.]

single-unit construction with a self-contained Ag-AgCl reference electrode. The entire device is isolated from the solution under measurement by a polythene membrane. This feature allows the electrode to be used for measuring oxygen tension in solutions of poor electrical conductivity or in the gas phase. The stability of response of the Clark electrode depends on the diffusion distance between the platinum surface and the membrane. Care must be exercised to ensure that the membrane is kept taut to maintain the diffusion distance constant.

In physiology the pO$_2$ electrode has been applied extensively to monitor the partial pressure of oxygen in biological fluids. Among the first to exploit the method were Davies and Brink (1942), who described the construction of a bare platinum electrode paired with a calomel cell polarized with 0.6 volt. Using this system they successfully recorded the oxygen tension changes in the arterioles of a cat's brain and in skeletal muscle during contraction. Their paper discusses the theory and electrode reactions as well as many of the practical details of the method. It is recommended reading for those wishing to enter the field. Kreuzer et al. (1958) compared the fidelity of the pO$_2$-electrode method with that of standard chemical procedures.

Two interesting and useful *in vitro* pO$_2$ electrodes were described by Tobias (1947, 1949). One was built into a hypodermic syringe barrel so that, upon withdrawal of a blood sample from a vessel into the syringe, the pO$_2$ tension was instantly read on a calibrated galvanometer; the other was built into a hypodermic needle which Tobias used to measure pO$_2$ in the eyelid, lip, and vagina.

Detailed descriptions of the use of the pO$_2$ electrode to measure the oxygen tension in the brain of a cat were presented by Davies and Brink (1942). Davies et al. (1943–1944) presented multichannel recordings of the EEG and local oxygen tension changes in experimental animals during convulsions. Using an ingenious occlusion method, Davies et al. (1948) recorded the rate of oxygen consumption on the surface of the cortex of cats before and after electrical stimulation of the brain. Clark (1956) developed a unique electrode assembly for monitoring oxygen tension in heart-lung machines. Clark et al. (1957, 1958) also achieved the remarkable feat of chronically implanting pO$_2$ electrodes in the brains of cats, and he recorded the local oxygen tension over a period of months to years.

The rate of oxygen consumption at synaptic endings of sympathetic ganglia was measured by Bronk et al. (1946), using the occlusion technique. They found that 90 seconds elapsed before the oxygen tension dropped to near-zero levels. Posternak et al. (1947), recording in the same region, found that the oxygen consumption was doubled when the ganglia were electrically stimulated at a rate of fifteen per second.

In frog and crab nerve fibers, pO$_2$ microelectrodes were used by Bronk et al. (1947) and Carlson et al. (1948) to record the oxygen consumption during stimulation. They found that oxygen consumption outlasted heat production by as much as $\frac{1}{2}$ minute.

Regional oxygen tensions have been measured on a variety of other tissues. Davies (1946) recorded the consumption of oxygen in frog skeletal muscle during and following a single twitch. He recorded a fall in the oxygen tension during the first half second and a return to the control level in 2 seconds. Oxygen tension measurements have also been recorded by Cater et al. (1957) in the intact lactating mammary gland and in tumors.

For the measurement of pO$_2$ in solution the oxygen electrode offers several advantages; among them are (a) the current obtained is linearly related to the concentration of oxygen, (b) the electrode can be made small enough to measure concentrations in highly localized areas, (c) when used *in vitro*, only a small sample of fluid is required, and (d) the measurement requires only seconds as compared to minutes for chemical determination. Electrode configurations have been developed with a response time short enough for continuous recording of transient changes.

Probably the greatest difficulty in the use of the pO_2 electrode is the size of the electrical signal produced. Although provision of a known stable polarizing voltage offers no difficulties, measurement of the current representing the partial pressure of oxygen presents special problems. The current measured by Tobias (1949) was 0.650 μa for a 500-mm Hg oxygen tension. The total range of the indicator used by Davies and Brink (1942) was 0.05 μa for an oxygen tension of 180 mm Hg. The recorder sensitivity employed by Kreuzer et al. (1958) was 0.96 μa, while that described by Clark et al. (1958) produced a full-scale deflection for 0.98 μa. The signal detected by Cater et al. (1957) was 0.01 μa.

9–9. THE COMBINED pO_2 AND pCO_2 ELECTRODE

With care in mechanical design, it is possible to combine the pO_2 and pCO_2 electrode in one assembly. Figure 9–11 shows an arrangement of a pO_2 electrode operating on the Clark principle and a pCO_2 electrode based on the Severinghaus principle, mounted in a temperature-controlled cell

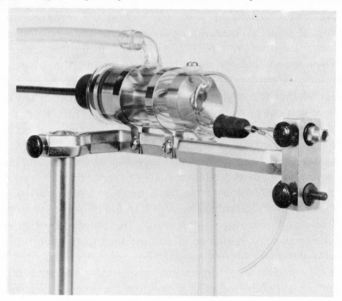

Figure 9–11. The combined pO_2 and pCO_2 electrode. (From Radiometer Catalog, 1967, Copenhagen. By permission.)

to continuously monitor a single stream of fluids or gases.[2] The following performance data are given for this combined electrode.

	pCO_2 Electrode	pO_2 Electrode
Response time	1.5 min (38°C)	30–60 sec (38°C)
Volume (minimum)	70 μl (with thermostatted cell)	
Accuracy	1% + error of adjustment	

The practical considerations of the routine use and maintenance of pH, pO_2, and pCO_2 electrodes in a cardiopulmonary physiology laboratory have been described by Purcell and Rodman (1965). These investigators compared the measurements obtained from these electrodes with those obtained from the classical procedures and emphasized the greater ease, convenience, and simplicity of use provided by the electrodes.

9–10. CATION ELECTRODES

The Nernst equation is the basis of all membrane electrodes, as was pointed out at the beginning of this chapter. Accordingly, the development of specific electrodes for a particular species of ions has logically centered upon finding selective membranes which allow the reversible transfer of only the desired ions. Membranes of this type are called permselective membranes, and the desirable characteristics that they should possess were summarized by Sollner (1958) as follows:

"1. The membranes should exhibit an extreme degree of ionic selectivity even at relatively high concentrations, so that the thermodynamically possible maximum of the concentration potential may be approached closely over wide concentration ranges.

"2. The absolute permeability of the membranes for the nonrestricted critical ions should be high, so that all ionic processes across them can occur at a rapid rate; this means the ohmic resistance of the membranes should be low.

"3. The membranes should come readily to equilibrium with electrolytic solutions, so that stable, well defined states (and potentials) may quickly be established across their thickness, this quality obviously being closely related to the thickness of the membranes and their ohmic resistance.

"4. The membranes should not deteriorate to a significant extent even on prolonged contact with electrolyte solutions.

[2] Radiometer Co., Copenhagen, Denmark.

"5. The membranes should be mechanically satisfactory, i.e., they should be smooth, uniform in thickness over their whole area, and strong enough for the purpose for which they are designed, high mechanical strength being a prerequisite for their successful industrial use.

"6. The preparation of the membranes should be easy and reproducible.

"7. For many scientific purposes the membranes should be of low ion exchange capacity per unit area."

In view of the considerable experience gained over the years in the development and use of the glass electrode for pH measurement, it was certainly to be expected that the possibility of making glass specific for other ions would be investigated. On the basis of the observation by von Lengyel and Blum (1934) that the addition of Al_2O_3 or B_2O_3 to sodium silicate glass caused the glass electrode potential to become strongly dependent on the concentration of several cations besides H^+, Eisenman et al. (1957) and Eisenman (1962), studied the relative cation sensitivities of various glasses as a function of their composition for the purpose of developing an electrode for measuring Na^+ activity in complex mixtures of ions. They constructed glass electrodes from various mixtures of oxides of sodium, aluminum, and silicon, and produced one having 250 times more sensitivity to sodium than potassium at pH $= 7.6$. They stated that the ultimate limits of specificity were unknown and that, in biological fluids containing $0.15M$ Na^+ or more, the electrode produced a sodium ion voltage with less than 0.2% error in the presence of potassium concentrations up to $30\,mM$ at any pH greater than 5.6. In addition the electrode was insensitive to calcium, magnesium, ammonia, and lithium ions except when they were present in unusual concentrations. Although data relating to the rapidity of response were not given, attention was called to the fact that the drift was less than 1.3% per hour. Moreover, the sodium-sensitive electrode could be used with any pH meter and was not poisoned by constituents of serum, cerebrospinal fluid, or brain homogenate even after it was soaked in these solutions for many hours.

Although the main concern of Eisenman and co-workers was the creation of an electrode for sodium ions, they found that certain mixtures of the oxides resulted in electrodes having a high specificity for potassium. They did not pursue this study further, but certainly this evidence promises a transducer for potassium ion.

Friedman et al. (1959), using a flow-through cuvette-type electrode, recorded continuously the concentration of sodium in the femoral arteries of dogs. They noted that in certain flow ranges the electrode was flow-sensitive, but not in others. Their striking records, made with a direct recorder, illustrate changes of a few milliequivalents per liter in sodium concentration produced by a variety of pressor and depressor drugs.

9–11. ELECTRODES FOR DIVALENT IONS

At least one manufacturer[3] markets a permselective electrode which is sensitive to certain divalent ions. The following material represents a summary of technical information released by this company.

The electrode depends upon the potential developed across a liquid ion-exchange membrane in which the conducting material is a water-immiscible liquid ion exchanger held by an extremely thin, porous, inert membrane disk. The liquid ion exchanger is a salt of an organophosphoric acid which exhibits a very high specificity for divalent ions. Electrical conductivity between the inner surface of the membrane and the Ag-AgCl reference cell is established by filling the electrode with calcium chloride solution. The calcium ion establishes a stable potential between the calcium chloride solution and the inner surface of the membrane, while the chloride ion provides a stable potential between the reference electrode and the solution. With all junction potentials stabilized, observed changes in potential are produced by changes in the activities of divalent ions in the sample under measurement. A comparison of the conventional glass electrode and the liquid-membrane divalent ion electrode is shown in Fig. 9-12.

This electrode has been designed to give almost identical response to calcium and magnesium ions on a molar basis, while providing slightly

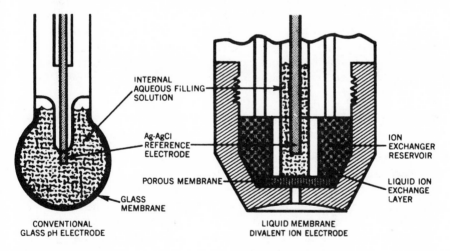

Figure 9–12. Glass electrode and divalent ion electrode. Just as the pH electrode measures hydrogen ion activity, the divalent ion electrode measures divalent activities. In the pH electrode the potential is developed across a glass membrane; in the calcium electrode the membrane is a thin layer of ion exchanger. (From "Divalent Cation Activity Electrode," Orion Research, Inc., Cambridge, Massachusetts, 1966. By permission.)

[3] Orion Research, Inc., Cambridge, Mass.

higher selectivity for Ni^{++}, Zn^{++}, Fe^{++}, and Ca^{++}. It is slightly less selective for Ba^{++} and Sr^{++}. The electrode shows negligible error in the presence of 10^{-2} mole/liter sodium or potassium down to 10^{-4} mole/liter calcium (or other divalent) ions. The selectivity is tenfold higher for Pb^{++} than Ca^{++}. The electrode detects calcium down to 10^{-5} mole/liter. It may be used over a range of pH from 5 to 11 with negligible error resulting from pH changes. The electrode can be employed with any modern expanded-scale pH meter and a conventional calomel reference electrode. It operates over a temperature range of 0 to 50°C and has an electrical resistance of less than 25 megohms at 25°C. The minimum sample size is less than 5 ml in a 50-ml beaker or 0.3 ml in a special microsample container. Under average operating conditions the minimum useful life of the electrode membrane and ion exchanger is 30 days without replacement.

Ross (1967) reported the development of a simple calcium-selective electrode capable of measuring calcium ion activity in the presence of many common interfering ions. The electrode utilizes a liquid ion- exchanger membrane containing the calcium salt of a disubstituted phosphoric acid and is able to measure free calcium ion activity in the presence of a thousand fold excess of sodium or potassium ions.

An electrode to measure sulfide ion activity is available commercially, and the following information has been supplied by the manufacturer.[4] This electrode is constructed of unbreakable plastic; because it is a solid-state device, it requires no renewal. No interference is obtained from a wide variety of other anions. The electrode will detect any level of sulfide for which stable standard solutions can be prepared. Its ultimate sensitivity is below 10^{-17} M, and it will follow sulfide activity over the pH range 1 to 12.

9–12. FLUORIDE ION ELECTRODE

The development of an electrode for measurement of fluoride ion activity has been announced by Frant and Ross (1966). The principle of construction of the electrode is similar to that of a conventional glass pH electrode except that the membrane material is a disk-shaped section of a single-crystal rare earth fluoride, such as LaF_3, NdF_3, or PrF_3. The disk-shaped section (1 cm in diameter and 1 to 2 mm thick) is cemented to the end of a rigid polyvinyl chloride tube filled with a solution containing both fluoride and chloride ions (typically $0.1M$ NaF and $0.1M$ KCl), and electrical contact is made by inserting a Ag-AgCl electrode into the solution. Electrical connection to the test sample is through a standard saturated calomel cell. Measurements were reproducible to within less than 1 mv.

[4] Orion Research, Inc., Cambridge, Mass.

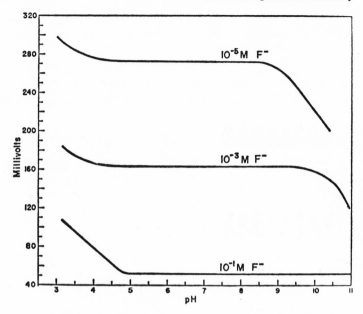

Figure 9–13. Sensitivity characteristics of the fluoride ion electrode. [From M. S. Frant and J. W. Ross, Science **154**: 1553–1554 (1966). Copyright, 1966, by the American Association for the Advancement of Science. By permission.]

Because the membrane is permeable only to fluoride ions, the potential developed is given by the Nernst equation. The only significant interference comes from the hydroxide ion, as would be expected on the basis of similarities in charge and ionic radii. The electrode response as a function of pH and fluoride concentration is shown in Fig. 9–13.

9–13.   CONTINUOUS MONITORING OF BLOOD CHEMISTRY

Gotoh et al. (1966), in a study of cerebral blood flow and metabolism, have reported the simultaneous use of several chemical transducers to monitor venous and arterial blood in more than eighty human subjects. The arrangement of equipment employed by these investigators is illustrated in Fig. 9–14. Arterial and venous blood was passed through similar transparent acrylic cuvettes, which were maintained at body temperature. Transducers mounted in the cuvettes monitored the values of pO_2, pCO_2, pH, Na^+, and K^+ in the circulating heparinized blood. Other physiological data, such as the EEG, ECG, blood pressure, temperature, expired pCO_2, and oxygen saturation, were also recorded. The primary advantage of this system lies in permitting the simultaneous detection of small

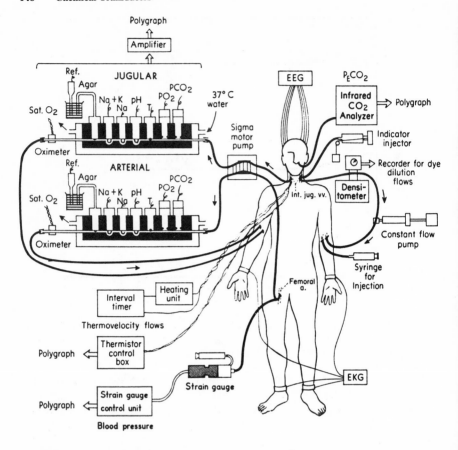

Figure 9–14. Continuous monitoring of blood chemistry. [From F. Gotoh et al., *Med. Res. Eng.* **5**:13–19 (1966). By permission.]

changes in blood chemistry as rapidly as possible, although Gotoh pointed out that the response times of all the chemical transducers are not the same, and that therefore the method is not suitable for studies in which time sequences within a second or two are important. The problems encountered with blood clotting were discussed; however, the use of an adequate amount of heparin appears to have eliminated these difficulties.

This study of Gotoh and co-workers indicates the possibility of continuous monitoring of blood chemistry for the whole body or specific organs. Besides the surgical techniques required, one of the chief technical limitations of this method at present is the relatively long response time of the chemical transducers.

REFERENCES

Band, D. M., and S. J. G. Semple. 1967. Continuous measurement of blood pH with an indwelling arterial glass electrode. *J. Appl. Physiol.* **22**:854–857.

Brems, N. 1962. Measurements of pH electrodes and pertinent apparatus. *Acta Anaesthesiol Scand.* **6** (Suppl. XI): 199–206.

Bronk, D. W., F. Brink, C. M. Connelly, F. D. Carlson, and P. W. Davies. 1947. The time course of recovery of oxygen consumption in nerve. *Fed. Proc.* **6**:83–84.

Bronk, D. W., M. A. Larrabee, and P. W. Davies. 1946. The rate of O_2 consumption in localized regions of the nervous system in presynaptic endings in cell bodies. *Fed. Proc.* **5**:11.

Bull, H. B. 1943. *Physical Biochemistry.* New York: John Wiley & Sons.

Bull, H. B. 1964. *An Introduction to Physical Biochemistry.* Philadelphia: F. A. Davis Co.

Carlson, F. D., F. Brink, and D. W. Bronk. 1948. A method for direct measurement of rate of O_2 utilization by nerve. *Fed. Proc.* **7**:18.

Cater, D. B., A. F. Phillips, and I. A. Silver. 1957a. Apparatus and techniques for the measurement of oxidation-reduction potentials, pH and oxygen tension *in vivo*. *Proc. Roy. Soc. (London)* **146B**:289–297.

Cater, D. B., A. F. Phillips, and I. A. Silver. 1957b. Induced changes in oxidation-reduction potentials, pH and oxygen tension in the intact lactating mammary gland. *Proc. Roy. Soc. (London)* **146B**:400–415.

Cater, D. B., A. F. Phillips, and I. A. Silver. 1957c. The measurement of oxidation-reduction potentials, pH and oxygen tension in tumors. *Proc. Ray. Soc. (London)* **146B**:382–399.

Clark, L. C. 1956. Monitor and control of blood and tissue oxygen tensions. *Trans. Am. Soc. Internal Organs.* **2**:41–48.

Clark, L. C., and G. Misrahy. 1957. Chronically implanted polarograph electrodes. *Fed. Proc.* **16**:22–23.

Clark, L. C., G. Misrahy, and R. P. Fox. 1958. Chronically implanted polarographic electrodes. *J. Appl. Physiol.* **13**:85–91.

Cooper, R. 1963. Electrodes. *Am. J. EEG Tech.* **3**:91–101.

Davies, P. W. 1946. Rapid bursts of oxygen consumption in stimulated muscle. *Fed Proc.* **5**:21–22.

Davies, P. W. 1962. In *Physical Techniques in Biological Research* (W. L. Nastuk, Ed.) Vol. IV: *Special Methods.* New York: Academic Press.

Davies, P. W., and F. Brink. 1942a. Direct measurement of brain oxygen concentration with platinum electrode. *Fed. Proc.* **1**:19.

Davies, P. W., and F. Brink. 1942b. Microelectrodes for measuring local oxygen tension in animal tissues. *Rev. Sci. Instrs.* **130**:524–532.

Davies, P. W., R. G. Grenell, and D. W. Bronk. 1948. The time course of *in vivo* oxygen consumption of cerebral cortex following electrical stimulation. *Fed. Poc.* **7**:25.

Davies, P. W., W. S. McCulloch, and E. Roseman. 1943–1944. Rapid changes in the O_2 tension of cerebral cortex during induced convulsions. *Am. J. Psychiat.* **100**:825–829.

de Bethune, A. J. 1964. Electrode potentials, temperature coefficients. In *Encyclopedia of Electrochemistry* (C. A. Hampel, Ed.) New York: Reinhold Publishing Corp.

Dole, M. 1935. *Theoretical and Experimental Electrochemistry.* New York: McGraw Hill Book Co.

Dole, M., R. M. Roberts, and C. E. Holley. 1941. The theory of the glass electrode. V. The influence of negative ions. *J. Am. Chem. Soc.* **63**:725–730.

Dubuisson, M. 1937a. A method for recording pH changes of muscle during activity. *J. Physiol.* **90**:47p–48p.

Dubuisson, M. 1937b. pH changes in muscle during and after contraction. *Proc. Soc. Exptl. Biol. Med.* **35**:609–611.

Dusser de Barenne, J. C., W. S. McCulloch, and L. F. Nims. 1937. Functional activity and pH of the cerebral cortex. *J. Cellular Comp. Physiol.* **10**:277–289.

Eisenman, G. 1962. Cation selective glass electrodes and their mode of operation. *Biophys. J.* **2**:259–323.

Eisenman, G. 1967. The origin of the glass-electrode potential. In *Glass Electrodes for Hydrogen and Other Cations—Principles and Practice* (G. Eisenman, Ed.) New York: Marcel Dekker.

Eisenman, G., D. O. Rudin, and J. U. Casby, 1957. Glass electrode for measuring sodium ion. *Science* **126**:831–834.

Frant, M. S., and J. W. Ross. 1966. Electrode for sensing fluoride-ion activity in solution. *Science* **154**:1553–1554.

Friedman, S. M., J. D. Jamieson, J. A. M. Hinke, and C. L. Friedman. 1959. Drug-induced changes in blood pressure and in blood sodium as measured by glass electrode. *Am. J. Physiol.* **196**:1049–1052.

Fruhling, G., and H. Winterstein. 1934. Registrierung der pH in stromenden Blut. *Arch. ges. Physiol.* **233**:475–485.

Gesell, R., A. B. Hertzman. 1926. Regulation of respiration. *Am. J. Physiol.* **78**:206–223.

Glasstone, S. 1946. *The Elements of Physical Chemistry*. Princeton, N.J.: D. Van Nostrand.

Gotoh, F., J. S. Meyer, and S. Ebihara. 1966. Continuous recording of human cerebral blood flow and metabolism: methods for electronic monitoring of arterial and venous gases and electrolytes. *Med. Res. Eng.* **5**(2):13–19.

Hertz, C. H., and B. Siesjö. 1959. A rapid and sensitive electrode for continuous measurement of pCO_2 in liquids and tissue. *Acta Physiol. Scand.* **47**:115–123.

Janz, G. J., and H. Taniguchi. 1953. The silver-silver halide electrodes. *Chem. Rev.* **53**:397–437.

Kolthoff, I. M., and J. J. Lingane. 1955. *Polarography*. New York: Interscience Publishers.

Kreuzer, F., T. R. Watson, and J. M. Ball. 1958. Comparative measurements with a new procedure for measuring the blood oxygen tensions in vitro. *J. Appl. Physiol.* **12**:65–70.

Lengyel, B. von, and E. Blum. 1934. The behavior of the glass electrode in connection with its chemical composition. *Trans. Faraday Soc.* **30**:461.

McClendon, J. F. 1915. New hydrogen electrode and rapid method of determining hydrogen ion concentrations. *Am. J. Physiol.* **38**:180–185.

Marshall, C., and L. F. Nims. 1937. Blood pH *in vivo*. 11. Effects of acids, salts, dextrose and adrenalin. *Yale J. Biol. Med.* **10**:561–564.

Mattock, G., and D. M. Band. 1967. Interpretation of pH and cation measurements. In *Glass Electrodes for Hydrogen and Other Cations—Principles and Practice* (G. Eisenman, Ed.) New York: Marcel Dekker.

Nims, L. F. 1937. Glass electrodes and apparatus for direct recording of pH *in vivo*. *Yale J. Biol. Med.* **10**:241–246.

Nims, L. F., and C. Marshall. 1937. Blood pH in *vivo*. 1. Changes due to respiration. *Yale J. Biol. Med.* **10**:445–448.

Nims, L. F., C. Marshall, and H. S. Burr. 1938. The measurement of pH in circulating blood. *Science* **87**:197–198.

Olson, R. A., F. S. Brackett, and R. G. Crickard. 1949. Oxygen tension measurement by a method of time selection using the static platinum electrode with alternating potential. *J. Gen. Physiol.* **32**:681–703.

Orion Research, Inc. 1966. Sulfide ion activity. *Electrode Bulletin*. Cambridge, Mass.

Posternak, J. M., M. A. Larrabee, and D. W. Bronk. 1947. Oxygen requirements of the neurones in sympathetic ganglia. *Fed. Proc.* **6**:182.

Purcell, M. K., and T. Rodman. 1965. Carbon dioxide and oxygen electrodes for arterial blood analysis in a cardiopulmonary physiology laboratory. *Am. J. Med. Electron.* **4**: 82–86.

Radiometer Co. *Bulletin* 21917E. Copenhagen, Denmark.

Reyes, R. J., and J. R. Neville. 1967. An electrochemical technic for measuring carbon dioxide content of blood. *USAF School Aerospace Med. Tech. Rept.* SAM-TR-67-23.

Ross, J. W. 1967. Calcium-selective electrode with liquid ion exchanger. *Science* 1ς6: 1378–1379.

Severinghaus, J. W. 1962. Electrodes for blood and gas pCO_2, pO_2, and blood pH. *Acta Anaesthesiol. Scand.* **6**(Suppl. XI):207–220.

Severinghaus, J. W., and A. F. Bradley. 1958. Electrodes for blood pO_2 and pCO_2 determination. *J. Appl. Physiol.* **13**:515–520.

Siggaard-Anderson, O. 1962. The pH-log pCO_2 blood acid-base nomogram revised. *Scand. J. Clin. Lab. Invest.* **14**:598–604.

Siggaard-Andersen, O., and K. Engel. 1960. A new acid-base nomogram, an improved method for the calculation of the relevant blood acid-base data. *Scand. J. Clin. Lab. Invest.* **12**:177–186.

Sollner, K. 1958. The physical chemistry of ion exchange membranes. *Svensk Kem. Tidsks.* **6–7**:267–295.

Stow, R. W., R. F. Baer, and B. F. Randall. 1957. Rapid measurement of the tension of carbon dioxide in blood. *Arch. Phys. Med. Rehabil.* **38**:646–650.

Tobias, J. M. 1949. Syringe oxygen cathode for measurement of oxygen tension in solution and respiratory gases. *Rev. Sci. Instrs.* **20**:519–523.

Tobias, J. M., and R. Holmes, 1947. Observation on the use of the oxygen cathode. *Fed. Proc.* **6**:215.

Voegtlin, C., F. F. De Eds, and H. Kahler. 1930. *Public Health Rept.* (*U.S.*) **45**:2223–2233; also: 1935. *N. I. H. Bull.* 164, Part II, pp. 15–27.

Vogel, J. H. K., R. F. Grover, and S. G. Blount. 1962. Detection of the small intracardiac shunt with the hydrogen electrode: a highly sensitive and simple technique. *Am. Heart J.* **64**:13–21.

10

Detection of Physiological Events by Impedance

Often it is necessary to measure a physiological event for which there is no specialized transducer. In many circumstances transduction can be carried out by means of the impedance method if the event can be caused to exhibit a change in dimension, dielectric, or conductivity. The technique is elegantly simple, requiring only the installation of two or four electrodes, and has been used successfully for many years to detect a remarkable variety of physiological events. It is extremely practical for those phenomena that produce a large change in one or more of the three quantities mentioned above. With the simplest of "transducers," that is, appropriately placed electrodes, the impedance between them may show seasonal variations or reflect the activity of the endocrine system or the functioning of the autonomic nervous system. Also, respiration, blood flow, the contraction of cardiac, skeletal, and smooth muscle, the activity of nerve cells, eye position, and a variety of other events—for example, heart sounds, the activity of salivary glands, the clotting of blood, and the number of cells in a specimen of blood—have all been detected by using the impedance technique. In some instances the impedance is dissected into its resistive and reactive components; in others, the total impedance is measured. Often only a change in impedance, with or without resolution into its components, conveys enough information to describe the physiological event. Many of the techniques which have been employed are described in this chapter.

The impedance method offers all of the advantages of the indirect techniques used in the biomedical sciences, the most important being that in many applications the integument need not be penetrated to make the measurement. Since electrodes are very easy to apply, practicality is an attractive feature of the method. Because a specialized transducer is not required, the same electrodes and the same impedance apparatus can often be used to detect a variety of events in man and animals. In the absence of a transducer, the response time is governed mainly by the event. If the electrodes are small enough, they offer little restraint to the subject and need not modify the phenomenon under study. Unlike many transducers, electrodes are affected little by temperature and barometric pressure changes. This property makes the impedance method practical for monitoring events under changing environmental conditions. In addition, because the usually bothersome galvanic potentials produced when metallic electrodes come into contact with electrolytes are not a part of the signal when the impedance method is employed, the problem of canceling these unwanted voltages is eliminated. A further advantage of the impedance method is obtained through employment of carrier-system techniques (see Chapter 13), which permit the use of narrow-band amplifiers with subsequent enhancement of the signal-to-noise ratio.

The impedance method is subject to the limitations inherent in many indirect techniques. Because frequently the signal is obtained at a distance from the phenomenon, resolution is compromised, and the signal is often difficult to calibrate in true physiological terms. It is to be noted, however, that uncalibratible signals which directly reflect a physiological event can have considerable value for monitoring changes under a variety of experimentally controlled conditions.

When current is passed through living tissue, special consideration must be given to the structures between the electrodes. Muscle (skeletal, cardiac, and smooth), nerve fibers, sensory receptors, glands, and body fluids form part of the current-carrying circuit. The parameters of stimulation for the irritable tissues in the current path can be found in their strength-duration curves. Physiologists customarily describe the strength-duration characteristics of an effective stimulus in terms of the chronaxie. From the strength-duration curve for a particular organ or tissue, chronaxie is defined as the duration of a stimulus having twice the intensity of a stimulus that would be just sufficient (threshold) to produce stimulation if allowed to remain on for an infinite time. The chronaxie is determined from the strength-duration curve by projecting to the vertical axis the value of intensity corresponding to a long duration, multiplying this value by 2, and projecting the latter value back to the curve. This value of time, corresponding to the stimulus of twice the threshold, is the chronaxie, which is found to be short in rapidly acting tissues and long in slowly responding ones. Stimuli with durations less than the chronaxie must be much higher in intensity to stimulate because typical strength-duration curves rise steeply in this region. Brazier (1960) gave chronaxies of 0.2 ms for mammalian nerve and 100 ms for smooth muscle. To minimize or avoid stimulation, pulses having durations many times shorter than the chronaxie must be employed. Sinusoidal current having a frequency of 5000 cps could conceivably stimulate the most rapidly responding tissues, indicating the need to use higher frequencies in the measurement of physiological events by impedance techniques.

In addition to consideration of stimulation of nerve and muscle, it is desirable to prevent stimulation of sensory receptors when surface electrodes are employed. Although the perception threshold is expected to vary widely with the richness of distribution of sensory receptors, the studies carried out to date are in good agreement and reveal the nature of the tolerance.

The perception of and tolerance to electric current of different frequencies attracted considerable attention at the dawn of the twentieth century when it became necessary to choose a frequency for the distribution of electrical energy. d'Arsonval, of galvanometer fame, showed in 1893 that when current was passed through the human body, no sensation was perceived as the frequency was increased beyond 2500 to 5000 cps. At much greater frequencies, even with a high intensity, there was no perception of the current. To prove his point in a most dramatic manner, d'Arsonval connected two human subjects (arm to arm) and a 100-watt light bulb in series to a high-frequency spark coil which delivered enough current (1 ampere) to cause the bulb to burn brilliantly. The subjects through whom the 1-ampere, 0.5-to-1-ma current flowed reported no sensation. In a later study d'Arsonval passed 3 amperes through his own body. These demonstrations, of course, paved the way for the use of high-frequency current for heating living tissues and in reality initiated medical diathermy.

When a-c generators capable of providing substantial electrical energy with frequencies up to 100,000 cps became available, further studies were carried out on the ability of human subjects to perceive and tolerate alternating current. Kennelly and Alexanderson (1910) reported on a series of experiments in which current was passed through subjects via buckets filled with 3% saline into which the hands were immersed. Using the limit of tolerance as the criterion, they plotted graphs of current versus frequency for five subjects. They found that the tolerance to current increased with rising frequency. At 60 cps the tolerance current varied between 4 and 100 ma. At 11 kc the tolerance current was 30 ma, and at 100 kc it varied between 450 and 800 ma. Even with these high currents the subjects reported only a slight tingling and a sensation of heat at the wrists.

Dalziel (1956) reported that the tip of the tongue is the most sensitive part of the body and determined the threshold for sensation on 115 subjects as 45 μa for both direct current and 60-cps alternating current. In another series of experiments he measured the ability of over 100 male subjects to perceive current flowing in the body through electrodes held in the hands. The threshold for sensation was 5.2 ma for direct current and 1.1 ma for 60-cps alternating current. Dalziel found that the threshold of sensation for women was two thirds that of the value for men.

In another series of studies using hand-held electrodes, he measured the threshold for sensation for different frequencies of sinusoidal current. The data he obtained are shown in Fig. 10–1.

In a study of the choice of frequency for impedance respiration Geddes (1962) determined the threshold of sensation for sinusoidal current with electrodes placed on the human thorax. The data obtained are in general agreement with those of Dalziel, that is, above about 300 cps the threshold of perception rises as frequency is increased. Both studies emphasize that frequencies high in the kilocycle region must be employed if stimulation of sensory receptors is to be avoided.

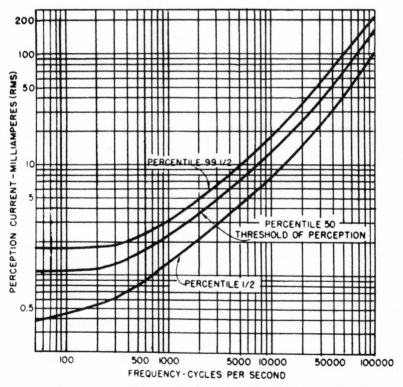

Figure 10–1.   Effect of frequency on perception of current, using hand-held electrodes. [From C. F. Dalziel, IRE Trans. Med. Electron. **5**: 48 (1956). By permission.]

The use of high frequencies is further emphasized when the parameters of myocardial stimulation are considered. The chronaxie of mammalian myocardium has been found to be around 2 ms (Brooks et al., 1955). Slowly repetitive stimuli of this duration evoke single ectopic contractions, but there is a real danger of ventricular fibrillation if the repetition rate is increased or if single stimuli of high intensity fall in the early phases of the relatively refractory period (the "vulnerable period" of the myocardium). To eliminate any possibility of such potentially lethal stimulation, pulses of low intensity and extremely short duration (i.e., high frequencies) are mandatory. Although a frequency of current can be chosen which will not stimulate, it is also important to employ an intensity low enough in value to prevent heating in the tissues. Even a small amount of heat alters blood supply and cellular metabolism.

The effect of current density on body fluids has not been adequately investigated. Most body fluids are not simple electrolytes but are suspensions of cells and large molecules. The extent to which these fluid components are modified by current awaits investigation. One study by Poppindieck (1964), pertinent to the techniques in which blood flow is measured by impedance change, showed that no detectable change occurred in canine blood when it sustained a current density of 0.5 ampere/cm^2 for 3 hours. Similar studies on other biological fluids will undoubtedly be carried out.

When electrodes are placed on living tissue, the current distribution between them is determined by the resistivities of the various intervening tissues and fluids. Many investigations have been carried out to determine the resistivities of the diverse structures that constitute the living organism. A review of the extensive literature in this field was presented by Geddes and Baker (1967). Although many biological specimens have been measured, some of the values appearing in the literature were determined without due regard to electrode polarization. In the opinion of the authors the resistivity figures appearing in Table 10–1 are the most representative values available at this time.

When the impedance technique is used to measure a physiological event, one of two methods is generally employed. With both, the physiological event is placed between the measuring electrodes in such a way that the event alters the current density distribution between the electrodes, thus manifesting itself as a change in impedance. In one method, the electrodes are in direct contact with the preparation and a relatively low impedance circuit is formed; in the other, they are insulated from the subject and a relatively high impedance capacitive circuit results.

Bipolar and tetrapolar electrode systems are currently employed to derive a signal from a physiological event by means of the impedance technique. With the bipolar arrangement two types of circuitry are

Table 10–1 Resistivities of Biological Specimens*

Specimen	Resistivity† (ohm-cms)	Species
Blood	150	Human
Plasma	63	Mammals
Cerebrospinal fluid	65	Human
Bile	60	Cow-pig
Urine	30	Cow-pig
Cardiac muscle (R)	750	Dog
Skeletal muscle (T)	1600	Dog
Skeletal muscle (L)	300	Dog
Lung	1275	Mammals
Kidney	370	Mammals
Liver	820	Dog
Spleen	885	Dog
Brain (R)	580	Mammals
Fat	2500	Mammals

* From L. A. Geddes and L. E. Baker, *Med. Biol. Eng.* **5**: 271–293 (1967).
† Average values for body temperature and the low-frequency region (< 1 mc).
R = Random orientation; T = transverse current; L = longitudinal current.

employed; with the tetrapolar system, only one circuit configuration is needed. All circuits require a source of alternating current and an amplifier with an input impedance which is high with respect to the impedance between the electrodes. The impedance signal is recovered by use of a detector, which may be a null indicator, a vacuum tube voltmeter, or a phase-sensitive circuit.

In many instances the physiological event changes the impedance by a small amount, and it is only the change which contains the useful information. Under these circumstances the voltage reflecting the change in impedance is amplified and displayed without dissection into resistive and reactive components. If separation of these components is desirable, phase-sensitive detecting systems are necessary.

Although the circuits to be described are those most frequently employed, in some cases in which movement has been converted into corresponding changes in capacitance, the variation in capacitance has been employed to frequency-modulate a carrier. On a few occasions a direct voltage was applied to the electrodes and the physiological event altered the conductivity and/or capacitance of the circuit, thereby modulating the direct current.

10–1. IMPEDANCE-MEASURING CIRCUITS

When two electrodes are employed, the impedance bridge circuit diagramed in Fig. 10–2 can be used. In such an arrangement, the oscillator

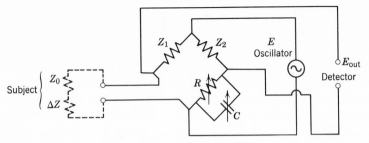

Figure 10–2.   Impedance bridge.

voltage E is applied to two opposite corners of the bridge and the detector is connected to the other two. When the ratio arms Z_1, Z_2 are resistors of equal value, the impedance bridge becomes a comparison bridge. The balancing arm RC may consist of parallel resistance and capacitance decade units which are adjusted to balance the bridge for the nominal impedance between the electrode terminals. At balance, the value of the balance arm gives the equivalent parallel resistive and reactive components of the tissue-electrode circuit. If R and C are placed in series and the bridge is balanced, the new values for R and C give the equivalent series circuit between the electrode terminals. These equivalents are valid only for the frequency employed. With some bridges the impedance is measured in terms of a parallel or a series equivalent, but not both. Often it is desirable to transform one equivalent into the other; for example, if in a given case R_s and C_s are the series resistance and capacitance at a particular frequency f, the parallel equivalents R_p and C_p at the same frequency are given by the following:

$$C_p$$

$$R_p$$ is equivalent to $$R_s \quad C_s$$

$$R_p = \frac{1 + (2\pi f C_s R_s)^2}{4\pi^2 f^2 C_s^2 R_s}, \qquad R_p = R_s + \frac{X_s^2}{R_s},$$

$$C_p = \frac{C_s}{1 + (2\pi f C_s R_s)^2}, \qquad X_p = X_s + \frac{R_s^2}{X_s}.$$

Frequently it is desirable to carry out the reverse process, that is, to express a series circuit in terms of a parallel one. Rearrangement of the expressions just given provides the following relationships:

$$R_s = \frac{R_p}{1 + (2\pi f C_p R_p)^2}, \qquad C_s = C_p \left[1 + \frac{1}{(2\pi f R_p C_p)^2} \right].$$

With the bridge circuit, the changes in impedance reflecting the physiological event produce a varying output voltage (E_{out}) which, after amplification and rectification, is displayed to produce a record related to changes in the physiological event. It must be emphasized that an output is obtained if there is a change in either the resistive or the reactive component or in both. If it is desired to examine the magnitude of each component individually, a phase-sensitive detector is required.

If the bridge is operated at the balance point and without the use of a phase-sensitive detector, an output voltage is obtained if the impedance being measured increases or decreases. Under this operating condition, direction indication is lost. However, if after the bridge has been initially balanced it is then unbalanced slightly by the addition of a small resistance in series with the impedance being measured, the output voltage from the bridge will increase and decrease in accordance with corresponding changes in the impedance being measured. The amount of resistance added is dictated by the maximum change in impedance required to drive the bridge toward the balance point.

The other bipolar electrode system is diagramed in Fig. 10–3. Current from the oscillator is fed to the electrodes symmetrically through two resistances R, R which are high in value with respect to the total impedance between the electrodes. With this circuit configuration the current through the subject is determined by these resistances and the oscillator voltage, and is relatively independent of the electrode impedance. The detector is connected across the electrodes, and the voltage present is a function of the nominal impedance between the electrodes and any change due to the physiological event. It can easily be shown that the voltage across the electrodes is given by the following expression:

$$E_{out} = \frac{E(Z_0 + \Delta Z)}{2R + Z_0 + \Delta Z}.$$

If R is made much greater than Z_0 and ΔZ is much less than Zo, then

$$E_{out} \doteq \frac{E(Z_0 + \Delta Z)}{2R}$$

$$\doteq \frac{EZ_0}{2R} + \frac{E\,\Delta Z}{2R}.$$

Rectification of these signals after amplification yields a large constant signal ($EZ_0/2R$) plus a smaller one ($E\Delta Z/2R$) proportional to the impedance change due to the physiological event. The larger signal, reflecting the nominal impedance of the subject, is often eliminated from the output by blocking this d-c component with a capacitance or by canceling it with an opposing voltage.

The third method for monitoring impedance changes employs four electrodes and is diagramed in Fig. 10–4. In this circuit the oscillator voltage (E) is fed to the current electrodes 1_1, 1_2, which are farthest apart on the preparation. Between them are the potential-measuring electrodes M_1, M_2, which receive a voltage determined by the current density distribution in the preparation. Amplification and rectification of this voltage (E_{out}) yield a signal related to the "resting" tissue impedance between the measuring electrodes and any changes associated with the physiological event.

Each of the three circuits has unique characteristics which are ideal for some applications and less suitable for others. Of the three, the bridge circuit has been the most commonly employed. The wide range of impedance that can be measured is an attractive feature of this configuration. With appropriate components it can be employed to detect the changes in capacitive reactance either when the electrodes do not touch the subject

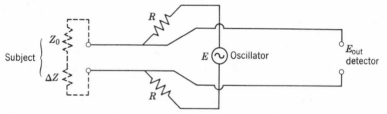

Figure 10–3. Symmetrical constant-current circuit. (For simplicity, the constant current circuit is diagrammed by the oscillator and two resistances R, R which are much larger than $Z_0 + \Delta Z$.)

or when they are in direct contact with the preparation. Calibration of the balance arm RC permits derivation of an equivalent circuit for the preparation between the electrodes at the frequency employed. A comparison of the magnitude of the oscillator and detector voltages and the phase angle between them permits dissection of the output signal into its reactive and resistive components.

One of the difficulties with the bridge circuit relates to isolation of the detector and oscillator circuits above ground potential. If the oscillator and subject are to be grounded, as by grounding their common point, the detector circuit must be lifted above ground by an appropriate isolating device. Practically this requires the use of a special low-capacitance transformer.

Another drawback to the bridge circuit involves its adaptation for physiological recording. If the impedance of the arm (Z_1) in Fig. 10–2 is not high with respect to the impedance of the tissue, the magnitude of the output signal produced by ΔZ will be dependent upon the nominal level of impedance (Z_0) between the electrodes. This situation arises when the amount of current flowing through the preparation is determined both by Z_1 and by the impedance between the electrode terminals. Should the latter change, the current will also change and the magnitude of the voltage produced by the physiological event will depend upon the value of Z_0. This undesirable feature of the bridge circuit can be minimized by a calibration technique in which a resistor of known value is switched into the circuit in series with the preparation. One method of obtaining an output which is not dependent on the electrode impedance is to make the arm of the bridge adjacent to the subject, (Z_1) high in resistance with respect to the impedance between the electrodes. Under these conditions the bridge circuit takes on the characteristics of the constant-current circuit. For a truly constant-current circuit, however, Z_1 must be controlled by a feedback circuit arranged so that the current through the subject is maintained at a constant value despite any change in Z_0.

The bridge circuit may be employed to measure the impedance between electrodes which are being used simultaneously to record bioelectric events

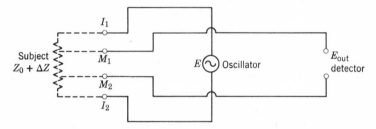

Figure 10–4.   Tetrapolar circuit.

if the oscillator and the detector are isolated from each other and ground and if the impedance of the arm of the bridge adjacent to the subject (Z_1) is made high as previously described. When the oscillator voltage is low and its frequency is beyond the frequency spectrum of bioelectric events, only simple filtering is required in the bioelectric recorder to eliminate the oscillator voltage.

Many of the practical inconveniences of the bridge circuit can be eliminated by use of the symmetrical constant-current circuit shown in Fig. 10–3. In essence, this circuit resembles that of the familiar shunt-type ohmmeter. With the constant-current circuit the oscillator voltage is applied to the electrodes through two series resistors, a thousand or more times the nominal impedance between the electrode terminals. In this circumstance the impedance of the electrodes and the biological material will not determine the current flowing through the preparation. Although the level of impedance between the electrode terminals will determine the size of the static signal presented to the detector, the same change in impedance, reflecting the physiological event, will always produce the same amplitude signal. The use of two resistors R,R to obtain the constant-current characteristic is strictly a practical expedient. For true functioning as a constant-current circuit the resistors R,R should be replaced by a constant-current source consisting of an amplifier connected for current feedback. Although this technique guarantees constant-current operation, the addition of transistors or vacuum tubes and the associated circuitry increases the distributed capacitance to ground, and unless care is exercised the low capacitance and symmetry to ground characteristically obtained with resistors are lost.

Another feature of practical value in the physiological application of the constant-current circuit is the few controls needed for its operation. If direct-coupled recording is required, only one control is needed to adjust the bucking voltage necessary to eliminate the large signal produced by the nominal impedance between the electrode terminals. A second control can regulate the amplitude of the display.

A less attractive feature of the constant-current circuit is its limited ability to measure events over a large range of impedance. With a wide range of nominal impedance, the amplifier and demodulator are presented with a wide range of voltage on which are superimposed the smaller changes due to the physiological event. This requires the use of an amplifier having a high input impedance and a wide dynamic range in order to guarantee linearity of reproduction. For this reason the constant-current circuit is most conveniently employed to detect physiological events when the impedance between the electrode terminals is low, that is, when there is direct electrolytic contact between the tissue and the electrodes.

The constant-current circuit shown in Fig. 10–3 constitutes a symmetrical system. A requisite which often presents practical difficulties is isolation of the oscillator and detector from each other and from ground. When proper isolation and symmetry are achieved; no change in operation will occur if either or neither side of the input is grounded. This feature permits connecting the circuit to electrodes which are connected to other devices for the measurement of bioelectric events.

When resistors are employed to obtain the constant-current characteristic, a prime requisite is high stability in oscillator voltage. Small variations in amplitude, such as noise or ripple, will appear with the output signal. When direct-coupled recording is employed, the stability requirements for the oscillator can be lessened by deriving the bucking voltage in the output circuit from the oscillator voltage.

With the constant-current circuit it is also possible to employ a detector which will permit dissection of the impedance into its resistive and reactive components. In most applications this is unnecessary. With the circuit shown in Fig. 10–3 a change in either capacitive reactance or resistance or both will alter the output of the system. If only the change in impedance, without its dissection, reflects the physiological event, the constant-current circuit, with its few controls and its freedom from the influence of nominal electrode impedance, is unusually practical for the measurement of a variety of physiological events.

The tetrapolar arrangement, shown in Fig. 10–4, is popular with those who measure peripheral pulses by impedance plethysmography. It was originally developed by Bouty (1884) to eliminate electrode polarization errors in the measurement of the specific resistance of electrolytes. Nyboer (1944, 1959) and Bagno (1959) have presented good accounts of the physiological application of this circuit. Because the current is admitted to the subject by electrodes that are distant from the measuring electrodes, with a homogeneously conducting medium there exists the possibility for a more uniform distribution of current density in the preparation between the measuring electrodes, despite a relatively large asymmetry in current density distribution in the vicinity of the current electrodes (see Fig. 10–16a,b). Inasmuch as variations in current density distribution are reflected at the surface of a volume conductor as changes in potential, one could expect artifact produced by movement of the current electrodes to be reduced when recording from potential electrodes located in a region in which the current density distribution remains more nearly uniform.

With a high-impedance detecting system, the voltage appearing across the potential-measuring electrodes M_1, M_2 (Fig. 10–4) is independent of their impedance. If the output impedance of the oscillator is made high with respect to the impedance between the current electrodes I_1, I_2 the constant-current feature is achieved. When these conditions are satisfied accurate measurement can be made of potential changes occurring between the potential electrodes, which reflect changes in the internal current density distribution.

In practice, the equipment used with the tetrapolar arrangement need not require more than three controls, two for balance and one for amplitude. If desired, it is possible to employ a phase-sensitive detector to dissect the impedance change into its resistive and reactive components. The tetrapolar method, when applied to the measurement of the resistivity of homogeneously conducting materials in an electrolytic cell, permits the creation of a uniform current density distribution between the potential electrodes. Therefore, resistivity measurements can be made without electrode polarization impedance errors. However, when the tetrapolar circuit is applied in the measurement of physiological events, uniform current density distribution is not likely to exist because of the differing resistivities of biological material and the relationship between the size of the electrodes and the extent of the volume conductor. Although a proper measurement of resistivity cannot be made under such circumstances, the tetrapolar circuit is useful in determining physiological events by impedance change. The primary disadvantage of the method is the requirement of four rather than two electrodes on the subject or preparation.

When the impedance being measured between the electrode terminals by any of the circuits just described is not dissected into its reactive and resistive components, it is not at all times clear which component contains the information related to the physiological event. When low frequencies are employed the impedance may be strongly reactive; with high frequencies the equivalent circuits are mainly resistive. Many investigations must still be carried out to discover whether, in a particular case, the resistive or the reactive component contains the more meaningful data.

10–2. SEASONAL VARIATIONS IN IMPEDANCE

The conducting properties of the body have been found to vary throughout the year. For example, Crile et al. (1922) discovered that the resistivity of excised samples of biological material depended on the time of the year when they were removed. Barnett (1940) noted that the 11.16-kc impedance measured between electrodes on the upper arms of 20 normal subjects varied cyclically over the period of a year. During the winter months the impedance was stable in the vicinity of 100 ohms; it increased from 140 to 250 ohms during the summer, an increase of 40 to 150%. There also occurred a 1-to 4-degree increase in phase angle during the summer. Similar changes were exhibited by the majority of 50 patients institutionalized and undergoing psychiatric care. Barnett explained the impedance change on the basis of alterations in epidermal thickness.

10–3. ENDOCRINE ACTIVITY

Because the composition and proportions of the body are profoundly affected by the endocrine system, changes in the levels of various circulating hormones would be expected to be revealed in the impedance between electrodes on subjects in which there are alterations in endocrine function. For example, in diseases of the thyroid gland, gross somatic changes occur. In hypothyroidism there is a characteristic increase in body proportions. The skin is thick, dry, coarse, yellowish in color, and characterized by heavy deposits of subcutaneous material. The hyperthyroid subject, on the other hand, is thin with a warm, soft, moist skin. Such gross differences in body composition have been found to alter the impedance measured by electrodes placed on the surface of the body.

Brazier (1935) presented two most provocative papers showing that in the intact human the phase angle[1] is directly related to thyroid function. In normal subjects, with both arms immersed up to the elbows in saline solutions serving as electrodes, she measured the impedance and phase angle at 20 kc and noted a difference in the phase angle between males and females. In 150 women with thyrotoxicosis she found that the phase angle was directly related to the metabolic rate and was independent of meals, muscular exercise, and the effect of autonomic drugs. Less correlation was found for hypothyroidism, but there was a measurable change when treatment of such subjects with thyroid-stimulating drugs or thyroid extract was begun.

Response to Brazier's paper was almost immediate. Horton and van Ravenswaay (1935) re-examined the data; they called attention to the fact that the ratio of reactance to resistance was the tangent of the phase angle but stated that for the small angles encountered the two were nearly equal. By strategically locating electrodes they were able to measure the impedance of the superficial and the deep layers of the arms separately. However, they were unable to establish a distinct correlation with thyroid function.

Barnett (1937) thoroughly investigated the problem and was able to obtain impedance values for the skin and deep tissue layers. The phase angle for normal skin was 71.5 degrees, and for deep tissue layers 5 to 10 degrees. He found that the important quantity was not the phase angle, which was almost constant, but the impedance value. He plotted the skin impedance for normal, hyperthyroid, and hypothyroid individuals in a range of frequencies extending from below 100 cps to above 40 kc. The three curves (Fig. 10–5) were significantly different, the curve for the hypothyroid subjects (3) lying above that for the normal (1) and the curve for the hyperthyroid (2) lying below. Choosing 11.15 kc, Barnett studied 458 cases and showed that a plot of basal metabolic rate (BMR) versus the reciprocal of the impedance (Fig. 10–6) correlated almost 80%. A BMR of -2% was equivalent to 109.7 ohms, and a range of 84 to 135 ohms represented a BMR spread of $+10$ to -13%.

Although the impedance method uncovers changes in the conducting properties of the skin which are related to thyroid function, in comparison to other thyroid tests it is not an adequately sensitive indicator for clinical use.

In the studies of impedance associated with thyroid dysfunction, small changes in impedance in the human being were observed to be related to age and sex (Brazier, 1935). The impedance changes reflecting estrogenic activity in the white rat were reinvestigated by Farzaneh (1953). Using

[1]Brazier used the tangent of the phase angle and the phase angle in radians interchangeably because the two were nearly identical at the frequency employed.

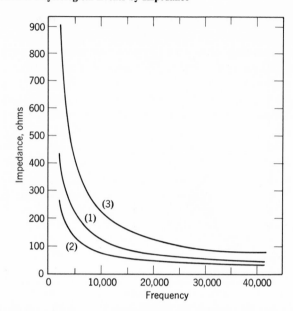

Figure 10–5. Skin impedance versus frequency for normal (1), hyperthyroid (2), and hypothyroid (3) subjects. [From A. Barnett, Western J. Surg. Obstet. Gynecol. 45 (October, 1937).]

approximately 100 animals and measuring the 15-kc impedance between the limbs, at estrous he observed a decrease in impedance of 20% and an increase in phase angle of approximately 5 degrees. In ovariectomized animals, the phase angle remained constant but the impedance varied slightly. Farzaneh also observed that thyroid activity altered the impedance. Much more remains to be investigated to discover the cause of the impedance changes which accompany changes in the level of estrogenic hormones in the circulation.

10–4. AUTONOMIC NERVOUS SYSTEM ACTIVITY

The terms galvanic skin reflex (GSR) [or psychogalvanic reflex (PGR)] and electrodermal response (EDR) designate two phenomena: the change in resistance and the appearance of a voltage measurable between one electrode in an area richly supplied by sweat glands and another in a region devoid of them. The change in resistance (the Fere effect) is now called the exosomatic response. The appearance of a voltage (the Tarchanoff phenomenon) is now termed the endosomatic response. Both events appear in response to an emotional stimulus and reflect a change in the activity of

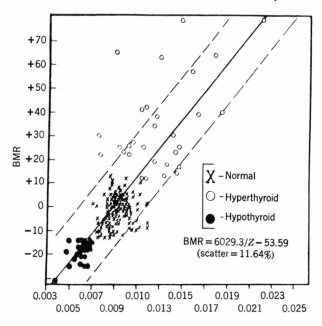

Figure 10-6. The relationship between the reciprocal of impedance at 11.15 kc and BMR for normal, hyperthyroid, and hypothyroid subjects. [From A. Barnett, Western J. Surg. Obstet. Gynecol. 45 (October 1937).]

the autonomic nervous system. Frequently, only the resistance change component is recorded.

Although direct current is usually employed to measure the resistance change, it is possible to observe the phenomenon by using the impedance method. The limiting frequency for its detection by impedance has not been established. McLendon and Hemingway (1930) observed that the GSR measured by d-c resistance change was forty-five times larger than the impedance change measured at 1.5 Mc. The two measurements were carried out simultaneously on human subjects. Using frequencies as high as 10 kc, Forbes and Landis (1935) were able to detect the GSR in a few subjects. They pointed out, however, that there were gross individual differences. In some subjects the upper frequency was 1 kc. Both Forbes (1936) and Montagu (1958) found a good correspondence between the potential change (endosomatic signal) and the impedance change in the low-frequency region below 100 cps. Nichols and Daroge (1955) and Taylor (1962) called attention to the advantages of using alternating current in minimizing electrode polarization problems in detecting the GSR. The former investigator employed 60 cps, and the latter 65 cps. Nichols and Daroge stated that the amplitude of the GSR decreased with increasing frequency and that with frequencies above 1 kc there is little response. At 60 cps they found the response to be half of that which is measured when using direct current. A similar decrease in the amplitude of the impedance change with increasing frequency was reported by Yokota and Fujimori (1962). More research must be carried out to correlate the effect of frequency on the impedance change with the resistive and voltaic components of the GSR. Because of the low-frequency nature of the GSR signal, high-gain direct-coupled amplifiers are traditionally used and drift has frequently been a problem. If the exosomatic component of the GSR can be adequately measured with alternating current, carrier amplifiers (see Chapter 13) can be used to provide a high stability and signal-to-noise ratio.

10–5. RESPIRATION

Mention was made in Section 5–2 of the studies by Atzler and Lehmann and Fenning, who employed the capacitance change principle to detect respiration. Other investigations have been carried out in which the impedance changes between two or four electrodes in direct contact with the chest wall have been employed to detect respiration. A good review of the circuits used in these studies was presented by Pacella (1966).

While recording cardiac impedance pulses with electrodes on the thorax, Nyboer (1944) noted variations in the baseline impedance which correlated with a simultaneously recorded spirogram. Schaefer et al. (1949) developed an impedance system for recording respiration in animals and man, using electrodes inserted subcutaneously in the chest wall. That such transthoracic impedance changes were related to the volume of air moved was demonstrated by Goldensohn and Zablow (1959), who passed a 10-kc constant current between electrodes on the wrists and detected the respiratory signal from similar electrodes placed farther up on each arm. Geddes (1962) described a two-electrode constant-current system in which respiration was detected by measuring the 50-kc impedance changes appearing between electrodes placed on the surface of the chest of animals and man. A high correlation between impedance change and volume of air breathed has been demonstrated by Goldensohn and Zablow (1959), Geddes (1962), Robbins and Marko (1962), Hanish (1962), Allison (1962), Allison et al. (1964), McCally et al. (1963), Kubicek et al. (1963–1964), Ax et al. (1964), Baker et al. (1965–1966), Pallett and Scopes (1965), and Hamilton et al. (1965).

Figure 10–7 shows a typical three-channel record of an electrocardiogram, an impedance pneumogram, and a spirogram in the human being, made

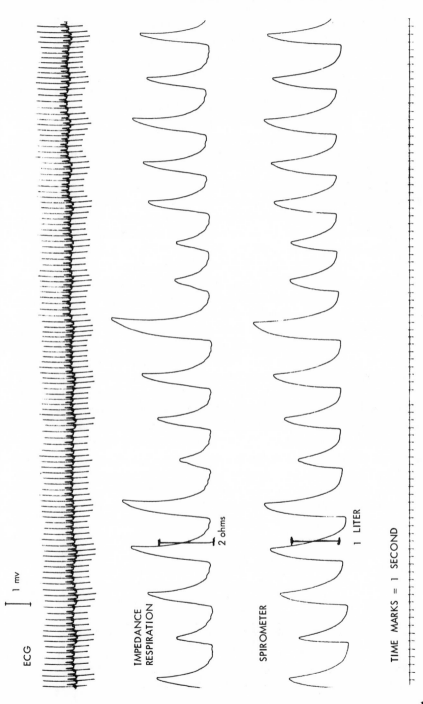

Figure 10-7. Impedance pneumogram, spirogram, and electrocardiogram.

167

with electrodes at the level of the xiphoid process and along the midaxillary lines. While the recording was being made, the subject was asked to vary his depth of respiration. The impedance and ECG recordings were made from the same pair of electrodes (Geddes, 1962). The excursions of the spirometer were detected by coupling a low-torque potentiometer to the pulley suspending the bell. Using the same impedance pneumograph, the authors have recorded respiration from horses, dogs, monkeys, cats, rabbits, rats, mice, alligators, and frogs. The magnitude of the impedance change encountered with respiration depends on the species and the location of the electrodes.

Throughout the years there has been some discussion concerning the importance of frequency for measurement of the respiratory impedance change. Apart from the considerations previously discussed, which require that a high-frequency current be used to avoid stimulation, there appears to be no particular advantage to the choice of one frequency over another. This fact is illustrated by Fig. 10–8, which shows the impedance change in a human subject produced by a vital capacity maneuver. It is noted that the change in transthoracic impedance from full inspiration to maximum expiration is practically the same in the frequency range of 50 to 600 kc. In this range the impedance change was almost entirely resistive.

The relationship between impedance change and volume of air moved is approximately linear under most circumstances. For the human being the coefficient $\Delta Z/\Delta V$ depends on the size of the subject and the location of the electrodes. In the studies carried out by Baker (1965), who used bipolar electrodes, a fairly good linearity was obtained for all electrode

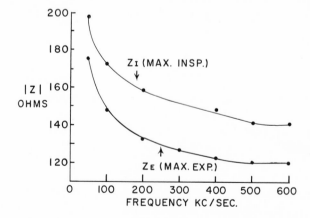

Figure 10–8. The relationship between impedance change and volume of air at different frequencies. [Redrawn from Baker et al., Am. J. Med. Electron. **4**:75 (1965). By permission.]

locations studied. In general he found coefficients ranging from 6.0 ohms per liter for adults of slight build to 1.0 ohm per liter for heavy subjects. Kubicek (1964) reported a coefficient of 1.2 ohms per liter of air breathed. The studies reported by Allison (1962), in which a tetrapolar electrode system was used, indicated a coefficient of 0.3 to 0.4 ohm per liter.

Figure 10–9, taken from Baker's investigation (1966), indicates the degree of linearity obtained in human subjects of differing builds with bipolar electrodes placed on midaxillary lines at different levels on the chest. Inspection of this illustration shows that the coefficient $\Delta Z/\Delta V$ is largest for adults of slight build. Figure 10–10 summarizes the data and illustrates the dependence of $\Delta Z/\Delta V$ on electrode location.

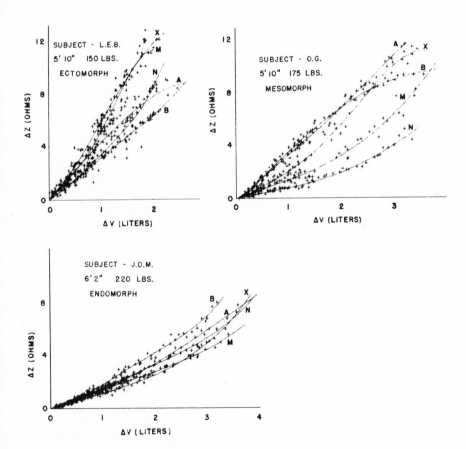

Figure 10–9. Transthoracic impedance changes (ΔZ) versus respired volume (ΔV) measured with bipolar electrodes. See Fig. 10–10 for electrode locations A, B, M, N, X. [From Baker and Geddes. *Med. Biol. Eng.* **4**:374 (1966). By permission.]

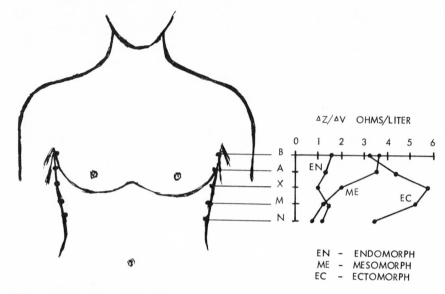

Figure 10-10. The relationship between respiratory impedance change and electrode location in the human being.

In the dog, the coefficient $\Delta Z/\Delta V$ varies with the size of the animal and the location of the electrodes. Geddes et al. (1962) obtained a coefficient of 20 ohms per liter. Baker and Geddes (1965) observed coefficients ranging from 50 to 70 ohms per liter. All of these studies were carried out with bipolar electrodes placed along midaxillary lines and at the level of the xiphoid process. With electrodes at other thoracic levels, the coefficient is considerably reduced. This relationship is shown in Fig 10–11.

Although the impedance pneumograph is widely used and many studies have been carried out to determine the relationship between the impedance change and the volume of air breathed, few studies have been directed toward identifying the factors which produce the impedance change. With a pair of electrodes on the thorax of the dog and by surgical interruption of the current pathways, Baker (1966) has found that approximately 80% of the injected current traversed the posterior thoracic path and 5% passed through the anterior path. Through the liver and diaphragm 10% of the current flowed, and through lung tissue only 5% passed.

Practicality is probably the most attractive feature of the impedance method for measurement of respiration. Nothing is simpler than affixing electrodes to a subject and connecting them to the recording equipment. The fact that the impedance change is related to the volume of air moved makes the method a calibratible one. Although calibration requires the

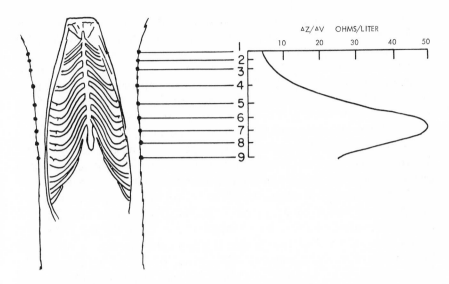

Figure 10–11. The relationship between respiratory impedance change per unit volume of air breathed and electrode location in the dog.

use of a spirometer or other volume-measuring instrument, the calibrating device can be removed and respiratory volumes measured without obstructing the air stream. Another attractive feature of the method is availability of the electrocardiogram from the same pair of electrodes.

Perhaps the most unattractive feature of the measurement of respiration by impedance is the need to calibrate each subject with a volume-measuring device. No single calibration factor can be specified for each species. However, once a calibration value has been obtained on a subject for electrodes in a given location, this factor remains remarkably constant.

As with any physiological event which is measured with electrodes, movement causes a variation in impedance and produces unwanted signals. Therefore precautions must be taken to avoid this complication.

10–6. BLOOD FLOW

When the impedance change technique is applied to the determination of blood flow, three methods are available. With the first, cardiac output (liters per minute) is determined by applying the dilution technique. With the second, stroke volume, that is, the systolic discharge from the left ventricle, is determined by measurement of the impedance change between electrodes placed on or in the heart. In the third method, which employs electrodes that encompass a segment of the body, attempts are made to calibrate the pulsatile impedance signal in terms of blood flow in the field between the electrodes. The various applications of each of these methods will be described.

One of the earliest studies to determine cardiac output employed the impedance method. By measuring transarterial impedance in dogs and by intravenously injecting 1.5% saline, Stewart (1897, 1921) was able to identify the time of arrival and the passage of the blood containing the injected saline. He accomplished this by using a simple impedance bridge, one arm of which was the transarterial impedance. The alternating current for the bridge was derived from an inductorium. The detector was a telephone receiver. Passage of the hyperconducting blood unbalanced the bridge and directed the investigators to collect blood at that moment for future determination of its salinity. Cardiac output was determined by use of the dilution formula. Continuous recording of the change in conductivity of the blood as it passed an arterial detector was accomplished by Romm (1924) and Gross and Mittermaier (1926). In both studies the conductivity curve was not calibrated because the information sought was circulation time. These two studies paved the way for Wigger's (1944) investigations, which employed a flow-through conductivity cell inserted in a femoral artery. Using the original Stewart constant-injection method, Wiggers obtained in anesthetized dogs cardiac output figures that were in good agreement with those measured by other observers. White (1947) refined the method by devising two types of hypodermic needle electrodes which were inserted directly into an artery. As the injected saline passed the electrodes, the intra-arterial impedance at 70 kc was continuously recorded on an oscilloscope. Despite certain practical difficulties, he obtained cardiac outputs differing between -12 and $+22\%$ from the values obtained by the Fick method.

When saline is employed as the injected material, some is lost from the vascular tree. Since this naturally affects the limit of accuracy attainable, the exact amount lost has been the subject of much debate which has questioned the precision of the saline method. Chinard (1962) stated that 5% of intravenously injected saline is lost in passing through the lungs. Saline is also removed from the circulation via the kidneys and capillaries. That the loss in one trip from vein to artery must be small can be deduced from studies in which the saline method has been checked against the Fick and dye-dilution methods. These studies, which were reviewed by Smith et al. (1967), indicate that the saline method gives values within approximately $\pm 5\%$ of those obtained with the dye-dilution and Fick methods.

To eliminate loss of the conducting material injected, Goodwin and Saperstein (1957) used autogenous plasma instead of saline. Blood from an artery was aspirated at a constant rate through a conductivity cell operated at 2,500 cps for conductivity measurements. In a series of 24 dogs Goodwin and Saperstein compared the conductivity method and the Evans blue technique and obtained remarkably similar results. The difference in the mean values was 0.3%.

Geddes and Hoff (1963) and Smith et al. (1967) have adapted the impedance method for the measurement of cardiac output by the dilution technique by employing specially designed electrodes placed on the surface of an intact artery. The electrodes were mounted in a retaining assembly which maintained them firmly in contact with the artery and prevented diameter changes in the artery caused by variations in blood pressure. Upon intravenous injection of 5% saline, a decrease in impedance was recorded as the hyperconducting solution passed the electrodes. Knowing the amount of saline injected and the calibration of the impedance curve, the investigators used the dilution formula to calculate cardiac output. Calibration was achieved by injecting a known concentration of saline in blood into the artery central to the extra-arterial electrodes. Figure 10–12 was made in this manner, employing an anesthetized dog as the experimental subject. At the mark on the time channel, an intravenous injection (3 cc of 5% saline) was administered. Approximately 15 seconds later the mixture appeared in the artery and altered the impedance being recorded. Calculation of cardiac output from the area under the curve gave a figure of 1.5 liters/minute.

In applying the saline conductivity method, the concentration of the

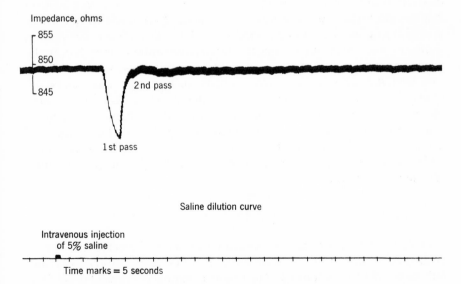

Figure 10–12.   Saline conductivity record.

injected material is an important consideration. Injection of a concentration only slightly different from that of blood requires the use of a high-gain recording system; a high concentration permits a much lower gain in the recording apparatus. It is possible to trade off gain and concentration over only a narrow range because very high concentrations produce physiological changes which alter cardiac output. Wiggers (1944) reported, "In preliminary experiments, such temporary disturbances [changes in cardiac output] occurred frequently when 5 percent saline was used and generally with a 10 percent solution." He chose a 3% sodium chloride solution as optimum. The authors have used 5% solutions in the dog without observable cardiovascular response.

The fractional emptying of the left ventricle of dogs was determined by Holt (1956–1962) and Holt and Allensworth (1957) using a modification of the saline conductivity technique. By injecting a known amount of saline into the left ventricle and continuously recording conductivity in the aorta, it was possible to calculate the volume of the left ventricle and the amount discharged per beat. Elegant as this technique is, it depends on the assumption that perfect mixing occurs. That this is not always the case was shown by Irisawa et al. (1960).

The mathematical expression for the aortic concentration of a material injected into the left ventricle can be derived if two assumptions are made. The first is that the weight (m gm) of the material injected into the left ventricle is contained in a volume which is small with respect to the diastolic volume of the ventricle (V ml), and the second is that uniform mixing takes place in the ventricle. The injection is made as quickly as possible just before systolic ejection. Then, if uniform mixing has occurred, and the stroke volume (v ml) remains constant for each beat, the aortic concentration (C mg/ml) will decrease in a stepwise fashion. For the first beat the aortic concentration will be m/V gm/ml. The number of grams ejected is mv/V, and the number remaining in the ventricle is $m - mv/V$ or $m(1 - v/V)$ gm. The ventricle then fills, and the diastolic volume is again Vml, into which this weight of material is diluted. The aortic concentration for the second beat is then $(1 - v/V)m/V$. The process continues to be repeated, and the general expression for the aortic concentration for the nth beat becomes

$$C_n = \frac{m}{V} \left(1 - \frac{v}{V}\right)^{n-1}.$$

Figure 10–13 illustrates the concentration as the injected material is cleared from the left ventricle for stroke volumes v equal to 40%, 50%, and 60% of the diastolic volume V. Thus, from calibrated records of these data, ventricular diastolic volume and stroke volume can be calculated. Cardiac

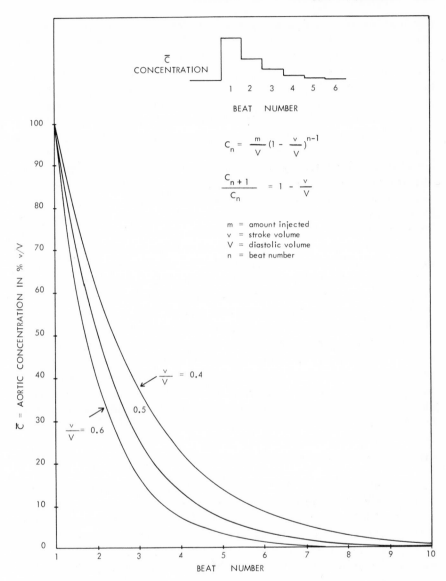

Figure 10–13. Fractional emptying of the left ventricle.

output can also be determined by multiplying stroke volume v by heart rate.

Sigman et al. (1937) noted that, in the measurement of the conductivity of blood samples, motion was an important factor. They therefore studied this phenomenon in flowing blood to discover that the conductivity to alternating and direct current increased slightly with flow when electrodes were placed along or across a tube. They further found that the increase was dependent on the percentage of red cells (hematocrit). The increase in conductivity approximated 5% with a flow range from 0 to 40 cm/sec. Similar observations were made by Velick and Gorin (1940), Coulter and Pappenheimer (1949), and Molnar et al. (1953), as well as by Liebman and Cosenza (1962–1963), who found a similar correlation with cell volume. The phenomenon has been put to practical use by Sugano and Oda (1960) and by Liebman and Cosenza to study changes in blood flow. The former investigators inserted electrodes into vessels and plastic tubes to measure flow; the latter team studied the flow of blood in canine teeth by measuring the impedance changes, using the tetrapolar electrode configuration implanted in a tooth cavity.

It must be noted that, although flow changes are easily detected by this method, calibration is difficult. The few impedance-flow calibrations made to date indicate a considerable degree of nonlinearity between these two quantities. However, the practical applicability of the method cannot be denied. Many careful investigations will be needed to quantitate the phenomenon in each instance where it is employed.

In explosive decompression studies, the tiny bubbles which appear in the venous system were recorded by Leverett (1962), using the impedance method. The impedance of blood flowing in a vein was measured by electrodes placed outside the vessel. The passage of air bubbles altered the impedance considerably, giving a semiquantitative indication of their presence.

10–7.   DIRECT IMPEDANCE CARDIOGRAPHY

Rappaport and Ray (1927) recorded the impedance changes in a tortoise heart as it was kept beating *in vitro*. In this study the heart, suspended in a beaker of saline, constituted one electrode; the other was placed nearby in the solution. The investigators noted a change in impedance of 10% with each heart beat. Rushmer et al. (1953) affixed electrodes to the interior walls of the right and left ventricles of dogs. In one animal they placed electrodes at the apex and the base of the right and left ventricles. They recorded a decrease in impedance during diastole and an increase during systole. Although the recordings resembled those made with cardiometers, their studies on models and animals led them to believe that the method contained variables which were difficult to quantitate, and they abandoned the technique in favor of others which appeared more promising at that time. Mello-Sobrinho (1963) and Geddes et al. (1965, 1966) reinvestigated the method, using electrodes (insulated except at the tip) inserted into the base and the apex of canine hearts. Accordingly, the cardiac chambers functioned as conductivity cells of varying dimensions; the impedance decreased with filling and increased with emptying. Because the resistivity of cardiac muscle is approximately five times that of blood, the current is largely confined to the ventricle. Figure 10–14 is a typical record of the 80-kc impedance changes recorded with this technique.

By injecting or withdrawing from the ventricle known amounts of blood with the outlet and inlet valves closed, it is possible to calibrate the impedance change in terms of volume. In preliminary studies with this method calibration factors of 3 to 6 ohms per milliliter were obtained for the left ventricles of 10-kg dogs. At present, dynamic calibration factors are being derived by recording impedance changes and simultaneously determining the cardiac output by means of the direct Fick method. Initial studies have yielded calibration factors slightly less than those determined by the injection and withdrawal method.

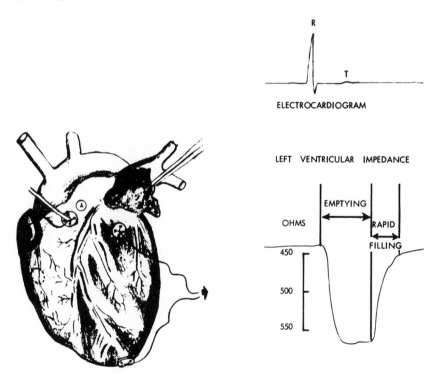

Figure 10–14. Left ventricular impedance cardiogram in the dog. [From Geddes et al., *Cardiovascular Res. Center Bull.* **4**(4) 118–130 (1966). By permission.]

This technique is very easy to apply to lower animals. Figure 10–15 illustrates the filling and emptying of a frog heart with two pin electrodes passed through the apex and the base of the ventricle. The ventricular electrogram was obtained from the same electrodes.

10–8.   IMPEDANCE PLETHYSMOGRAPHY

The use of the impedance change technique for recording peripheral volume pulses was first described by Mann (1937). In a few years there appeared numerous papers on the subject, and the technique soon became known as impedance plethysmography. Pioneering in this field were Nyboer (1943, 1944, 1950, 1959), Brook and Cooper (1957), Polzer et al. (1960), and Polzer and Schuhfried (1961). Nyboer became the advocate of the tetrapolar electrode method, while most of the other investigators cited employed two-electrode systems. Although the literature shows that the impedance change is mainly resistive at the frequencies presently employed (20 to 200 kc), Mann (1953) demonstrated the existence of a reactive component at 10 kc when the impedance was measured between electrodes on each forearm. With either the two- or the four-electrode system it is easy to obtain impedance changes strikingly similar to those recorded with capsule plethysmographs. The real difficulty lies in the lack of accurate methods to relate the impedance change to a volume change.

The basis for impedance plethysmography as applied to body segments is the decrease in impedance when a volume of blood is introduced between the measuring electrodes. The expression most frequently employed to relate the measured impedance change to the volume change can be derived by assuming that there is a homogeneous conducting material and a uniform current density distribution between the measuring electrodes. Obviously these requirements are never satisfied in practical situations, and to minimize some of the resulting errors, current is introduced to the specimen by widely spaced electrodes. Figure 10–16a,b illustrate the current distribution between electrodes placed on homogeneous conducting cylinders of differing lengths. Note that in both cases there is the same distortion of the lines of equal current at each electrode, but in the central region a–a' (Fig. 16b) the current distribution is more uniform.

To illustrate how a volume change can be identified by a resistance change, we remove the conducting cylinder a–a' and place electrodes over its ends. For a length L, area A_0, and resistivity ρ, the resistance is $R_0 = \rho L / A_0$. Consider now the addition of a volume ΔV of conducting material to the segment without producing a change in length. The cross-sectional area will increase uniformly to A_1, and the resistance measured between

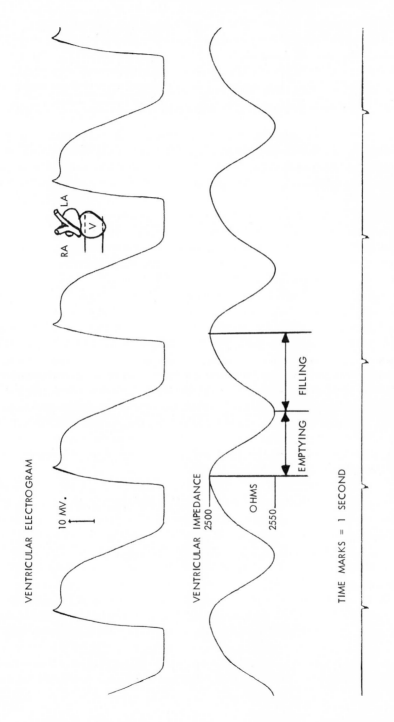

Figure 10-15. Frog ventricular electrogram and impedance cardiogram.

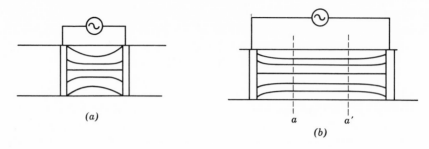

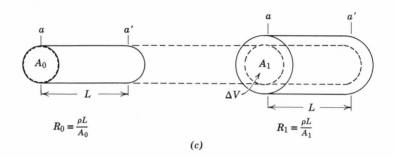

Figure 10–16. Simplified basis for impedance plethysmography: (*a*) current distribution with closely spaced electrodes: (*b*) current distribution with widely spaced electrodes; (*c*) the result of adding a volume ΔV to the conducting cylinder $a - a'$. $R_1 - R_0 = \Delta R = - (pL^2/V_0^2)\, \Delta V$.

the electrode covering the ends will be $R_1 = \rho L/A_1$. The difference in resistance reflects the volume change; therefore:

$$\Delta R = R_1 - R_0 = \frac{\rho L}{A_1} - \frac{\rho L}{A_0} = \rho L\left(\frac{1}{A_1} - \frac{1}{A_0}\right),$$

but

$$V_0 = LA_0 \quad \text{and} \quad V_1 = LA_1.$$

Substituting,

$$\Delta R = \rho L\left(\frac{L}{V_1} - \frac{L}{V_0}\right)$$

$$= \rho L^2\left(\frac{V_0 - V_1}{V_1 V_0}\right) = -\frac{\rho L^2(V_1 - V_0)}{V_1 V_0}.$$

If V_1 is not appreciably larger than V_0 (i.e., the volume added, $\Delta V = V_1 - V_0$, is small),

$$\Delta R \doteq -\left(\frac{\rho L^2}{V_0^2}\right)\Delta V.$$

Thus it can be seen that an increase in the volume of conducting material of resistivity ρ will be accompanied by a decrease in resistance appearing between electrodes separated by a distance L. Sometimes, instead of calculating the volume V_0 between the electrodes, the impedance value is used. This can be inserted into the formula by multiplying the expression $R_0 = \rho L/A_0$ by L/L to obtain $R_0 = \rho L^2/V_0$. Substitution of this relationship in the above equation gives

$$\Delta R = -\left(\frac{R_0^2}{\rho L^2}\right)\Delta V.$$

It is important to recall that these expressions were derived assuming a uniform current distribution through a homogeneous conductor of uniform cross-sectional area. In the physiological application of these expressions, these requirements are rarely fulfilled. In addition, when a pulsatile impedance change is recorded with the impedance method applied to a body segment, the amplitude of the change reflects the difference between arterial inflow and venous outflow. Inflow occurs during only a portion of the cardiac cycle; outflow from the vascular tree exists throughout the cardiac cycle. If venous outflow is occluded just before an inflow to the region between the electrodes, the stepwise change in baseline reflects the pulsatile arterial inflow. Because such an occlusion is difficult to achieve without artifact, graphical constructions have been applied to the impedance plethysmogram to obtain the impedance change which reflects the true flow into a body segment. Powers (1958) and Allison (1966) have presented a discussion of these constructions as they apply to the circulation in the limbs and digits; Kubicek et al. (1966) reviewed them for studies of the thoracic impedance pulse.

Impedance plethysmography has been applied to virtually every region of the body, including the digits, limbs, head, thorax, kidney, and eye. Although the contour of the impedance pulses is almost identical with that obtained with a simultaneously recorded capsule plethysmograph, the real drawback of the method is that it is difficult to calibrate the impedance pulse accurately in terms of blood flow. Van der Berg and Alberts (1954) studied the relationship between the volumes calculated on the basis of the pulsatile impedance changes at 60 and 185 kc and the pulsatile volume changes as measured by capsule plethysmographs applied to the digits of normal subjects. They found that the ratio of the former to the latter was 1.5 with a deviation from the mean value of 2 to 35%. When the two methods were compared while occluding the venous outflow, inconclusive results were obtained.

Although true calibration of the impedance pulse is not always possible, a two-channel record from homologous body segments provides a good indication of the patency of vessels supplying the region between the electrodes. In addition, changes in the amplitude of the impedance pulses reflect changes in the circulation in the area examined.

Variations in the impedance between electrodes encompassing the kidney were described by Lofgren (1951). He found that when a solution of dextran was forced into the rat kidney a decrease in the 2- and the 200-kc impedance occurred. He then proceeded to employ the method to study the change in kidney volume in response to injections of drugs.

Pulsatile impedance changes have been recorded from canine and human eyes by Bishop and Nyboer (1962). The meaning of the pulses recorded awaits correlation with the movement of fluids within the eye.

Underwood and Gowing (1965) reported that the impedance between widely spaced electrodes on experimental animals reflected blood volume changes. In their studies on dogs and cats, they used a bipolar electrode arrangement; one electrode was placed on the sternal notch and the other in the lumbar region. A 10-kc square wave of current was employed, and the impedance change was measured as blood was withdrawn from the animals. A 10% change in blood volume was found to produce a 1.5-ohm change in resistance.

The authors have verified these observations, using a tetrapolar electrode arrangement applied to dogs. The current electrodes were placed on the right forelimb and left hind limb, and the potential electrodes on the left forelimb and right hind limb. A 50-kc constant-current system was used. Withdrawal of blood increased the impedance; the addition of blood decreased it. A coefficient of 0.16% change in resistance for a 1% change in blood volume was obtained. A nearly linear relationship was observed for a $\pm 30\%$ change in blood volume (calculated on the basis of blood constituting 7% of body weight) and impedance change. The addition of isotonic saline, which has a lower resistivity than blood, produced smaller changes in impedance.

Despite the attractiveness of the method of total body impedance to indicate blood loss or addition, it cannot identify translocation of blood or fluid from one body compartment to the other. Furthermore, because the signal is so small, electrodes of high electrical stability are required.

With two pairs of electrodes placed over a superficial artery, the pressure pulse can be recorded. Measurement of the time difference between the pulses permits calculation of the approximate pulse wave velocity. This technique was embodied in an instrument devised by Schmitt for Simonson and Nakagawa (1960).

10–9. RHEOENCEPHALOGRAPHY

There is available an instrument called the rheoencephalograph (REG), which records impedance changes between electrodes placed on the scalp. Rheoencephalography was introduced in 1950 when Polzer and Schuhfried placed electrodes on the heads of several subjects and recorded the fluctuations in impedance during the passage of a 20-kc alternating current. In a patient with a carotid occlusion, the pulsatile amplitude was diminished on the affected side, indicating a possible relationship with cerebral blood flow. Since that time various studies have been carried out and several different electrode configurations have been employed. Investigations with forehead-to-mastoid, mastoid-to-occiput, transparietal, trans-occipital, and vertex electrodes have all been described. Reviews of this field have been presented by Jenkner (1962), Lifshitz (1963), Geddes (1964), and McHenry (1965).

Jenkner (1959, 1962) studied the pulse waves obtained with electrodes placed on the forehead and behind the ears on the mastoid processes and was able to show that the amplitude of the pulsatile impedance changes reflected blood flow to the cortex. This extensive study involved 4000 patients in all. He noted that on the side of a hemispherectomy no pulsations were recordable. Respiratory changes were recorded, and with hyperventilation the amplitude of the pulses decreased. If the subjects breathed air mixtures containing carbon dioxide, the pulsations increased. It is well known that reduction in the amount of carbon dioxide in the blood lowers the cerebral blood flow, while an increase produces the opposite effect. A lack of oxygen in the respired air altered the contour of the pulse, while amyl nitrite increased and histamine decreased the size of the pulsatile impedance change.

Certain maneuvers decrease cerebral blood flow and at the same time increase the amplitude of the impedance changes, making it difficult to read flow information from the size of the pulses. For example, occlusion of the venous outflow or performance of the Valsalva maneuver decreases cerebral blood flow and increases the amplitude of the impedance pulses.

When electrodes are placed on the head, both the extracranial and intracranial vascular beds carry current. The extracranial vascular bed is free to expand; the intracranial bed is in a rigid container, the skull. There is as yet no agreement on the exact contribution of each bed to the pulsatile impedance change.

Markovich and Namon (1965) called attention to the importance of the size and spacing of the electrodes. They pointed out that small electrodes detect impedance changes in their immediate vicinity, while larger electrodes have increased sensitivity to impedance changes deeper within the brain. Their studies also indicated that the amount of impedance change contributed by the vascular bed of the scalp could be altered by changing the size and spacing of the electrodes. From the results of their experiments, these investigators preferred measuring the REG by using transtemporal current electrodes connected to a constant-current generator. Recordings were made between an indifferent monopolar electrode on the vertex and electrodes on or near the current electrodes.

A typical REG from a normal subject is shown in Fig. 10–17. The electrodes were arrayed as shown, forehead to mastoid, and the impedance changes were measured at 70 kc. The first and fifth channels are the EEG; the second and fourth, the REG. Lead II ECG was included for reference purposes. The EEG and REG recordings were made from the same pair of electrodes.

In this record, it is observed that the REG's from the right and the left sides are slightly different in waveform. This is a fairly common finding in normal subjects. The pulse transmission time from the heart to the head is evident from the relationship between the QRS complex of the ECG and the onset of the impedance pulse. This interval is often described as the appearance time. It is customary to measure the peak amplitude (usually 20 to 200 milliohms) and the rate of rise of the impedance pulse (ohms per second). At present these parameters constitute the quantitative measurements derived from the rheoencephalogram. Although dramatic alterations can be produced in the REG by a variety of factors, the clinical value of this signal awaits further investigation.

10–10. THORACIC IMPEDANCE CARDIOGRAPHY

If electrodes are placed to encompass the thorax, impedance changes reflecting cardiac activity are recordable with ease. Bipolar and tetrapolar electrode arrangements have been placed on the arms, on either side of the thorax, on the back, and around the neck and chest at the level of the diaphragm. Clear cardiac impedance pulses can be recorded with any of these electrode configurations. Figure 10–18 illustrates the type of recording made with two electrodes on a human subject. The electrocardiogram, made from the same pair of electrodes, is presented to identify the location of the impedance pulse in the cardiac cycle.

A number of investigators have studied the thoracic impedance cardiogram and hoped to calibrate it in terms of the systolic discharge

(A decrease in impedance is shown upward.)

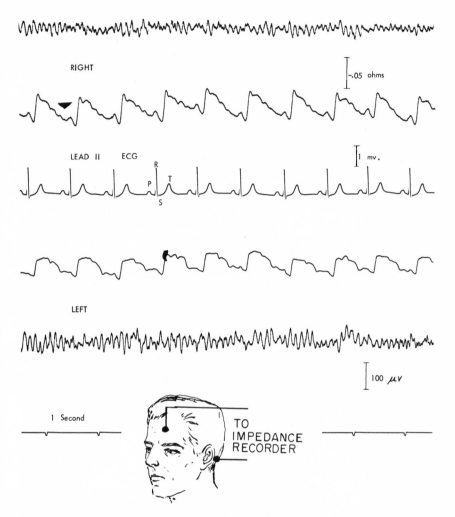

Figure 10–17.   Rheoencephalogram.

from the heart. Probably the earliest were Atzler and Lehmann (1932) and Atzler (1933, 1935), who placed electrodes in front of and behind the thorax and detected ultrahigh-frequency impedance changes synchronous with cardiac activity. Because their circuit was mainly capacitive, they called the method "Dielektrographie." Later Nyboer et al. (1940) described precordial impedance changes which also reflected cardiac activity.

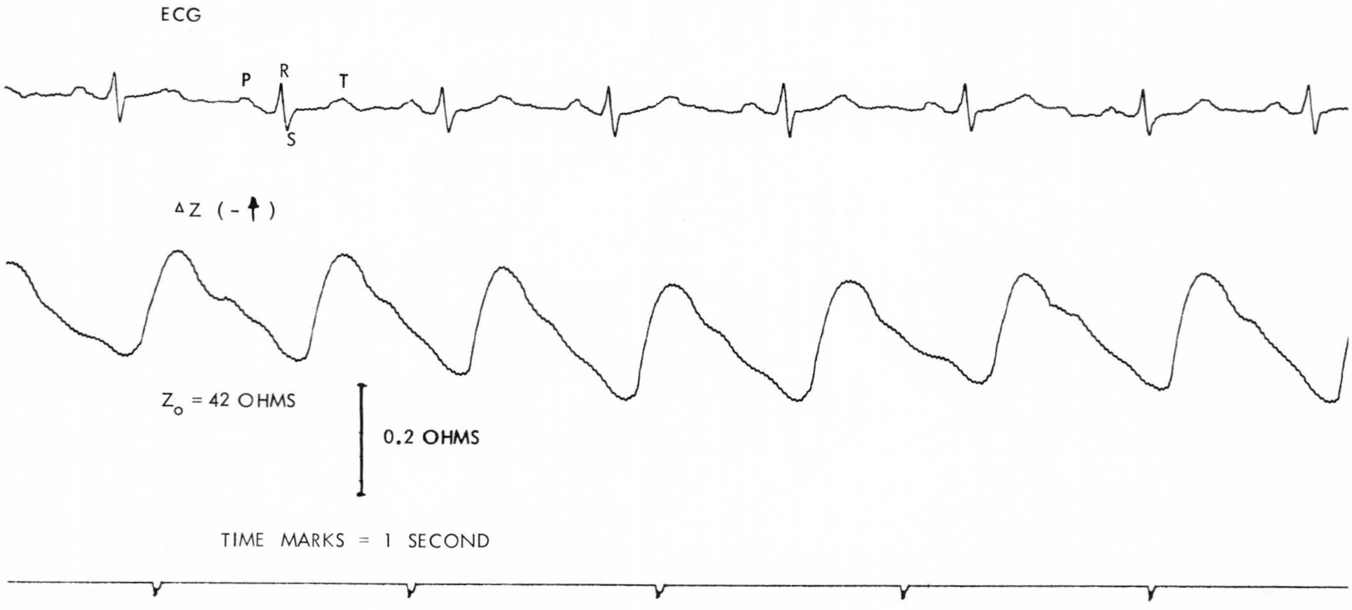

Figure 10-18. Thoracic impedance cardiogram.

ECG

P R T S

ΔZ (- ↑)

Z_o = 42 OHMS

0.2 OHMS

TIME MARKS = 1 SECOND

Probably in an attempt to standardize electrode placement, Holzer et al. (1945) measured the 14-kc cardiac impedance pulses appearing between electrodes placed on the arms and legs. Their study examined the impedance pulses in human subjects in health and disease, measuring impedance changes by means of the standard electrocardiographic lead configurations. They called their method "Rheokardiographie."

Improving the capacitive method of Atzler and Lehmann, Whitehorn and Pearl (1949) employed a 10.7-mc current and were able to record impedance pulses with high fidelity, stating: "Values for stroke volumes, cardiac output and cardiac indices calculated from such records, on the basis of preliminary calibration of the instrument by introduction of known volumes of saline between the plates, fall within the range of accepted normal values, but conclusions as to the validity of the method are not yet possible."

Mann (1953), using his 10-kc capacigraph, which recorded only the capacitance changes between single electrodes placed on each forearm, believed that these changes were due mainly to blood volume changes within the thorax, although he admitted the presence of smaller changes in the arms. Zajic et al. (1954), using 270 kc, applied to one electrode on the neck and another either in the pelvic area or on the thighs, observed changes in the impedance pulse with maneuvers which were known to change stroke volume. In one study Nyboer (1959) presented records called "radiocardiograms," taken at several levels on the precordium with his tetrapolar electrode system.

The thoracic impedance cardiogram is at present being studied in an effort to creat an indirect method of measuring stroke volume in human subjects. The extensive four-electrode studies being carried out by Kubicek et al. (1964, 1966), Kinnen et al. (1964), and Patterson et al. (1964) show considerable promise in this direction. Using two band electrodes around the neck and two around the thorax, they recorded impedance pulses and corrected their amplitudes by a geometric method to obtain a value for ΔZ to substitute in the expression $\Delta Z = -\Delta V Z_0^2/\rho L^2$, in which Z_0 is the impedance, L is the distance between the potential electrodes, and ρ is the resistivity of blood (150 ohm-cm). Patterson compared the direct Fick method with the impedance method in subjects with and without cardiac defects and obtained a surprisingly good correlation in both groups. In a series of 35 unselected patients with cardiovascular disease, 60% had impedance estimates of blood flow which checked within 20% of the conventionally determined values. Patients in atrial fibrillation and those with atypical impedance waveforms provided impedance measurements with the poorest correlation.

One investigation has been made to identify the phenomena underlying the transthoracic cardiac impedance pulse. Bonjer et al. (1952), in a series of ingenious experiments which consisted of wrapping first the heart and then the lungs in rubber sheeting and perfusing each with a stroke pump, concluded that the transthoracic impedance changes were due mainly to perfusion of the pulmonary vascular circuit by the output from the right ventricle and that only a small component was due to direct volume changes of the heart. Bonjer's work appears to indicate that it may be possible to derive an impedance signal related to stroke volume. It must be remembered, however, that thorax-encompassing electrodes detect impedance changes caused by extra- and intrathoracic circulations. In addition within the thorax there may appear an impedance change which reflects the output of both ventricles. Until current pathways have been defined, it is not possible to identify the origin of the impedance change. If it turns out that the major portion of the current traverses the pulmonary vascular bed, there exists the possibility of obtaining an impedance signal related to the systolic discharge from the right ventricle.

10–11. BLOOD PRESSURE

A very interesting application of the impedance method to measure blood pressure in tiny vessels is due to Wiederhelm and Rushmer (1964), who employed a micropipette (0.5 to 5 microns in diameter) as the sensor. It was filled with 2 M saline and connected to an electrical actuator which could apply pressure to the saline. The saline in the pipette and the blood in a tiny blood vessel of frog mesentery constituted an electrical resistance, the value of which depended on the position of the saline-blood interface in the micro tip. The micropipette-animal resistance constituted one arm of a 1000-cps impedance bridge. The detector consisted of an amplifier connected to the actuator. The bridge was then balanced and set to hunt for a fixed position of the meniscus. The current driving the actuator, which constantly rebalanced the bridge, was proportional to the blood pressure. The system exhibited a response time of 35 ms to a step function of pressure. The remarkably clean and faithful records revealed a blood pressure of 20/15 mm Hg in the microcirculation of the frog mesentery.

10–12. MUSCULAR CONTRACTION

Cardiac Muscle
The contraction of the three types of muscle can easily be recorded by the impedance method. Previous mention was made of recording the filling and emptying of the ventricles. The isometric contraction of cardiac

muscle has been demonstrated to produce an impedance change. Rosenbleuth and del Pozo (1943) measured this change between electrodes inserted into a tortoise ventricle which was prevented from shortening. An impedance change of approximately 10%, which appeared coincident with contraction and outlasted it, was measured. The precise relationship of this impedance change to the action potential awaits further investigation.

Skeletal Muscle

In many studies it is necessary to detect the contraction of skeletal muscle without gaining access to the tendon. Traditionally the electromyogram has been employed as an indicator of muscular contraction. Although this signal is related (but not proportional) to muscular contraction, in some instances it cannot be conveniently employed. Another method, described by Geddes (1966), consists of using a caliper myograph to measure the amount of lateral force development at the belly of the muscle. In some instances this method is not practical. In situations where it is not possible to measure tension directly or to use the EMG or caliper myograph, it may be advisable to investigate application of the impedance method to derive a signal related to muscular contraction.

The position of the tongue was transduced to an electrical signal by Petrovick and Brumlik (1961–1962) via the impedance method. With the tongue acting as one plate of a capacitor and the other plate embedded in a denture, they were able to record movements of the tongue during speech. This technique may offer promise for speech therapy studies. The same authors employed the method to detect the muscular tremor in Parkinson's disease.

Dubuisson (1933) employed the impedance method to indicate muscular contraction by measuring the impedance between electrodes directly on the surface of an exposed frog gastrocnemius muscle. A record of the decreasing impedance accompanying contraction, made with needle electrodes passed through the ends of the muscle, is shown in Fig. 10–19 (Geddes and Hoff, 1963). With this particular electrode arrangement, contraction moves the electrodes closer together and increases the cross-sectional area of muscle between them. Both factors contribute to a reduction in impedance. Electrodes placed across the belly of the muscle do not give a reliable impedance change with contraction.

The authors have detected the contraction of skeletal muscles in human subjects by measuring the impedance change between electrodes placed on the skin above the muscle. This change was used to control a solenoid valve and to operate an artificial muscle affixed to an orthesis.

To illustrate the type of signal obtainable with the contraction of skeletal muscle in man, two pairs of electrodes were placed on the skin over the

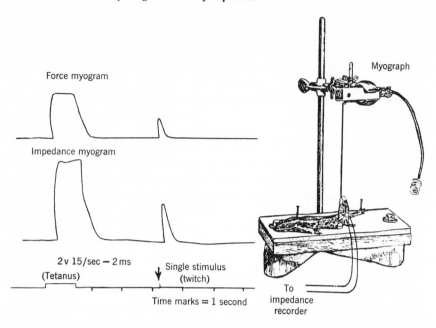

Figure 10–19. Frog muscle myogram and impedance myogram. (From Geddes and Hoff, Proceedings of the San Diego Symposium for Biomedical Engineering, 1963, p.119. By permission.)

biceps muscle. One pair was placed over the origin and insertion; the other, across the belly of the muscle. Impedance changes were recorded at 50 kc while the subject contracted the muscle voluntarily. The records obtained are shown in Fig. 10–20. With the electrodes placed along the muscle, a standing subject lifted and lowered a 5-pound weight from a position of full extension of the elbow through an angle of approximately 90 degrees. The EMG and impedance changes were recorded from the same electrodes. In the lower part of the record below the time line are the recordings obtained from electrodes over the belly of the muscle. In the first portion of the record the weight was clamped, resulting in isometric contraction of the muscle. Just past the middle of the record, the weight was released and the muscle contracted isotonically.

When the impedance method is employed to record muscular contractions, great care must be exercised in interpreting the records. The impedance change is not necessarily proportional to the force or the amount of shortening. The electrodes measure only the impedance between them, which during muscular contraction may vary with many factors. Furthermore, the greatest impedance change may occur at the beginning, at the

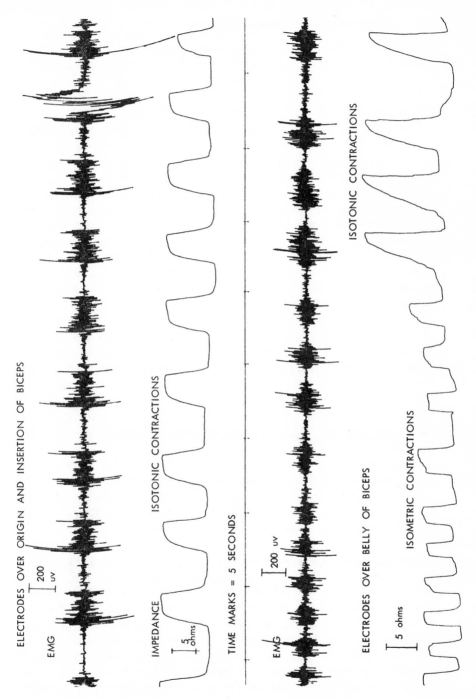

Figure 10–20. Impedance myograms and the EMG.

middle, or near the end of contraction. However, despite the lack of direct correlation with muscular contraction, the impedance method can provide an easily obtainable signal indicative of muscular activity.

Smooth Muscle

Electrodes placed on, in, or over smooth muscle can be employed to detect contractions. Electrodes appropriately inserted into the stomach, bladder, etc., can serve to monitor the impedance change during a volume change or deformation. Kornmesser and Nyboer (1962) used surface electrodes to detect impedance changes reflecting contractions of the human uterus during labor. Gastrointestinal motility can be detected by measuring the impedance change between electrodes placed around the wall of the small intestine of a dog. The record shown in Fig. 10–21 was made with a pair of electrodes mounted in a split rubber sleeve, which was placed around the proximal small intestine of an anesthetized dog. An impedance change of a few ohms was encountered when segmentation contractions occurred. Respiratory artifacts usually accompany the recording of gut motility by other techniques. To demonstrate the absence of such artifacts when the impedance method is used, respiration was recorded simultaneously with gut motility. In the first portion of the record it can be seen that the frequency of the two events is different. In the center of the record a small dose of epinephrine was given to arrest both respiration and gut motility; thereafter, the two phenomena reappeared at different times. In this study respiration started ahead of gut motility, and during this period no respiratory artifacts are identifiable in the gastrointestinal recording.

The impedance change described above is obviously due to alterations in the amount of conducting material between the electrodes. Accurate calibration in terms of volume change is, of course, not possible; however as an indirect indicator of gastrointestinal motility the impedance method exhibits many possibilities.

10–13. NERVOUS ACTIVITY

Perhaps the most familiar example of biological impedance change is that which accompanies the physiological activity of nerve. Cole and Curtis (1939) showed that, as an impulse travels along a nerve fiber, the membrane exhibits a transient decrease in impedance. Similar studies on dendritic layers deep within the brain made by Adey et al. (1962) give promise of providing a method of studying neuronal activity. Employing coaxial electrodes and less than 30 μv to measure the impedance at 1000 cps, they found that, with electrodes in the hippocampal area of cats, arousal

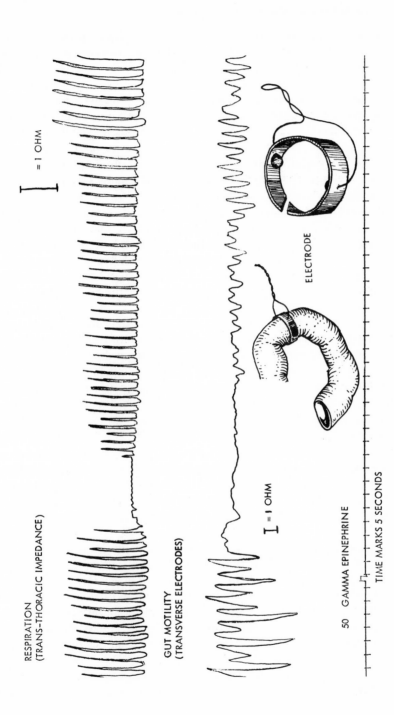

RESPIRATION
(TRANS-THORACIC IMPEDANCE)

$\mathbf{I}$ = 1 OHM

GUT MOTILITY
(TRANSVERSE ELECTRODES)

$\mathbf{I}$ = 1 OHM

ELECTRODE

50 GAMMA EPINEPHRINE

TIME MARKS 5 SECONDS

Figure 10–21. Gastrointestinal motility detected by impedance change.

193

decreased the resistive component of the impedance by 1 to 2%. On the other hand, sleep, and anesthesia produced by pentobarbital, increased the impedance by as much as 6%. In addition to these baseline shifts, rhythmic oscillations in impedance occurred in a frequency range extending from 0 to 20 cps. More recently Kado and Adey (1965) reported dissection of the impedance changes into resistive and reactive components. While recording impedance in the amygdala, hippocampus, and midbrain reticular formation in the cat, they observed that brief alerting stimuli decreased the resistance and increased the capacitance measured between electrodes in these regions. These interesting impedance changes await correlation with other parameters of nervous activity.

The impedance changes accompanying anoxia of the brain and spinal cord of cats have been demonstrated by Van Harreveld and Biersteker (1963). By clamping blood vessels and causing cats to breathe nitrogen, they produced tissue anoxia that in both cases resulted in an increase of impedance amounting to 16 to 25%. Such changes were completely reproducible and reversible. Their significance at the cellular level awaits explanation.

An early study by Grant (1923) appeared to indicate some promise of applying the impedance method for locating brain tumors. Using a thin, bipolar probe electrode connected to an impedance bridge, he found that, as the probe was advanced into the brain, the impedance was constant until the tumor was encountered. When glioma tissue surrounded the electrodes, the impedance decreased by one half to one third.

10–14.   EYE MOVEMENTS

The position of the eye and the characteristic movements it executes are often factors of interest. A record of these events is called an electro-oculogram (EOG). Two methods have been employed to measure eye position. In one technique pairs of electrodes placed either above and below or at the inner and outer canthis of one eye detect a position-dependent component of the corneo-retinal potential (Kris, 1960). The other method requires that the eye be placed in a strong magnetic field and uses the voltage induced in coils embedded in a contact lens or affixed to the sclera as the position-indicating signal. With the first technique Robinson (1963) detected signals corresponding to vertical, lateral, and rolling movements of the eye. Fuchs and Robinson (1966) mounted a three-turn search coil to the sclera of a monkey eye and detected signals proportional to vertical and horizontal components of eye movement.

Each of the methods has its advantages and difficulties. The method described by Kris provides a small signal which is often accompanied by muscle action potentials and galvanic electrode potentials. Furthermore, Byford (1962) has reported that for horizontal eye movement there is a lack of agreement between this voltage signal and one measured by optical tracking of the eye. The more difficult method of using search coils offers high precision but requires exacting techniques for fabrication of the coils and complex equipment.

Sullivan and Weltman (1963) have shown that eye movements can be recorded by using the impedance method. Geddes (1965) has verified their observations on man and the horse. Because a signal free from electrode potentials and muscle artifacts can be obtained with open or closed eyes, the technique has some attractive features. To illustrate the type of signal obtained, a pair of electrodes was placed above and below one eye of a human subject. The electrodes were connected to a direct-coupled impedance recorder and to a high-gain preamplifier to permit recording the electro-oculogram along with the impedance oculogram. Figure 10–22 illustrates the record obtained. The upper trace shows the impedance oculogram (ZOG): the lower, the EOG. The subject was instructed to gaze from one object to another, both in a vertical plane. In the center of the record he was told to clench his jaw. The EOG record illustrates the muscle action potentials which are absent from the impedance tracing.

Figure 10–23 is an impedance oculogram made on a horse during the induction of anesthesia. In this species there are conspicuous oscillatory

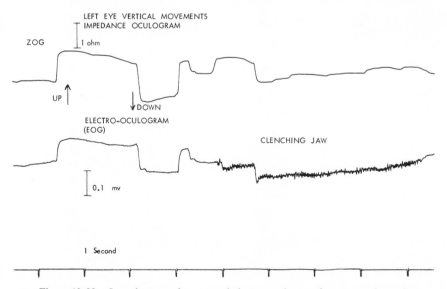

Figure 10–22. Impedance oculogram and electro-oculogram from same electrodes.

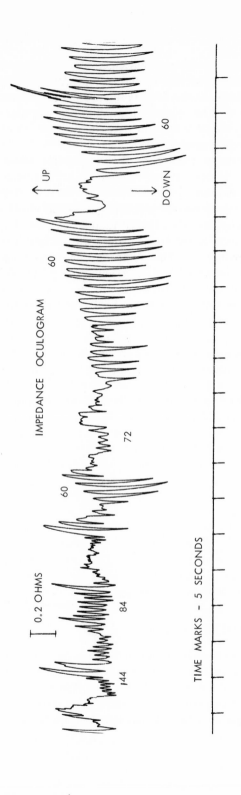

Figure 10-23. Impedance oculogram in the horse. [From Geddes, Southwestern Vet. **19**:23–25 (1965). By Permission.]

eye movements under anesthesia. The figures on the record indicate the frequency of the eye movements in oscillations per minute. Although the phenomenon is somewhat dependent on the type of anesthesia employed, many veterinarians use the eyeball movements as indicative of the depth of anesthesia. A record of them can serve as a means of identifying the depth of anesthesia while graphic recordings of other events are being made.

Sullivan and Weltman (1963) described a nearly linear relationship between impedance change and eye position in the vertical plane. The authors have verified these observations. When the impedance method is employed to detect horizontal eye movements, the size of the signal and the linearity appear to be less. No studies have as yet been conducted to determine the optimum location of two pairs of electrodes for obtaining purely orthogonal signals, nor have any investigations been carried out to identify the origin of the impedance change. Presumably impedance changes are due to changes in current distribution resulting from movement of the eyeball, which contains materials of a different resistivity from that of the surrounding tissue.

10–15.   HEART SOUNDS

The manner in which impedance has been employed to detect heart sounds was described in Chapter 5. Briefly two techniques have been used. In one, the impedance changes between an intracardiac and an external electrode were recorded. In the other, the capacitance changes due to vibration of the chest wall were recorded continuously. Both methods are capable of detecting the full spectrum of vibrations caused by cardiac action.

10–16.   SALIVATION

That an increase in the impedance of the canine submaxillary salivary gland accompanied secretion was noted by Bronk and Gesell (1926). Nervous stimulation and drug-induced salivation produced an impedance change of slightly more than 10% just before the appearance of saliva.

10–17.   BLOOD CLOTTING

Impedance changes have been shown to accompany the clotting of blood. Rosenthal and Tobias (1948) measured such changes at 1 kc in a thermostatically controlled chamber in which a blood sample was placed. They noted an increase in resistivity after 5 minutes as the blood clot was forming. Blood samples treated with anticoagulants exhibited no such changes within a 1-hour period. They called attention to the fact that with this technique the changes in clotting time which occur with motion of the blood were absent. Henstell (1949) continued these studies, using 60 cps, with particular interest in the configuration of the electrodes. He found a circular loop with a horizontal crossbar to be the optimum shape. Using these electrodes he plotted impedance versus time curves over a 48-hour period. He reported that with his electrode the normal clot resistance for adult white males is 311 ± 44.4 ohms and for adult white females 179 ± 33.5 ohms. The resistance clotting time was found to be 10.3 ± 1.0 minutes for normal males and 9.5 ± 0.94 minutes for normal females. He also noted changes in the impedance-clotting relationship in diseases of the blood.

A different approach to determine clotting time was taken by Richardson and Bishop (1957). In their instrument the blood was contained in a tube fitted with two rod electrodes, and the assembly was placed on a platform which oscillated ± 45 degrees from the horizontal, six times per minute. A record of the 60-cycle impedance change showed a sharp transition at the time that the clot was formed.

Mungall et al. (1961) continued studies of the impedance changes in clotting blood. Using 100 kc and a thermostatically controlled conductivity cell, they recorded resistive and reactive changes in blood over a 100-minute period. Their records, made on normal subjects and patients with blood disorders, revealed several transitional points which await clarification.

10–18. THE VOLUME OF CELLS IN A BLOOD SAMPLE

Over a century ago, Maxwell made theoretical studies on the conductivity of a solution containing insulating spheres. Since that time studies have been carried out with a view to applying this theory to the practical determination of the volume of cells in a blood sample by applying a form factor correction to Maxwell's equation. In this connection the analytical studies of Fricke (1924) must be cited.

Because the red cells are usually more numerous than other types, the total cell volume is often used to determine the hematocrit, which by definition is the percentage of red cells. The electrical methods to be described recognize the total volume of cells, regardless of type, but in many cases it is permissible to designate the cell percentage determined in this way as the hematocrit.

Rosenthal and Tobias (1948) chose an appropriate form factor and employed a variation of Maxwell's formula to calculate the cell volume fraction from measurements of the plasma and blood resistivities. They checked their data with centrifuged samples and stated, "A comparison of the results obtained by the two methods revealed that the resistance determinations were 7.7% lower than the centrifuge values in normal subjects and 7.8% lower in patients with polycythemia vera." A similar study by Okada and Schwan (1960) supports this early work. The latter investigators constructed an instrument in which the hematocrit was determined in a blood sample of 0.02 cc. The frequency employed was 10 kc, and their calibration curve of conductivity and erythrocyte volume was linear up to 15×10^6 cells/mm^3. Okada and Schwan called attention to two important considerations in using this method. They demonstrated that the specific resistance of plasma is relatively constant but that appreciable variations in the size of the red cells can occur in certain pathological conditions.

10–19. CONCLUSION

The flexibility of the impedance method to detect a wide variety of physiological events is its chief attribute. Its chief drawback is the difficulty encountered in calibrating the impedance in true physiological terms. At present many studies are underway which aim to establish the relationship between impedance values and physiological events. In many, the signals are being dissected into their resistive and reactive components with a view to establishing which component contains the more meaningful information. It is as yet too soon to draw conclusions regarding the true value of the impedance method for the measurement of physiological events.

In conclusion, a word of caution is addressed to those who will investigate the use of impedance or impedance changes as a means of transduction. In every study adequate care must be exercised to guarantee that the change in impedance measured between the electrodes is due to the physiological event investigated and is not an artifact caused by changes in impedance at the electrode-electrolyte-tissue interface.

REFERENCES

Adey, W. R., R. T. Kado, and J. Didio. 1962. Impedance measurements in brain tissue using microvolt signals. *Exp. Neurol.* **5**:47–60.

Allison, R. D. 1962. Volumetric dynamics of respiration as measured by electrical impedance. Ph. D. Thesis, Wayne University, Detroit, Michigan.

Allison, R. D. 1966. Arterial-venous volume gradients as predictive indices of vascular dynamics. *Instrumentation Methods for Predictive Medicine.* T. B. Weber, and J. Poyer, (eds.). Instr. Soc. America, 215 pp.

Allison, R. D., E. L. Holmes, and J. Nyboer. 1964. Volumetric dynamics of respiration as measured by electrical impedance plethysmography. *J. Appl. Physiol.* **19**:166–173.

Allison, R. D., and J. Nyboer. 1965. The electrical plethysmography determination of pulse volume and flow in ionic circulatory systems. *New Istanbul. Contr. Clin. Sci.* **7**:281–306.

d'Arsonval, A. 1893a. Action physiologique des courants alternatifs a grande fréquence. *Arch. Physiol. Norm. Path.* **5**:401–408 and 789–790.

d'Arsonval, A. 1893b. Influence de la fréquences sur les effects physiologique des courants alternatifs. *Comptes Rendus.* **116**:630–633.

Atzler, E. 1933. Neues Verfahren zur Funktionsbeurteilung des Herzens. *Deut. Med. Wochschr.* **59**:1347–1349.

Atzler, E. 1935. Dielektrographie. *Handbuch der Biolog. Arbeitsmethoden* **5**:1073–1084.

Atzler, E., G. Lehmann. 1932. Über ein neues Verfahren zur Darstellung der Herztätigkeit. (Dielektrographie) *Arbeitsphysiologie* **5**:636–680.

Ax, A. F., R., Andreski, R. Courter, C. DiGiovanni, S. Herman, D. Lucas, and W. Orrick 1964. Measurement of respiration by telemeter impedance strain gauge and spirometer *Proc. ISA Second National Biomed. Sci. Instr. Symp.* pp. 1–12.

Bagno, S. 1959. Impedance measurements of living tissue. *Electronics* **32**:62–63.

Baker, L. E. 1962. Impedance spirometry. SWIRECO Conference, Houston, Texas, April.

Baker, L. E., and L. A. Geddes, 1965. Quantitative evaluation of impedance spirometry in man. *Am. J. Med. Elect.* **4**:73–77.

Baker, L. E., and L. A. Geddes. 1966. Transthoracic current paths in impedance spirometry. *Proc. Symp. Biomed. Eng.*, Marquette University, Milwaukee, Wisconsin, **1**:181–186.

Baker, L. E., L. A. Geddes, and H. E. Hoff. 1966. A comparison of linear and non-linear characterizations of impedance spirometry. *Med. Biol. Eng.* **4**:371–379.

Baker, L. E., L. A. Geddes, H. E. Hoff, and C. J. Chaput. 1966. Physiological factors underlying transthoracic impedance variations in respiration *J. Appl. Physiol.* **21**: 1491–1499.

Barnett, A. 1937. The basic factors involved in proposed electrical methods for measuring thyroid function (parts I-IV). *Western J. Surg. Obstet, Gynecol* **45**:322–326, 380–387, 540–554, and 612–623.

Barnett, A. 1938. The phase angle of the normal human skin. *J. Physiol.* **93**:349–366.

Barnett, A. 1940. Seasonal variations in the epidermal impedance of human skin. *Am. J. Physiol.* **129**:306–307.

Bishop, S., and J. Nyboer. 1962. Electrical impedance plethysmography of canine and human eyes. *Harper Hosp. Bull.* **20**:142–151.

Bonjer, F. H., J. van der Berg, and M. N. J. Dirken. 1952. The origin of the variations of body impedance occurring during the cardiac cycle. *Circulation* **1**:415–420.

Bouty, E. 1884. Sur la conductibilité électrique de dissolutions salines très étendues. *J. Physique.* **2**:325–355.

Brazier, M. A. B. 1960. *The Electrical Activity of the Nervous System.* New York, The Macmillan Co., 273 pp.

Brazier, M. A. B. 1935. The impedance angle test for thyrotoxicosis. *Western J. Surg. Obstet. Gynecol.* **43**:429–441 and 514–527.

Bronk, D. W., and R. Gesell. 1926. Electrical conductivity, electrical potential, and hydrogen ion concentration measurements on the submaxillary gland of the dog recorded with continuous photographic methods. *Am. J. Physiol.* **77**:570–589.

Brook, D. L., and P. Cooper. 1957. The impedance plethysmograph—its clinical application. *Surgery* **42**:1061–1070.

Brooks, C. McC., B. F. Hoffman, E. E. Suckling, and O. Orias. 1955. *Excitability of the Heart. New York*, Grune and Stratton. 373 pp.

Burns, R. C. 1950. Study of skin impedance. *Electronics* **23**:190–196.

Byford, G. H. 1962a. Non-linear relations between the corneo-retinal potential and horizontal eye movements. *J. Physiol.* **168**:14P–15P.

Byford, G. H. 1962b. A sensitive contact lens photoelectric eye movement recorder. *IRE Trans. Bio-Med. Electron.* **4**:236–243.

Chinard, F. P., T. Enns, and M. F. Nolan. 1962. Indicator-dilution studies with "diffusible" indicators. *Circulation Res.* **10**:473–490.

Cole, K. S., and H. J. Curtis. 1939. Electric impedance of the squid giant axon during activity. *J. Gen. Physiol.* **22**:649–670.

Coulter, N. and J. R. Pappenheimer. 1949. Development of turbulence in flowing blood. *Am. J. Physiol.* **159**:401–408.

Crile, G. W., H. R. Hosmer, and A. F. Rowland. 1922. The electrical conductivity of animal tissues under normal and pathological conditions. *Am. J. Physiol.* **60**:59–106.

Dalziel, C. F. 1956. Effects of electric shock on man. *IRE Trans. Med. Electron.* **PGME–5**: 44–62.

Dubuisson, M. 1933. Recherches sur les modifications que surviennent dans la conducibilité électrique du muscle au cours de la contraction. *Arch. Int. Physiol.* **37**:35–57.

Farzaneh, T. 1953. Endocrine factors influencing impedance and impedance angle. Ph. D Thesis, Ohio State University, 124 pp.

Fenning, C. 1936–1937. A new method for recording physiological activities, I. *J. Lab. Clin. Med.* **22**:1279–1280.

Fenning, C., and B. E. Bonnar. 1936–1937. A new method for recording physiological activities, II. *J. Lab. Clin. Med.* **22**:1280–1284.

Fenning, C., and B. E. Bonnar. 1939. Additional recordings with the oscillato-capacitograph. *J. Lab. Clin. Med.* **25**:175–179.

Forbes, T. W. 1936. Skin potential and impedance response. *Am. J. Physiol.* **117**:189–199.

Forbes, T. W., and C. Landis. 1935. The limiting AC frequency for the exhibition of the galvanic skin (psychogalvanic) response. *J. Gen. Psychol.* **13**:188–193.

Fricke, H. 1924 A mathematical treatment of the electrical conductivity of colloids and cell suspensions. *J. Gen Physiol.* **6**:375–384.

Fuchs, A. F., and D. A. Robinson. 1966. A method for measuring horizontal and vertical eye movement chronically in the monkey. *J. Appl. Physiol.* **21**:1068–1070.

Geddes, L. A., H. E. Hoff, D. M. Hickman, M. Hinds, and L. E. Baker. 1962. Recording respiration and the EKG with common electrodes. *Aerospace Med.* **33**:791–793.

Geddes, L. A., and L. E. Baker. 1967. The specific resistance of biological material—A compendium of data for the biomedical engineer and physiologist. *Med. Biol. Eng.* **5**: 271–293.

Geddes, L. A., and H. E. Hoff. 1962. Hales, Marey, and Chauveau. Annual Report, NIH Grant HTS 5125—*Classical Physiology with Modern Instrumentation*—The Heart Institute, National Institutes of Health, 53 pp.

Geddes, L. A., and H. E. Hoff. 1963. The measurement of physiological events by impedance change. *Proc. San Diego Symp, Bio-Med. Eng.* **3**:115–122. La Jolla, Calif. See also *Am. J. Med. Electron.* 1964, **3**:16–27.

Geddes, L. A., and H. E. Hoff. 1965. Continuous measurement of stroke volume of the left and right ventricles by impedance. Sixth Int. Conf. on Med. Elect. and Biol. Eng. Tokyo, 1965. *Japan. Heart J.* **7**:556–565.

Geddes, L. A., H. E. Hoff, C. W. Hall, and H. D. Millar. 1964. Rheoencephalography. *Cardiovascular Res. Center Bull.* **2**:112–121.

Geddes, L. A., H. E. Hoff, D. M. Hickman, and A. G. Moore. 1962. The impedance pneumograph. *Aerospace Med.* **33**:28–33.

Geddes, L. A., H. E. Hoff, A. Mello, and C. Palmer. 1966. Continuous measurement of ventricular stroke volume by electrical impedance. *Cardiovascular Res. Center Bull.* **4**: 118–130.

Geddes, L. A., H. E. Hoff, A. Moore, and M. Hinds. 1966. An electrical caliper myograph. *Am. J. Pharm. Ed.* **30**:209–211.

Geddes, L. A., J. D. McCrady, and H. E. Hoff. 1965. The impedance nystagmogram—a record of the level of anesthesia in the horse. *Southwestern Vet.* **19**:23–25.

Goldensohn, E. S., and L. Zablow. 1959. An electrical impedance spirometer. *J. Appl. Physiol.* **14**:463–464.

Goodwin, R. S., and L. A. Saperstein. 1957. Measurement of the cardiac output in dogs by a conductivity method after a single intravenous injection of autogenous plasma. *Circ. Res.* **5**:531–538.

Grant, F. C. 1923. Localization of brain tumors. *J. Am. Med. Assoc.* **8**:2168–2169.

Gross, R. E., and R. Mittermaier. 1962. Untersuchungen über das Minutenvolumen des Herzen. *Arch. ges. Physiol.* **212**:136–149.

Hamilton, L. H., J. D. Beard, and R. C. Kory. 1965. Impedance measurement of tidal volume and ventilation. *J. Appl. Physiol.* **20**:565–568.

Hanish, H. 1962. Telemetry of respiration and the electrocardiogram from the same pair of electrodes. 15th Annual Conf. Eng. Med. Biol., Chicago. Carl Gorr Ptg. Co., 66 pp.

Henstell H. H. 1949. Electrolytic resistance of the blood clot. *Am. J. Physiol.* **158**:367–387.

Holt, J. P. 1956. Estimation of the residual volume of the ventricle of the dog's heart by two indicator dilution techniques. *Cir. Res.* **4**:187–195.

Holt, J. P. 1962. Left ventricular function in mammals of greatly different size. *Circ. Res.* **10**:798–806.

Holt, J. P. and J. Allensworth. 1957. Estimation of the residual volume of the right ventricle of the dog's heart. *Circ. Res.* **5**:323–326.

Holzer, W., K. Polzer, and A. Marko. 1945. *RKG, Rheokardiographie*. Wein, Verlag Wilhelm Maudrich, 46 pp.

Horton, J. W., and A. C. Van Ravenswaay. 1935. Electrical impedance of the human body. *J. Franklin Inst.* **20**:557–572.

Irisawa, H., M. F. Wilson, and R. F. Rushmer. 1960. Left ventricle as a mixing chamber. *Circ. Res.* **8**:183–187.

Jenkner, F. L. 1959. Rheoencephalography. *Confinia Neurol.* **19**:1–20.

Jenkner, F. L. 1962. *Rheoencephalography*. Springfield, Ill, Charles. C. Thomas, 81 pp.

Kado, R., W. R. Adey. 1965. Method for the measurement of impedance changes in brain tissue. *Digest 6th Int. Cong. Med. Electron Biol. Eng.*, Tokyo, Okamura Publ. Co., 638 pp.

Kado, R., W. R. Adey, and D. O. Walter. 1966. Regional specificity of impedance characteristics of cortical and subcortical structures evaluated in hyperapnea and hypothermia. Abstracts of Papers, XXIII Int. Cong. of Physiological Sci. Tokyo, 549 pp.

Kennelly, A. E., and E. F. W. Alexanderson. 1910. The physiological tolerance of alternating-current strengths up to frequencies of 100 kilocycles per second. *Electron World* **50**: 154–156.

Kinnen, E. 1965. Estimation of pulmonary blood flow with an electrical impedance plethysmograph. School of Aerospace Medicine, Tech. Rep. SAM TR-65–81.

Kinnen, E., and Kubicek, W. 1963. Thoracic cage impedance measurements. Impedance product system. School of Aerospace Medicine, Tech. Rep. Sam TDR-63–69.

Kinnen, E., W. Kubicek, and R. Patterson, 1964. Thoracic cage measurements. Impedance plethysmographic determination of cardiac output. School of Aerospace Medicine, Tech. Rep. TDR-64–15.

Kinnen, E., W. Kubicek, and D. Witsoe. 1964. Thoracic cage impedance measurements. Impedance plethysmographic determination of cardiac output. School of Aerospace

Medicine, Tech. Rep. TDR-64–23.

Kornmesser, J. G., and J. Nyboer. 1962. Electrical and dynamic changes in uterine activity during labor. *Harper Hosp. Bull.* **20**:248–261.

Kris, C. 1960. *Vision: Electro-oculography in Medical Physics.* Vol. 3. Chicago, Year Book Publishers, Inc., 754 pp.

Kubicek, W. G., J. N. Karnegis, R. P. Patterson, D. A. Witsoe, and R. H. Mattson. 1966. Development and evaluation of an impedance cardiac output system. *Aerospace Med.* **37**:1208–1212.

Kubicek W., E. Kinnen, and A. Edin. 1963. Thoracic cage impedance measurements. School of Aerospace Medicine, Tech. Rep. TDR-63–41.

Kubicek, W. G., E. Kinnen, and A. Edin. 1964. Calibration of an impedance pneumograph. *J. Appl. Physiol.* **19**:557–560.

Leverett, S. 1962. Personal communication. School of Aerospace Medicine, Brooks Air Force Base, Texas.

Liebman, R. M., and F. Cosenza. 1962–1963. Study of blood flow in the dental pulp by an electrical impedance technique. *Phys. Biol. Med.* **7**:167–176.

Lifshitz, K. 1963a. Rheoencephalography: I. Review of the technique. *J. Nervous Mental Disease* **136**:288.

Lifshitz, K. 1963b. Rheoencephalography: II. Survey of clinical applications. *J. Nervous Mental Disease* **137**:285.

Lofgren, B. 1951. The electrical impedance of a complex tissue and its relation to changes in volume and fluid distribution. *Acta Physiol. Scand. Suppl. 81*, **23**:1–51.

McCally, M., G. W. Barnard, K. E. Robins, and A. Marko. 1963. Observations with an electrical impedance respirometer. *Am. J. Med. Electron.* **2**:322–327.

McHenry, L. C. 1965. Rheoencephalography. *Neurology* **15**:507–517.

McLendon, J. F., and A. Hemingway. 1930. The psychogalvanic reflex as related to the polarization-capacity of the skin. *Am. J. Physiol.* **94**:77–83.

Mann, H. 1937. Study of the peripheral circulation by means of an alternating current bridge. *Proc. Soc. Exp. Biol. Med.* **36**:670–673.

Mann, H. 1953. The capacigraph. *Trans. Amer. Coll. Cardiol,* **3**:162–175.

Markovich, S. E., and R. Naman. 1965. Theory and facts concerning rheoencephalography. *Trans. 4th Conf. Cerebrovascular Diseases,* 1964. New York, Grune and Stratton, pp. 68–86.

Mello-Sobrinho, A. 1963. Impedance plethysmography of the canine ventricles. M. S. Thesis, Baylor University College of Medicine. Houston, Texas, 85 pp.

Molnar, G. W., J. Nyboer, R. L. Levine. 1953. The effects of temperature and flow on the specific resistance of human venous blood. U.S. Army Med. Res. Lab., Fort Knox. Kentucky. Rep. 127.

Montagu, J. D. 1958. The psychogalvanic reflex. *J. Neurol. Neurosurg. Psychiat.* **21**:119–128.

Mungall, A. G., D. Morris, and W. S. Martin. 1961. Measurement of the dielectric properties of blood. *IRE Trans. Bio-Med. Electron.* **BME-8**:109–111.

Nichols, R. C., and T. Daroge. 1955. An electric circuit for the measurement of the galvanic skin response. *Am. J. Psychol.* **68**:455–461.

Nyboer, J. 1944. Electrical impedance plethysmography, in O. Glasser. *Medical Physics,* Vol. 1. Chicago, Year Book Publishers, 744 pp.

Nyboer, J. 1950. Electrical impedance plethysmography. *Circulation* **2**:811–87.

Nyboer, J. 1959. *Electrical Impedance Plethysmography.* Springfield, Ill., Charles C. Thomas, 243 pp.

Nyboer, J. S. Bagno, A. Barnett, and R. H. Halsey. 1940. Radiocardiograms. *J. Clin. Invest.* **19**:773.

Nyboer, J., S. Bagno, and L. F. Nims. 1943. The impedance plethysmograph, an electrical volume recorder. *Off. Sci. Res. and Dev.* Comm. on Aviation Med. Report 149, 12 pp.

Okada, R. H., and H. P. Schwan. 1960. An electrical method to determine hematocrits. *IRE Trans. Med. Electron.* **ME-7**:188–192.

Pacella, A. F. 1966. Impedance pneumography—a survey of instrumentation techniques. *Med. Biol. Eng.* **4**:1–15.

Pallett, J. E., and J. W. Scopes. 1965. Recording respirations in newborn babies by measuring impedance of the chest. *Med. Biol. Eng.* **3**:161–168.

Patterson, R., W. G. Kubicek, E. Kinnen, G. Noren, and D. Witsoe. 1964. Development of an electrical impedance plethysmograph system to monitor cardiac output. *Proc. 1st Ann. Rocky Mt. Conf. Biomed. Eng.*, Colorado Springs, Colo. pp. 56–71.

Petrovick, M. S., and J. Brumlik. 1961–1962. Clinical measurements of biological vibrations in normal and disease states. Symposium on Recent Developments in Research Methods and Instrumentation, National Institutes of Health, October 9–12, 1961. *15th Ann. Conf. Eng. Med. Biol.* Chicago, Carl Gorr Ptg. Co., 66 pp.

Plutchik, R., and H. R. Hirsch 1963. Skin impedance and phase angle as a function of frequency and current. *Science* **141**:927–928.

Polzer, K., and F. Schuhfried. 1950. Rheographische Untersuchungen am Schädel. *Z. Nervenheilkunde.* **3**:295–298.

Polzer, K., F. Schuhfried, and H. Heeger. 1960. Rheography. *Brit. Heart J.* **22**:140–148.

Polzer, K., and F. Schuhfried, 1961. Application of rheography in vascular disease. *Spec. Issue, J. Oester. Krank-Zeitung.* **8–9**:5.

Poppendiek, H. E., G. L. Hody, N. D. Greene, J. L. Glass, and J. E. Hayes 1964. In vivo study of the effects of alternating currents on some properties of blood in dogs. *Phys. Med. Biol.* **9**:215–217.

Powers, S. R., C. Schaffer, A. Boba, and Y. Nakamura. 1958. Physical and biologic factors in impedance plethysmography. *Surgery* **44**:53–61.

Rappaport, D., and G. B. Ray. 1927. Changes of electrical conductivity in the beating tortoise ventricle. *Am. J. Physiol.* **80**:126–139.

Richardson, A. W., and J. C. Bishop. 1957. A new accurate and reliable method to record blood coagulation times using an AC bridge principle. *J. Am. Pharm. Assoc.* **46**:553–555.

Robbins, K. C., and A. Marko. 1962. An improved method of measuring respiration rate. *15th Ann. Conf. Eng. Med. Biol.* Chicago, Carl Gorr Ptg. Co., 66 pp.

Robinson, D. A. 1963. A method of measuring eye movements using a scleral search coil in a magnetic field. *IEEE Trans. Biomed. Eng.* **BME-10**:137–145.

Romm, S. O. 1924. Zur Bestimmungsmethode der Umlaufzeit des Blutes im Kreislauf. *Arch. ges. Physiol.* **202**:14–24.

Rosenbleuth, A., and E. G. del Pozo. 1943. The changes of impedance of the turtle ventricular muscle during contraction. *Am. J. Physiol.* **139**:514–519.

Rosenthal, R. L., and C. W. Tobias. 1948. Measurement of the electric resistance of human blood use in coagulation studies and cell volume determination. *J. Lab. Clin. Med.* **33**:1110–1122.

Rushmer, R. F., T. K. Crystal, C. Wagner, and R; Ellis. 1953. Intracardiac plethysmography. *Am. J. Physiol.* **174**:171–174.

Schaefer, H., E. Bleicher, and F. Eckervogt. 1949. Weitere Beitrage zur elektrischen Reizung und zur Registrierung von elektrischen Vorgangen und der Atmung. *Arch. ges. Physiol.* **251**:491–503.

Schwan, H. P. 1955. Electrical properties of body tissues and impedance plethysmography. *IRE Trans. Bio-Med. Electron.* **PGME-3**:32–46.

Schwan, H. P. 1963. Determination of biological impedances, in *Physical Techniques in Biological Research*, Vol. 6, Part B. New York and London, Academic Press, 425 pp.

Schwan, H. P., and C. F. Kay, 1957. Capacitative properties of body tissues. *Circ. Res.* 5: 439–443.

Schwan, H. P., and K. Li. 1953. Capacitance and conductivity of body tissues at ultra high frequencies. *Proc. IRE* 41:1735–1740.

Sigman, E., A. Kolin, L. N. Katz, and K. Jochim. 1937. Effect of motion on the electrical conductivity of the blood. *Am. J. Physiol.* 118:708–719.

Simonson, E., and K. Nakagawa. 1960. Effect of age on pulse wave velocity and ejection time in healthy men and in men with coronary heart disease. *Circulation* 22:126–129.

Smith, McK., L. A. Geddes, and H. E. Hoff 1967. Cardiac output determined by the saline conductivity method using an extra-arterial conductivity cell. *Cardiovascular Res. Center Bull.* 5:123–134.

Stewart, G. N. 1897-1898. Researches on the circulation time and on the influences which affect it. *J. Physiol.* 22:158–183.

Stewart, G. N. 1921. The output of the heart in dogs. *Am. J. Physiol.* 57:27–50.

Sugano, H., and M. Oda. 1960. A new method for blood flow measurement. *Japan. J. Pharmacol.* 10:30–37.

Sullivan, G., and G. Weltman. 1963. The impedance oculogram—a new technique. *J. Appl. Physiol.* 18:215–216.

Tasaki, I. 1952–1953. Properties of myelinated fibers in frog sciatic nerve in spinal cord as examined with microelectrodes. *Japan. J. Physiol.* 3:73–94.

Taylor, D. H. 1962. The measurement of galvanic skin response. *Electron. Eng.* 34:312–315.

Tomberg, V. T. 1963. The high frequency spirometer. *Proc. Int. Cong. Med. Electron* Liege. Belgium.

Tomberg, V. T. 1964. Device and a new method of measuring pulmonary respiration. *17th Ann. Conf. Biol. Med.* Washington, D.C., McGregor and Werner, 129 pp.

Underwood, R. J., and D. Gowing. 1965. An electronic method of detecting blood volume changes. *Anesthesiology* 26:199–203.

Van der Berg, J., and A. J. Alberts. 1954. Limitation of electrical impedance plethysmography. *Circ. Res.* 2:333–339.

Van Harreveld, A., and P. A. Biersteker. 1963. Acute asphyxiation of the spinal cord and other sections of the nervous system. *Am. J. Physiol.* 206:8–14.

Velick, S., and M. Gorin. 1940. The electrical conductance of suspensions of ellipsoids and its relation to the study of avian erythrocytes. *J. Gen. Physiol.* 23:753–771.

White, H. L. 1947. Measurement of cardiac output by a continuously recording conductivity method. *Am. J. Physiol.* 151:45–57.

Whitehorn, W. V., and E. R. Pearl. 1949. The use of change in capacity to record cardiac volume in human subjects. *Science* 109:262–263.

Wiederhelm, C. A., and R. F. Rushmer. 1964. Pre and post-arteriolar resistance changes in the blood vessels of the frog's mesentery. *Bibliotheca Anat.* 4:234–243.

Wiggers, H. C. 1944. Cardiac output and total peripheral resistance measurements in experimental dogs. *Am. J. Physiol.* 140:519–534.

Yokota, T., and B. Fujimori. 1962. Impedance change of the skin during the galvanic skin reflex. *Japan. J. Physiol.* 12:210–224.

Zajic, F., Z. Fejfar, L. Franc, and J. Brod. 1954. Impedance plethysmography. *Physiol. Bohemoslov.* 3:355–361.

11

Recording Electrodes

11–1. INTRODUCTION

In presenting a bioelectric event to an amplifier, a pair of electrodes plays the role of a transducer. As such the electrodes must transfer the bioelectric event to the amplifier input circuit, which had been designed to accommodate the characteristics of the electrodes. The event, its anatomical location, and the dimensions of the bioelectric generator dictate the type of electrodes to be used, and the electrical characteristics of the electrodes specify the type of amplifier input circuit required. When large-area electrodes are employed, the restrictions on input impedance are not too severe and most vacuum tube and high-input impedance transistor amplifiers suffice. However, when small electrodes and, in particular, when microelectrodes with their inherently high impedance are employed, special low-capacitance, high-resistance input circuits are needed to transfer the bioelectric event to the amplifying system. Distortionless insertion of the event into the recording apparatus requires, therefore, special consideration of the electrical characteristics of the electrodes and the input impedance of the amplifier. These subjects will be discussed in this chapter.

11–2. ELECTRODE POTENTIAL

Although a truly remarkable variety of electrodes has been used to detect bioelectric events, there exists a fundamental component which is common to all. This component is a metal-electrolyte interface: the metal is the material of the electrode; the electrolyte may be an electrolytic solution or paste, such as is used with surface electrodes, or it may be the tissue fluids which come into contact with an electrode inserted below the integument. When a metal electrode comes into contact with an electrolyte, there is a tendency for the electrode to discharge ions into solution and for ions in the electrolyte to combine with the electrode. The net result is the creation of a charge gradient, the spatial arrangement of which is called the electrical double layer. Although it is known to be complex in organization and occupies a region immediately adjacent to the electrode, in its simplest form the double layer has been pictured as two parallel sheets of charge of opposite sign. Parsons (1964) has described electrodes in terms of the reactions at the double layer. Electrodes in which no net transfer of charge occurs across the metal-electrolyte interface are designated by him as perfectly polarized. Those in which unhindered exchange of charge is possible are called perfectly nonpolarizable. Real electrodes have properties that lie between these idealized limits.

In practical electrodes the electrode-electrolyte interface resembles a voltage source and a capacitance in parallel with a resistance. The exact values of these components are not constant and are nonlinearly dependent on many factors, which include the kind of metal, the type and concentration of the electrolyte, the temperature, the frequency, and the current density. The nature of the double layer and the voltages associated with it are discussed in Chapter 9. The equivalent capacitances are remarkably large for most metals; a typical example is mercury, which exhibits a capacitance of 10 to $70 \mu f/cm^2$ when in contact with saline (Grahame, 1941, 1952).

The voltage developed at an electrode-electrolyte interface is designated as the half-cell potential. The total voltage between a pair of electrodes is therefore the difference in the two half-cell potentials. Because it is impossible to measure the potential developed at a single electrode, an arbitrary standard electrode has been chosen and electrode potentials are measured with respect to it. The standard electrode is the hydrogen electrode; it consists of a specially prepared platinum surface in contact with a solution of hydrogen ions (of unit activity) and dissolved molecular hydrogen; the activity of the latter is specified by requiring it to be in equilibrium with hydrogen at 1 atmosphere of pressure in the gas phase (Janz and Kelly, 1964).

The potentials of many of the metals used for electrodes are shown in Table 9–1. Inspection of this table indicates that an appreciable voltage can be produced when dissimilar metals are employed. When such electrodes are connected together through the input impedance of the measuring device, a current will flow. The consequences of this situation are discussed later. The table also indicates that a galvanic cell of zero potential will be created if the metals are identical. In practice, even if the same material is used for both electrodes, some potential difference can be measured between the pair. In many instances the presence of a potential would not be objectionable if it were stable. In practice it is not, and its variations constitute a source of artifact.

Many investigators have carried out studies of the stability of electrode potentials. Forbes (1934) studied the potential difference between amalgamated lead-mercury electrodes in contact with a lead chloride solution which was applied to a chamois in contact with the skin. In ten electrodes, potential differences ranging from 0 to 600 μv were measured. The spontaneous voltage variations ranged between 1.3 and 6.8 μv. A more extensive study was carried out by Greenwald (1936), who measured the potential difference and resistance of pairs of calomel, zinc, and zinc-zinc sulfate electrodes used for recording the electrodermal response. The calomel and zinc electrodes were measured with saline as the electrolyte. The zinc-zinc sulfate electrodes consisted of a zinc plate in contact with a kaolin paste made with zinc sulfate. Between them was a saline solution. The potential difference between the calomel electrodes, before passage of direct current to measure resistance, ranged between 1 to 20 μv and became considerably higher after the d-c resistance had been measured. The zinc plates exhibited a potential difference of 450 μv, which quadrupled after the passage of direct current. The potential difference for the zinc-zinc sulfate electrodes was 180μv, which tripled after the passage of a direct current.

In a similar study Lykken (1959) investigated the potentials developed by many of the electrodes used for the measurement of electrodermal phenomena. He measured the potential difference between pairs of stainless steel, zinc, zinc-mercury, silver, silver-mercury, silver-silver chloride, lead, lead-mercury, and platinum electrodes; in each case the electrolyte was saline. Pairs of zinc and zinc-mercury in contact with zinc sulfate and saline were also measured. During the first hour of measurement the various electrodes exhibited the following voltages: stainless steel, 10 mv; zinc, 100 mv; zinc-mercury, 82 mv; silver, 94 mv; silver-mercury, 90 mv; silver-silver chloride, 2.5 mv; and platinum, 320 mv. For the others listed, the voltage difference was approximately 1 mv. Edelberg and Burch (1962), while conducting GSR studies, reported that stainless steel and aluminum produced high random noise levels. Solder, silver, and copper produced slow wave artifacts. O'Connell et al. (1960) examined the galvanic potentials developed by various electrodes made from silver, lead, and zinc. The highest potential (13 mv) was produced by the zinc-zinc chloride pair and the lowest (0.2 mv) by the silver-silver chloride electrodes affixed to a sponge.

A pair of electrodes made from the same piece of metal, when placed in 0.9% saline and joined through a resistance, will frequently produce a fluctuating "noise" current which can often be eliminated by connecting the electrodes together and allowing them to reach a stable equilibrium with the electrolyte. This technique has been employed by electrophysiologists. A related observation has been that newly prepared electrodes are often noisy when placed in an electrolyte, but with the passage of time the noise decreases. Another method of quieting electrodes is to deposit electrolytically, from a large electrode, a uniform film of material covering both recording electrodes. In this way the minute differences in electrode material are virtually eliminated, and a pair of electrodes having a very small and stable potential difference can be made.

The principle just described is frequently applied when silver electrodes are first made. The authors have demonstrated that a new set of cortical electrodes (Fig. 11–8b, 1-mm silver balls) which were scraped to remove surface contaminants, when placed in 0.9% saline and connected to the recording system, produced an unstable random noise signal of several hundred microvolts. Figure 11–1a illustrates the type of record obtained. The noise was diminished by maintaining all of the electrodes positive by about 3 volts with respect to a 1 × 2 inch silver plate in the saline for 2 minutes and reconnecting them to the recording equipment without changing their position in the saline. This process is known as chloriding. The noise record obtained is shown in Fig. 11–1b.

To further demonstrate the phenomenon, the electrodes were scraped to remove the coating, and they became noisy again (Fig. 11–1c). The electroplating current was reapplied, but this time in reverse (electrodes negative by 3 volts for 3 minutes), and much of the electrode noise disappeared (Fig. 11–1d). Finally, the electrodes were most effectively quieted by the simple procedure of chloriding them after the electrolytic cleaning. The polarity was then reversed (electrodes positive), and with a milliammeter in the circuit the current was turned on and interrupted when it started to fall. After the electrodes were connected to the amplifier, the noise record shown in Fig. 11–1e was obtained. To illustrate that all of the noise cannot be attributed to the electrodes, Fig. 11–1f shows the inherent noise level of the amplifying channel under open-and short-circuit conditions.

An ingenious method of stabilizing chlorided silver electrodes while they are in storage was described by Cooper (1956). The method serves to maintain the electrodes short circuited to each other and at the same time keeps them in a chlorided condition. These two actions are brought about by mounting the electrodes with their silver-silver chloride surfaces immersed in a dish of saline in which is mounted a carbon rod projecting out of the solution. At the tip of the carbon rod, Cooper affixed a stainless steel plate to which all of the electrode terminals were connected. Thus all electrodes were joined together, and because carbon is slightly electronegative with respect to silver-silver chloride, a small chloriding current was maintained. Therefore during storage the electrodes were maintained at the same potential to each other and were continuously chlorided. Cooper

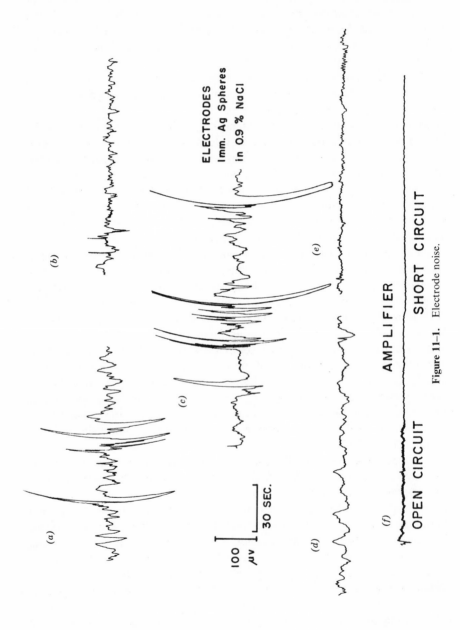

Figure 11-1. Electrode noise.

reported that electrodes treated in this way were adequately stable for use with high-gain d-c amplifiers.

Undeniable evidence throughout all of the literature indicates that silver-silver chloride electrodes appear to be the most stable electrochemically. However, there is a paucity of information on their proper preparation. An excellent review of the properties and method of preparation of such electrodes has been presented by Janz and Taniguchi (1953). This authoritative paper is recommended reading for those who desire to employ silver-silver chloride electrodes.

One of the chief advantages of chloriding a silver electrode is stabilization of the half-cell potential. Initial studies by the authors (1967) have also shown that chloriding reduces the low-frequency electrode-electrolyte impedance.

Another useful piece of information derives from a consideration of the double layer, namely, the effect of its mechanical disturbance. It has been found that electrodes relatively free of movement artifacts are of the floating type, in which the electrode-electrolyte interface is removed from direct contact with the subject. Because the double layer is a region of charge gradient which is a source of potential, disturbance of it gives rise to a change in voltage which, although small electrochemically, is often large with respect to the size of the bioelectric events. Movement artifacts produced by disturbance of the electrical double layer are in the frequency range of many of these events. Hence filtering techniques can seldom be employed with success. Therefore the electrical stability of an electrode is considerably enhanced by stabilization of the electrode-electrolyte interface. This fact has been demonstrated practically when attempts have been made to measure bioelectric events on moving subjects; for example, Forbes et al. (1921) were perhaps the first to record such measurements when they employed a type of floating electrode to obtain electrocardiograms and electromyograms on an elephant. When standing, elephants sway from side to side, making it difficult to obtain artifact-free records with plate electrodes. Forbes employed a zinc electrode in the neck of a funnel filled with zinc sulfate. The opening of the funnel was covered with a permeable membrane soaked in saline. Two rubber-gloved assistants held these electrodes against the inner surfaces of the forelimbs of the animal. The electrocardiogram was successfully recorded by a string galvanometer.

In a study of the electrocardiograms of perspiring miners Atkins (1961) found that the main source of artifacts was contact variations between the electrode metal and the skin. When the electrodes were separated from the skin by a layer of filter paper or gauze soaked with an electrolyte, electrode artifacts virtually disappeared.

Roman and Lamb (1962), using miniature floating electrodes applied to the skin over each end of the sternum, presented some truly remarkable records of the ECG in which no artifacts were to be observed when the electrodes were tapped or struck or when the subject was jumping or engaged in vigorous activity. These electrodes were employed for monitoring ECG changes in pilots flying in high-performance aircraft. Lucchina and Phipps (1962) similarly demonstrated that their electrodes (Fig. 11-6*d*) were free from artifacts when pressure was applied or when the electrodes were displaced. To prove their point, high-quality electrocardiograms were recorded from ambulatory subjects. Similar floating electrodes have been employed successfully to record the ECG of astronauts, laborers, swimmers, and a variety of other subjects exercising strenuously.

To record the EEG on moving subjects Kado et al. (1964) et al. constructed interesting electrodes in which the metal was tin in contact with a tin chloride solution contained in a small ceramic chamber. Contact between the ceramic chamber and the skin was made via a sponge soaked in physiological saline. Other than removing oil from the scalp, no special precautions were required for the installation of the electrodes. When carefully applied, these electrodes produced remarkably stable EEG recordings in subjects who were moving their heads rapidly.

In summary, the electrical stability of an electrode is related to the stability of the regions of charge gradient. With all electrodes there is a metal-electrolyte interface. Stabilization of this interface prevents the development of variable electrochemical voltages which have become known as "movement artifacts." With surface electrodes, however, the metal-electrolyte interface is only one of the regions of charge gradient. Others exist between the electrode electrolyte and the skin and underlying the tissue fluids. Disturbance of these regions also produces electrochemical voltages of appreciable magnitude. The skin-drilling technique of Shackel (1959), by decreasing the ionic gradient, attenuates movement artifacts produced by disturbance of this region.

The preceding discussion of electrode potentials was presented to alert the reader to the possibility of the presence of voltages of nonphysiological origin. In order to have confidence in the magnitude of the voltage appearing between the electrode terminals, electrodes should be routinely checked for voltage without the bioelectric event interposed.

Often relatively little attention is given to the large unstable potentials developed when the electrode wires come into contact with electrolytes. Special precautions should be taken after a carefully prepared electrode is joined to the wire connected to the recording apparatus. In the early days of electrocardiography, Pardee (1917) recommended that the connecting wire be riveted to the electrode and the use of solder avoided. Henry

(1938) called attention to the fact that, if the solder connection joining the electrode to the interconnecting wire became wet with an electrolytic solution, there was produced a multimetal electrolytic cell that developed unstable voltages and caused eventual corrosion and breakage of the connection. The simple practice of covering the wire connection at the electrode with a waterproof coating will result not only in a more stable electrode but one that will last longer.

11–3.   ELECTRODE IMPEDANCE

In addition to developing a half-cell potential, each electrode exhibits an impedance which is dependent on the nature of the electrical double layer. This impedance is often called the polarization impedance. Through the impedance of both electrodes and the input impedance of the recording apparatus flows a small current derived from the bioelectric event. Because the input impedance of most bioelectric recorders is high, the current is small and the voltage drop caused by the electrode impedance is usually negligible. As pointed out later, however, this situation does not always obtain, and under such circumstances, in addition to a loss of amplitude, undesirable waveform distortion of a bioelectric event can occur.

Electrode impedances are complex and can be difficult to measure with high accuracy on living subjects. The term electrode impedance really refers to the impedance at each electrode interface and does not include the impedance of the biological material between the electrodes. Frequently, however, the term is used to describe the total impedance of the circuit between the electrode terminals. Such an impedance of course includes the impedance at both electrodes and that of the biological material between them. If the total impedance between the electrode terminals is measured at different frequencies, the nature of the circuit created by the electrode-electrolyte interface will manifest itself, for the resistivity of most body segments and large samples of biological material is fairly constant in the low- and audio-frequency regions.

Conceptually an electrode-electrolyte interface resembles a capacitance shunted by a resistance, with this combination in series with a voltage that represents the half-cell potential E of the electrode (Fig. 11–2a). Another popular equivalent is shown in Fig. 11–2b. Clearly evident is the fact that the impedance is reactive and exhibits a decrease in magnitude with increasing frequency. The authors hasten to point out that for any particular electrode the values of the resistances and capacitances are not constant and are dependent on the frequency and current density used to measure them.

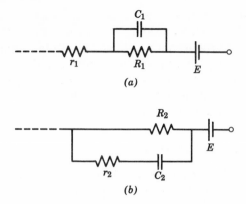

Figure 11–2. Approximate equivalent circuits for electrode-tissue interface.

11–4. TYPES OF ELECTRODES

Many types of electrodes have been employed to detect bioelectric events. A few of the more familiar types are sketched in Figs. 11–3 to 11–8, 11–10 to 11–12, 11–14, 11–15, 11–20, and 11–22. A practical basis for their comparison is the electrode area,[1] and an important characteristic is the impedance measured between the electrode terminals. When large-area electrodes are used, it is customary to measure the d-c resistance between the electrode terminals. Direct-current resistance, however, does not by itself describe the electrical circuit constituted by the electrodes and the biological material. To adequately describe this circuit, it becomes necessary to know the resistive and reactive components at all frequencies. In general, the smaller the electrode, the higher the interface impedance. The frequency-impedance characteristic of electrodes of various sizes will be discussed in some detail in this section.

Among the largest recording electrodes are those used for electrocardiography (Fig. 11–3a), consisting of two rectangular (3.5×5 cm) or circular (4.75 cm) plates of German silver,[2] nickel-silver, or nickel-plated steel. When these electrodes are applied to a subject with electrode jelly, typical d-c resistance values are in the range of 2 to 10 kilohms; the high-frequency impedance amounts to a few hundred ohms. In 1910 James and Williams reported that such plate electrodes replaced the more cumbersome immer-

---

[1] The area referred to here is calculated from the physical dimensions of the electrodes and not the effective area, which, in the case of many specially prepared electrodes, is much greater.

[2] German silver is an alloy of nickel, copper, and zinc and contains no silver.

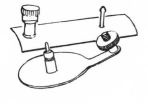
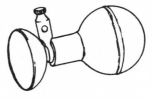

A.   METAL PLATES   B. SUCTION ELECTRODE

Figure 11–3.   Electrodes for electrocardiography: (*a*) metal plates; (*b*) suction electrode.

sion (bucket) electrodes traditionally used for recording the ECG. The metal plate electrodes were separated from the subject by cotton or felt pads soaked in concentrated saline. Pardee (1917) indicated that the electrodes used then were 12 × 25 cm, and the saline was described as "strong."[3] The plate electrodes and the electrolytes developed were so practical for electrocardiography that they quickly displaced the immersion electrodes, which had been observed to have serious practical defects that made the taking of an ECG a time-consuming procedure: (a) the subject had to remove his boots, (b) the subject had to be seated, and hence the ECG's of many bedridden patients could not be obtained, and (c) spillage of the electrolytes made it difficult to keep the subject insulated from ground.

A very useful type of electrode is the suction-cup electrode (Fig. 11–3*b*), the forerunners of which were described by Roth (1933–1934) and Ungerleider (1939). Such an electrode is extremely practical as an ECG chest electrode and is well suited for attachment to flat surfaces of the body and to regions where the underlying tissue is soft. Although physically large, this electrode has a small area because only the rim is in contact with the skin.

A variant of the electrocardiograph electrode which permits quick application is contained in a strip of adhesive tape. This electrode, shown in Fig. 11–4, consists of a lightweight metallic screen backed by a pad for electrolytic paste. Measuring approximately $1\frac{1}{2}$ inches square, it adheres well to the skin and exhibits a relatively low resistance. The adhesive backing holds the electrode in place and retards evaporation of the electrolyte. These electrodes are commercially available.[4]

A most interesting type of electrode, which was described by Lewes (1965), is shown in Fig. 11–5. This very practical ECG electrode, now

[3]The authors estimate that the concentration of saline was between 5 and 30%.
[4]Telemedics, Inc., United Aircraft, Southampton, Pa.

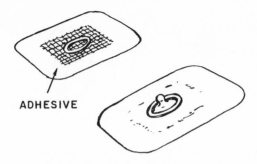

ADHESIVE

Figure 11–4. Adhesive tape electrode. (Courtesy Telemedics Dept., Vector Division of United Aircraft Corp., Southampton, Pa.)

designated as the multipoint electrode,[5] consists of a 6 × 5 cm segment of a standard nutmeg grater made of stainless steel or tin-plated soft iron. It is slightly curved to fit over fleshy parts of the body; the abrasive side is placed against the skin. Approximately 1000 fine, active contact points are obtained when the electrode is applied to the skin with a very slight rotary movement that causes the multipoints to penetrate the stratum corneum, the layer responsible for the major part of the skin resistance. When penetration occurs, a low-resistance contact is established with the subject. Lewes reported that the multipoint electrode resistance was similar to that obtained with plate electrodes and jelly. The impedance-frequency curves obtained by Lewes and Hill (1966) over a frequency range of 1 cps to 1 kc closely resemble those produced with plate electrodes and electrode jelly. With a smaller 1-inch circular chest electrode, the d-c resistance was slightly higher (6 kilohms).

Multipoint electrodes are of special value in some unusual recording circumstances; for example, for screening the ECG in large numbers of human subjects, the short time required for application and removal is a most attractive feature. In a demonstration on one of the authors, installation, recording three standard leads, and removal of the electrodes required only 80 seconds. In circumstances in which it is not possible to prepare the skin for conventional electrodes, multipoint electrodes are ideal. For example, with hairy animals, when it is not permissible to remove the hair, coarse multipoint electrodes can be readily employed. Using such electrodes applied directly to the unprepared skin of the horse, Hill (1967) recorded the ECG and impedance respiration. Multipoint electrodes also see useful service in extreme environmental conditions. In situations of low temperature and barometric pressure, it is difficult to store electrode

[5]U.K. Patent Application 52,253/64. Now available from Cardiac Recorders, London, EC1. U.K.

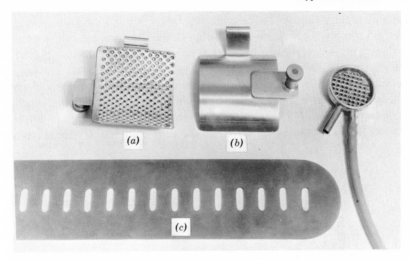

Figure 11–5. Multipoint electrodes: (a) limb electrode; (b) suction electrode; (c) rubber strap. (Courtesy D. Lewes, Bedford, England.)

pastes and jellies in their containers. The use of multipoint electrodes eliminates the need for these substances and permits easy recording under field conditions.

An electrode popular in aerospace studies and frequently used on exercising subjects is the floating electrode, occasionally referred to as the liquid-junction electrode. In this type the metal does not contact the subject directly; contact is made via an electrolytic bridge. The principle embodied in the floating electrode was used by the electrophysiologists of the nineteenth century, when it was customary to employ a metallic electrode in contact with an aqueous solution of one of its salts contained in a porous plug. Surrounding the plug was a saline solution which made contact with the subject. As time passed, the awkwardness of this type of electrode led investigators to contain the salt of the electrode metal in a kaolin plug or paste which adhered to the electrode. Between the kaolin and the subject was a film of saline. Occasionally the saline was omitted, and contact with the subject was made via the salt of the electrode metal.

The modern version of the floating electrode takes many forms. It appears to have originated with investigators of the galvanic skin reflex. One form, consisting of a zinc electrode recessed in a holder and contacting the palm via a film of jelly, was described by Haggard and Gerbrands (1947). A similar design was reported by Clark and Lacey (1950). Shackel (1958) embodied the principle in an interesting suction-cup floating electrode consisting of a silver-silver chloride rod mounted centrally in a rubber cup filled with electrode jelly. This electrode, shown in Fig. 11–6a, was found to have remarkably high electrical stability despite movement of the cup on the skin. The d-c resistance between a pair of these electrodes applied to the forearm was 2000 to 7000 ohms.

A similar high-stability floating electrode, consisting of a silver-silver chloride sponge in a small enclosure resembling a top hat, was described by O'Connell et al. (1960). This electrode, illustrated in Fig. 11–6b, was designed for GSR measurements. A type of floating electrode which has

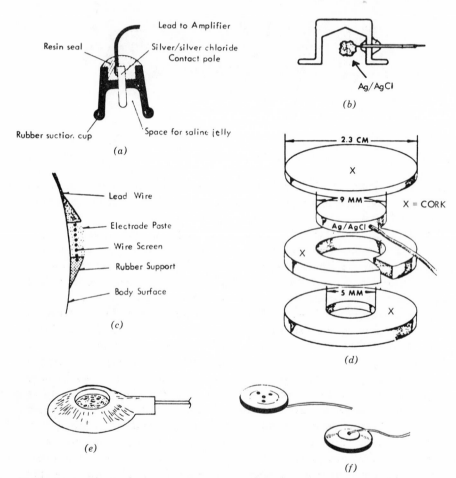

Figure 11–6. Floating or liquid-junction electrodes: (a) B. Shackel, *J. Appl. Physiol.* **13**:153–158(1958); (b) O'Connell et al., *Arch. Gen. Psych.* **3**:252–258(1960); (c) E. Hendler and N. J. Santa Maria, *Aerospace Med.* **32**:126–133(1961); (d) G. G. Lucchina and C. G. Phipps, *Aerospace Med.* **33**:722–729(1962); (e) J. Day and M. Lippitt, *Psychophysiol.* **1**: 174–182(1964); (f) A. Kahn, personal communication, 1964.

become popular in aerospace medicine and is now employed extensively for recording bioelectric events on moving subjects was described by Hendler and Santa Maria (1961). In this electrode, shown in Fig. 11-6c, the metallic conductor is mounted in a flat rubber or plastic washer which is cemented to the skin by special adhesives.[6,7] The washer holds the electrode away from the skin, and contact is established via a thick film of electrolytic paste. Choice of the electrode materials and electrolytes depends on the event and the circumstances of measurement. Monel wire screens (Hendler and Santa Maria 1961), crossed tinned copper wires in a segment of rubber tubing (Rowley et al., 1961), stainless steel screens (Roman and Lamb, 1962; Mason and Likar, 1966), silver disks (Boter et al., 1966), chlorided silver screens and plates (Day and Lippitt, 1964, Fig. 11-6e; Skov and Simons 1965), and disks of a compressed mixture of silver and silver chloride (Lucchina and Phipps, 1962, 1963, Fig. 11-6d; Kahn, 1964, Fig. 11-6f) have been employed with considerable success. With these electrodes applied to the human thorax the d-c resistance varies with the method of preparing the skin, the type of conducting electrolyte, and the area of the electrodes. In practice d-c resistances varying from about 2 to 50 kilohms are typical.

Lucchina's and Kahn's investigations merit special consideration, for they focus attention on important factors relative to the stability of floating electrodes. Lucchina's (1962) electrode, shown in Fig. 11-6d, consisted of a disk of equal parts of silver and silver chloride made by first grinding and then compressing the mixture under a pressure of 20,000 psi. The disk was then mounted in a cork ring which held the electrode away from the skin. With a pair of these electrodes applied to the abraded human thorax, the authors reported a d-c resistance of 500 to 2000 ohms.

Lucchina and Phipps (1963) made a series of electrodes having different amounts of silver and silver chloride. They measured the voltage difference and resistance between similar electrodes in contact with Graphogel[8] in a test jig and found that reducing the amount of silver chloride decreased the d-c resistance but increased the voltage difference. Although they noted that the presence of a minute amount of silver chloride reduced the potential difference between a pair of electrodes, they recommended a 30% silver and 70% silver chloride mixture as the best compromise between voltage difference and resistance.

The electrodes described by Kahn (1964), which are commercially available,[9] are illustrated in Fig. 11-6f. In these electrodes a disk of silver-

[6] Eastman 910: Eastman Kodak Co., Rochester, N. Y.

[7] Stomaseal: 3M Manufacturing Co., St. Paul 6, Minn.

[8] Tablax Corp., New York, N. Y.

[9] Beckman Instruments, Spinco Division, Palo Alto, Calif.

silver chloride is mounted behind a stiff baffle in which holes have been drilled. Contact between the electrode and the skin is made via electrode jelly which fills the holes. The combination of a stiff baffle and the use of silver-silver chloride results in an electrode of high mechanical and electrical stability with which remarkably clean electrocardiographic records can be obtained from subjects exercising vigorously.

When recordings are to be made on subjects experiencing large vibration or acceleration forces, it is important to make the electrodes as small and light as possible. Thompson and Patterson (1958), Sullivan and Weltman (1961), Roman and Lamb (1962), Lucchina and Phipps (1962), and Simons et al. (1965) have described such electrodes and demonstrated their value. Sullivan and Weltman's electrode weighed 2 mg and consisted of Mylar 0.001 inch thick on which was deposited a metallic film. The center was filled with electrode jelly, and Eastman 910 adhesive[10] was employed to cement the electrode to the subject. Remarkably clean electromyograms were obtained on exercising subjects. Thompson's electrodes consisted of small pieces of silvered nylon applied to an area of skin which had been lightly sanded. The electrodes were applied with a special conducting adhesive. Although the electrodes were small and performed remarkably well during vigorous movement, the d-c resistance between pairs was in the vicinity of 100,000 ohms, a characteristic which demanded the use of an amplifier with a very high input impedance.

Edelberg (1963) described an efficient low-mass electrode made by electrodeposition of silver into the layers of the skin. The resistance between a pair of silver depositions was remarkably low, and no electrolytic paste was required; the silver spots were virtually terminals on the subject. The only drawback to these remarkable electrodes is their relatively short life. As time passes, the silver undergoes chemical changes and the spot eventually disappears. Nonetheless, the obvious advantages of these electrodes indicate that investigation of their use will continue.

A most interesting low-mass dry electrode, designed for aerospace research, was described by Roman (1966), with technical details being presented by Patten et al (1966). This electrode, which exhibits many desirable characteristics for human use, can be applied to the skin in only a few minutes. With a pair of these electrodes on the thorax remarkably clean ECG and impedance respiration recordings can be obtained. To date 500 hours of in-flight and 700 hours of ground recording of the ECG have been logged successfully on Air Force personnel. The electrodes are applied by first rubbing electrode jelly into the skin with a toothbrush and then wiping the skin dry with gauze. Next a film of conducting adhesive[11] is

[10]Eastman Kodak Co., Rochester, N. Y.

[11]43 gm of Duco Household Cement (Dupont S/N 6241), 23 gm of silver powder (Handy and Harman Silflake 135), and 125 cc of acetone.

painted or sprayed on the skin, forming a conducting spot about 20 mm in diameter. Then a silver-plated copper wire is placed in the conducting adhesive glue and is captured as drying occurs. When dry, a coat of insulating cement is applied to cover the electrode. The process is illustrated in Fig. 11–7. The impedance of these electrodes is dependent upon their area. In the sizes customarily used, the low-frequency impedance is in the range of 50 kilohms, so that an amplifier with an input impedance of 2 megohms or more is required if distortion-free ECG's are to be recorded.

When some of the small-area, high-resistance electrodes just described are used for electrocardiography, in addition to the obvious need for amplifiers with an adequately high input impedance,[12] attention must be given to the conditions existing when high-resistance electrodes are connected to resistance networks, such as those constituting the V-terminal (Wilson et al 1934) or those employed with the various vectorcardiographic lead systems. Schwarzschild et al (1954), Dower et al (1959), and King (1964) have challenged the validity of records taken under such circumstances. Although the magnitudes of the distortions encountered in the various situations have not always been critically examined, they are calculable from measured values of electrode resistance and the values of the resistances in the networks to which the electrodes are connected. Rappaport et al (1949) presented a mathematical analysis of this problem. Schwarzschild's suggestion of using cathode followers ahead of the averaging resistors merits consideration when high-resistance electrodes are to be employed with such resistance networks. Emitter or source follower circuits will achieve the same end with fewer components.

When special electrodes are used for electrocardiography, their location is often chosen to minimize artifacts. For example, slight differences in electrode materials, variable contact resistance, and action potentials from contracting muscle masses between the electrodes all produce spurious signals. To obtain ECG's free from muscle artifact, Geddes et al. (1960) developed the MX lead, in which one electrode was placed on the manubrium and the other over the xiphoid process. Standard EEG electrodes (1-cm silver disks), jellied and attached to the skin with adhesive tape, were employed. To attain the same goal Carbery et al. (1960) introduced two electrode placements. In both they used 1-inch stainless steel wire-mesh electrodes. In one configuration three electrodes were employed; one was placed over the manubriosternal junction, another over the vertebral column at the lumbrosacral junction, and the third over the vertebral column at the level of the eighth thoracic vertebra. In the other configuration electrodes were placed at the lower margin of the rib cage on the midaxillary lines. The third electrode was placed over the vertebral column at

[12]See Section 11–9.

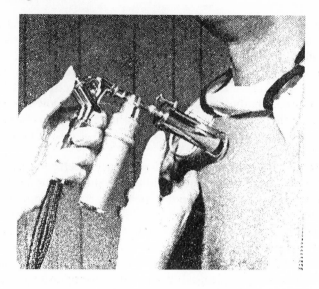

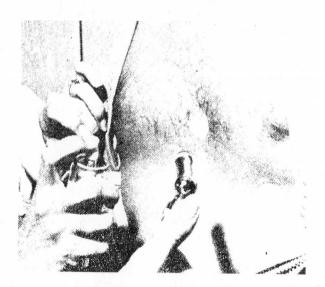

Figure 11–7. Spray-on electrode. [From *Aerospace Med.* **37**:790–795 (1966). By permission.]

the level of the lumbrosacral junction. In addition they employed a band-pass filter to select only the frequencies of importance in the ECG. They reported that with the first electrode array they obtained satisfactory

ECG's on 95% of the subjects tested; the only difficulties occurred with truly hyperasthenic subjects. For the latter group the second electrode array was satisfactory.

Recognizing that ECG's taken on the exercising subject by using limb leads always produces movement artifacts, Mason and Likar (1966) investigated electrode locations on the thorax, which produced records nearly identical with those derived from leads 1, 11, 111. Two electrodes were located on the right and left chest below the clavicles, and the third was on the anterior axillary line halfway between the costal margin and the crest of the ilium.

Rose (1963) reported that if ECG changes are sought which are indicative of the metabolism of the myocardium, such as alterations in the T wave and S-T segment, the location of the electrodes merits special consideration. In his experience he found that locating one electrode over the manubrium and the other at the left fifth or sixth interspace at the anterior axillary line produced better results than any of the other possibilities investigated. A similar electrode location was adopted by Gibson et al. (1962) and designated as the T lead by Davis and Thornton (1965). Rose reported that electrodes placed along the sternum, while relatively free from movement artifact, were of little value in indicating ischemic S-T segment shifts.

Thus, when taking the ECG with special electrodes placed in nonstandard locations, it is important to examine the type of information to be obtained from the recordings. If only heart rate is desired, the choice of electrodes and their location presents no problem. If clinically acceptable records are sought, it is necessary to make careful comparison of the results with those obtained with clinically accepted instruments and standard lead configurations. If changes in cardiac metabolism are to be determined, attention to placement is paramount; the location for ECG electrodes which permits recording with a minimum of artifacts is not necessarily the optimum for identification of subtle changes occurring with alterations in the metabolism of cardiac muscle.

In electroencephalography, solder pellets a few millimeters in diameter are sometimes applied to the cleaned scalp and contact is established via electrode paste. Small needles inserted subcutaneously are also used. In most studies, however, small silver disks approximately 7 mm in diameter, such as those shown in Fig. 11–8a, are employed. Sometimes the disks are chlorided, and occasionally they are separated from the scalp by a washer of soft felt. Contact with the cleaned scalp in both cases is made via an electrolytic paste. In practice the d-c resistance measured between a pair of these electrodes on the scalp varies between 3 and 15 kilohms.

The impedance measured between pairs of the electrodes just described

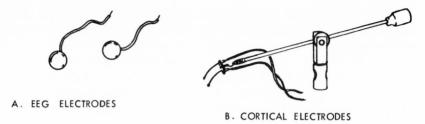

A. EEG ELECTRODES

B. CORTICAL ELECTRODES

Figure 11–8. (*a*) Scalp and (*b*) cortical electrodes for electroencephalography.

was determined by the authors in the frequency range extending from 0 to 100 kc. The electrodes were applied to human subjects in the manner typical for each event recorded. The measurements were made with the same current density at each frequency. To examine the importance of current density, currents of 0.1 and 1.0 ma were employed. Impedance-frequency curves were obtained by using pairs of ECG plates (Fig. 11–3*a*), EEG disks (Fig. 11–8*a*), and ECG screens (Fig. 11–6*c*) of two sizes.

Often there were appreciable differences between individual electrodes of the same type. When this occurred, many electrodes were tested and the data averaged. The effect of current density, although detectable, was smaller than the variability between electrodes of the same kind. The values plotted included the impedance of the electrodes and that of the subject between them. In each case d-c resistance was measured, using a low-current ohmmeter. Figure 11–9 summarizes the data obtained.

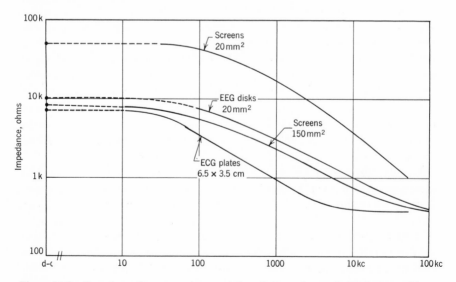

Figure 11–9. Impedance-frequency characteristics of electrodes applied to human subjects.

For all electrodes the d-c resistance was greater than the high-frequency impedance, indicating that, if a low-current ohmmeter is used to measure the resistance, the value obtained, although indicative of circuit continuity, only approximates the low-frequency impedance of the circuit. In the 10- to 100-cps region, the impedance approximated the d-c resistance. Above 100 cps the impedance decreased progressively, reaching values many times smaller than the magnitude of the d-c resistance.

Although the figures given for the impedances of large-surface electrodes can be called typical, considerable variation which is dependent on the quality of application to the subject may be encountered. To demonstrate this point, Schmitt et al. (1961) measured the 60-cps impedance between standard ECG electrodes on subjects before taking routine electrocardiograms. Although a median value of 2400 ohms was obtained, even under well-controlled conditions impedances forty times this large were encountered. In this investigation, which employed technicians familiar with attaching electrodes to human subjects impedances as high as 100,000 ohms were occasionally measured.

Although the physical size of the electrode appears to be the property most directly determining its impedance, a factor worthy of note is that the effective area of the electrode is increased by wetting the skin with electrolytic solutions (e.g., electrode paste or perspiration). Blank and Finesinger (1946) directed attention to the importance of this factor when measuring the resistive component of the galvanic skin reflex. Effective area can also be increased by special treatment of the electrode metal. Electro-deposition of a spongy layer of metal greatly increases the area and reduces the impedance. Use of this technique was described by Marmont (1949), Svaetichin (1951), and Dowben and Rose (1953).

When the electrical activity of the exposed cortex is recorded, it is customary to employ silver ball electrodes approximately 1 mm in diameter, bare or chlorided and sometimes covered with a small cotton pad. Geddes (1948–1949) described the preparation and use of these electrodes, which are illustrated in Fig. 11–8b. The d-c resistance between a pair of these electrodes spaced a few centimeters apart on the human brain is in the kilohm range.

Because electrodes placed on the scalp or cortex detect mainly the electrical activity of the neurons in the superficial layers of the brain, the need has arisen to find a method of detecting the electrical activity of subcortical nerve cells. Two types of highly successful depth electrodes have been developed; one, due to Delgado (1955), is shown in Fig. 11–10a, and the other, due to Ray (1966), in Fig. 11–10b. Delgado's electrode consists of a bundle of Teflon-insulated stainless steel wires (0.005 inch in diameter) of differing lengths bonded to a central supporting wire

(0.007 inch in diameter) by an insulating varnish. The end of the supporting wire is rounded for ease of insertion into the brain. The ends of the individual wires are staggered 3 mm, and their 1-mm exposed surfaces constitute the individual electrodes. The active area of each electrode is in the vicinity of 0.5 mm². The end of the central supporting wire often serves as an indifferent electrode.

Ray's electrode, which is commercially available,[13] consists of a bundle of 18-gauge insulated wires bonded to a length of 24-gauge stainless steel needle tubing with a high-temperature varnish. Each wire is platinum (90%)—iridium (10%) and is 0.0035 inch in diameter, and the active electrodes are made by scraping the varnish from the

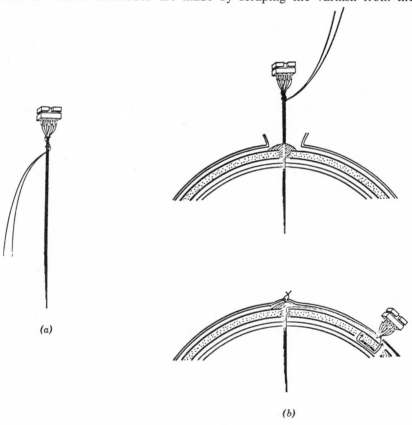

(a)

(b)

Figure 11–10A. (*a*) Delgado's depth: electrode; (*b*) method of insertion. [From J.M.R. Delgado EEG Clen. *Neurophysical* 7:637–644 (1955). By permission.]

[13]Medical Applications Dept., Advanced Systems Development Division, I. B. M., Rochester, Minn.

wires at the desired places. The scraped area is then platinized to reduce the tissue-electrode impedance by about one hundred-fold. The contact area employed by Ray was 0.075 × 1.00 mm.

The depth electrodes described by Delgado and Ray have been implanted into the brains of animals and man and left there for prolonged periods for recording the electrical activity of subcortical neurones under a variety of normal and abnormal states. Ray reported that the central stainless steel needle that supports the electrodes could be used for the injection of materials into the brain or the passage of a guarded microelectrode. He also stated that his electrodes could serve to measure localized impedance

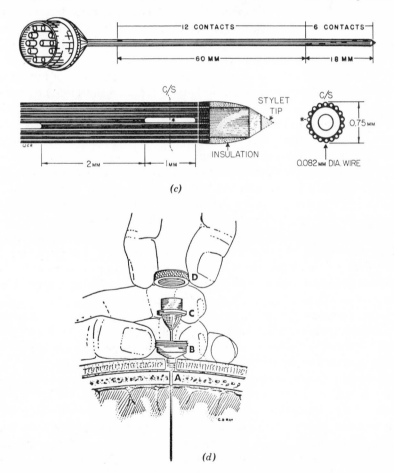

(c)

(d)

Figure 11–10B. Ray's depth electrode: (c) method of insertion; (d) now available from Medical Applications Dept. 249, IBM Corp., Rochester, Minn. [From C. D. Ray, *J. Neurosurg* **24**:911–921 (1966). By permission.]

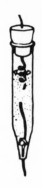

Figure 11–11.
Wick electrode.

changes and that by the application of the proper polarizing voltage they are suitable for the continuous recording of oxygen tension.

In some studies it is necessary to employ a pair of what have come to be known as nonpolarizable electrodes. One frequently employed type, illustrated in Fig. 11–11, is often made from a medicine dropper. A cotton wick is placed in the tapered end, and a cork in the large end holds a chlorided silver wire in contact with the electrolyte in the dropper. These electrodes were described and thoroughly investigated by Burr (1944, 1950). They are frequently used for d-c recording because a pair can be made having a voltage difference as small as 10μv or less. The d-c resistance of two cotton wick electrodes in saline is in the kilohm range. Kahn (1965) described electrodes of this type in which the metal consisted of a compressed mixture of silver and silver chloride. The electrolyte employed was saline and in some instances plasma. The voltage difference between a saline-filled pair varied between 5 and 10μv.

A similar type of medicine dropper electrode, which was developed for total implantation, was described by Rowland (1961). The stem of his electrode measured 15 mm in length and 6 mm in diameter, and in it he placed a coiled-coil electrode made from 30-gauge silver wire which was in contact with saline. The coiled coil was made by first winding 5 inches of wire around a 20-gauge needle and then removing and stretching the coil slightly so that the individual turns did not contact each other. The coil was then wrapped around a needle of the same size and inserted into the stem of the small medicine dropper. This technique permits obtaining a large electrode-electrolyte junctional area in a small space. Rowland reported that the d-c resistance range of such electrodes was 30 to 50 kilohms with a potential difference in the millivolt range between pairs. He demonstrated their value in recording six channels of EEG in the cat.

Electromyographers often find it convenient to use a variety of electrodes; some are placed on the skin, whereas others are inserted directly into the muscle being examined. For precise localization, steel needle electrodes are inserted directly into the muscle. Usually the electrodes are coated with an insulating varnish and are bare only at the tip. Frequently one needle electrode is paired with a metallic plate on the surface of the skin. Figure 11–12a illustrates this type of electrode, which was described by Jasper et al. (1945). When the shaft of the needle electrode is coated with insulating varnish, the area of the electrode in contact with active tissue

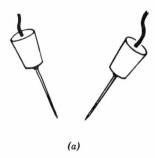

(a)

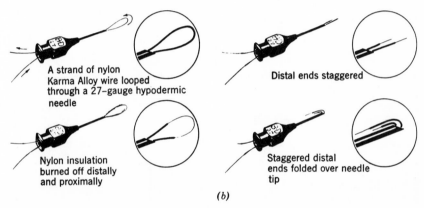

A strand of nylon
Karma Alloy wire looped
through a 27–gauge hypodermic
needle

Distal ends staggered

Nylon insulation
burned off distally
and proximally

Staggered distal
ends folded over needle
tip

(b)

Figure 11–12.   Electrodes for electromyography: (a) needle electrodes; (b) steps in making new bipolar electrode assembly before sterilization. [From Basmajian and Stecko, J. Appl. Physiol. **17**:894 (1962). By permission.] (c) Scott's electrode; (d) Parker's electrode.

is quite small. In the case of Jasper's needle electrode the area was approximately 0.2 mm^2.

Over the past several years there has arisen the need for EMG electrodes which can be left in place for prolonged periods. To meet this requirement, many interesting electrodes have been developed. The main goals have been ease of insertion, freedom from pain during insertion, mechanical and electrical stability during muscular contraction, minimal interference with muscular movement, and freedom from pain while *in situ*. Although few types have attained all of these goals, some very promising electrodes have been constructed. For example, a bipolar fine-wire (25 microns in diameter) electrode was developed by Basmajian and Stecko (1962), which is easily inserted and remains well anchored in the muscle. The steps in construction

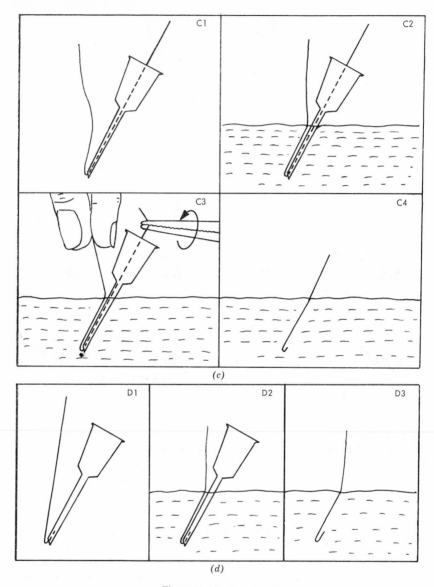

Figure 11–12. (*continued*)

of this electrode are shown in Fig. 11–12*b*. In the lower right-hand corner of the figure, the electrode is shown ready for insertion into the muscle by advancing the hypodermic needle. When the depth desired is reached, the needle is withdrawn, leaving the electrode in the muscle.

The bent ends serve as hooks to prevent the electrode from coming dislodged.

In a similar fine-wire electrode described by Scott (1965) the insulated wire[14] is passed through the lumen of the needle and bent back to pass along the outside of the needle [Fig. 11–12c (1)]. The hypodermic needle and wire are then inserted to the desired depth in the muscle [Fig. 11-12c(2)]. With the outside wire held firmly, a pair of forceps is applied to the inner wire, and by winding the wire on the forceps [Fig. 11-12c(3)] it is cut by the sharp edge of the hypodermic needle. Then the needle is withdrawn, leaving the outer wire in the tissue [Fig. 11–12c(4)]. The active surface of the electrode is approximately the cross-sectional area of the wire.

Another method of inserting fine-wire electrodes was developed by Parker (1966). A short length at the end of a fine wire is bent back upon itself. The bent-back portion is then inserted into the tip of the hypodermic needle [Fig. 11–12d(1)] and the needle and wire are advanced into the muscle [Fig. 11–12d(2)]. At the desired depth the needle is withdrawn, leaving the electrode hooked into the muscle [Fig. 11–12d(3)]. With this technique, monopolar or bipolar electrodes can be installed. The active surface of the electrode is the cross-sectional area of the wire.

The authors have measured the impedance-frequency characteristics of a variety of pairs of stainless steel needle electrodes, similar to those illustrated in Fig. 11–12a. The electrodes were insulated down to the tip, which was left bare. The area of each pair of electrodes was carefully measured before insertion into the left hind limb and right forelimb of an anesthetized dog. After 5 minutes impedance-frequency curves were determined. The procedure was repeated for each pair of electrodes. Current density was maintained at the same level at each frequency.

The impedance-frequency curves for the various pairs of needle electrodes are presented in Fig. 11–13. Clearly evident at all frequencies is the inverse relationship between electrode area and impedance. Also apparent is a decrease in impedance with increasing frequency. The contours of the impedance-frequency curves of the various electrodes examined are similar to those obtained by Barnett (1937), Offner (1942), Burns (1950), Gray and Svaetichin (1951-1952), Tasaki (1952-1953), Gesteland et al. (1959), Plutchik and Hirsch (1963), and Schwan (1963).

Occasionally, when it is necessary to record from animals with thick dry hides, the use of plate electrodes is impractical and conventional needle electrodes cannot be easily inserted. To solve this problem, Geddes et al. (1964) developed two types of cutting electrodes shown in Figs. 11–14a,b. These electrodes are made from surgical cutting needles and have beveled sharpened shanks which permit easy insertion through the hide.

[14]Karma Wire, Driver-Harris Co., Harrison, N. J.

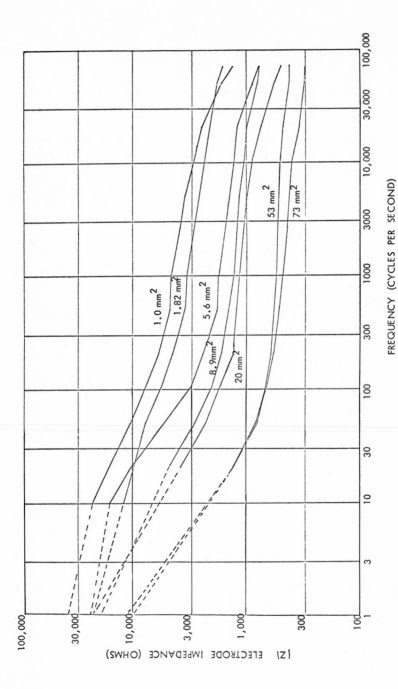

Figure 11-13. Impedance-frequency curves for needle electrodes. [From L. A. Geddes and L. E. Baker, *Med. Biol. Eng.* **4**:439–450 (1966). By permission.]

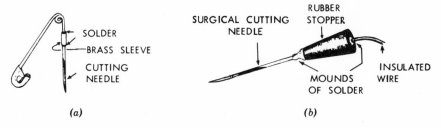

Figure 11-14. Cutting electrodes: (a) safety pin electrodes; (b) needle electrodes. [From L. A. Geddes et al., *Southwestern Vet.* **18**:56–57 (1964). By permission.]

When cutting electrodes are used, movement artifacts can be minimized by inserting the needles in a manner such that the area of the bare metal electrode in contact with the tissues is constant. The safety pin electrode should be inserted through a pinch of skin and fastened. When the pinch is released, the skin will press against the head and spring of the safety pin. The connecting wire is soldered to the brass sleeve, and the sleeve and solder connection are all covered with insulation to prevent their contact with body fluids. To provide strain relief for the solder joint, the connecting wire is passed through the coils of the spring and tied. Similarly, with the needle electrode, it is advisable to insulate the soldered portions of the electrode and the part of the shank above the cutting edge and to insert the electrode into the animal far enough so that no bare needle protrudes.

To record the electrical activity of small groups of cells, monopolar and bipolar hypodermic electrodes are often used. Such types, first described by Adrian and Bronk (1929), are shown in Figs. 11–15*a,b*. The monopolar electrode was made with 36-gauge wire (190 microns in diameter), and the bipolar electrode contained two 44-gauge wires (80 microns in diameter). These electrodes exhibit d-c resistances in the range of tens of kilohms.

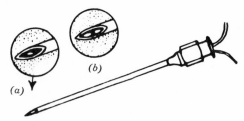

Figure 11-15. (*a*) Monopolar and (*b*) bipolar hypodermic needle electrodes.

11-5. ELECTRODE ELECTROLYTES

When metallic electrodes are placed on the surface of the body, contact is made via electrolytic solutions. If the electrodes are to be left in place for extended periods, evaporation of the solution takes place. To prevent such an occurrence, it is possible in some cases to locate the electrodes in body cavities and use the fluids in these regions as electrolytic conductors; sometimes the cavities can serve as containers for the electrolytes. Although not all of the body cavities can be employed in unanesthetized subjects, consideration should be given to using the nose, ear, mouth, axilla, navel, rectum, vagina, and urethra. Often electrodes in these and other areas can be combined with other transducers, such as electrical thermometers or heart sound pickups. Sometimes the metallic cases of these devices can serve as active, indifferent, or ground electrodes. The fluid in some fluid-coupled pressure transducers makes direct contact with the metallic case of the transducer, which is usually grounded. If this occurs, a ground connection is automatically placed on the subject. Although this may be desirable in many instances, it may constitute a hazard. For example, if the subject comes into contact with the "hot" side of a voltage which is ground-referred, the low-resistance ground path through the transducer may result in the passage of a sizable current through the subject if the voltage is high. In some instances, in which catheter electrodes are employed for measuring blood pressure or for pacemaking and when other devices (such as EEG or ECG instruments) are connected to the subject, there is a real danger of the existence of multicircuit loops in which currents intense enough to precipitate ventricular fibrillation may flow. An excellent review of the practical considerations in this area was presented by Whalen et al. (1964).

Electrode jellies and pastes were developed during the early string galvanometer days of electrocardiography when there was a need to eliminate the cumbersome immersion electrodes, which required that the subject be seated with both hands and feet in saline-filled buckets. To eliminate this requirement investigators began to study the behavior of electrodes consisting of sheets of metal wrapped in saline-soaked bandages and applied to the skin. Experience with the immersion electrodes indicated that the ECG was distorted if the electrode resistance was high. Under these conditions, the string tension had to be reduced in order to obtain adequate sensitivity, and, as a consequence, the response time of the string was prolonged. Thus to obtain a satisfactory ECG a tight string was required, which meant that the electrode resistance could not exceed a certain value. Large electrodes and strong electrolytes were needed to obtain a low resistance contact with the subject.

James and Williams (1910) were the first to introduce plate electrodes made of German silver. The electrodes were wrapped in saline-soaked gauze and applied to the subject. Cohn (1920) described a more practical electrode of soft lead (22 × 7 cm) backed by a rubber sheet. The electrode was applied to the skin which had been rubbed with a saline solution. The ECG's taken with German silver electrodes and lead electrodes were essentially the same as those taken with the immersion electrodes, probably because the resistance in all cases was comparable.

About 1935, when electrode pastes and jellies began to replace the saline-soaked pads, the characteristics of several of the earliest electrode jellies were investigated by Bell et al. (1939). Using lead electrodes (14 × 5 cm) on human subjects, they measured the d-c resistance and 300-cps impedance with the following substances under the electrodes: (a) 1% saline; (b) a paste of saline, glycerine, water, and pumice; (c) soft green soap; and (d) a recently introduced electrode jelly which contained crushed quartz. They found that, when the electrodes were wrapped in gauze, soaked in 1% saline, and applied to the subjects, the d-c resistance was highest (3080 ohms). With the other three preparations in direct contact with the electrodes and skin, the resistances were 2010, 2040, and 1100 ohms, respectively. By analyzing their results they quickly found that the presence of an abrasive reduced the resistance considerably. They were able to show that the resistance with green soap was divided by 3 when crushed quartz was added and the mixture rubbed into the skin. They also found that by lightly rubbing the dry skin with glass paper (fine sandpaper), "so that it lost its sheen and white color," and then applying the electrolyte they could obtain d-c resistance and impedance values that were very low and extremely stable. This early observation demonstrated the need for abrasives in electrode pastes and jellies.

A novel method for obtaining a low resistance, which Shackel (1959) described and called the skin-drilling technique, is painless when properly employed. The area of skin where the electrode is to be placed is first cleaned with an antiseptic solution. The region is then abraded with a dental burr in a hand tool. Only the epidermis is eroded and no blood is drawn. The amount of abrasion required depends on the type of skin. Kado (1965) reported that deeply pigmented skin requires more abrasion. In a few seconds, tissue fluid can be seen seeping into the drilled depression. The area is then cleaned with alcohol or acetone. If the skin has been drilled to the proper depth, the subject should feel a slight tingling sensation when the region is cleaned with either of these solutions. The electrode jelly is then applied and the electrode secured.

To test the value of the technique, Shackel compared the resistance values obtained with and without drilling. The drilled sites consistently exhibited values one-fifth to one-tenth of those of undrilled areas. When the electrodes are removed, the drilled site is again cleaned with an antiseptic solution. Lanolin cream is then rubbed in, and the site soon becomes invisible.

A modern reappraisal of traditional electrode jellies for recording the ECG was presented by Lewes (1965), who called attention to the fact that strong electrolytes were essential in the string galvanometer days, when the electrode-subject resistance had to be in the low-kilohm range, but that with the advent of electronic instruments with high input impedance the need for a low electrode resistance had disappeared. To prove his point he recorded more than 4000 ECG's with instruments of high input impedance (2 to 4 megohms), using a remarkable variety of substances as electrode jellies. The recordings made with each substance were compared with those obtained with standard electrode jelly. The substances used were lubricating compounds (K-Y jelly, Lubrifax), culinary compounds (mayonnaise, marrons glacés, French mustard, tomato paste), and toilet preparations (hand cream and tooth paste). All of these substances are poor conductors, and all produced ECG's indistinguishable from those taken with standard electrode jelly.

To emphasize his point further, Lewes employed dry polished electrodes (15 cm^2) on dry skin and in 6 minutes obtained entirely satisfactory ECG's indistinguishable from those taken with standard jelly. Examination of the skin under each electrode revealed the presence of a small amount of sweat, which on analysis was found to contain approximately 6 mg of sodium chloride. Additional evidence that strong electrolytes are unnecessary was provided by obtaining entirely satisfactory ECG's within 15 seconds after placing a single drop of distilled water under each electrode.

Lewes's studies prove that, when instruments of high input impedance are employed to record the ECG, a low electrode-subject resistance is not necessary. His findings, however, relative to the relationship between amplifier input impedance and high-impedance electrodes produced by electrolytic solutions of low ionic content have not received widespread acceptance as yet. For single-or multiple-channel recording with bipolar electrodes the facts adduced by Lewes are clear. However, King (1964) pointed out that, when monopolar recording techniques are employed in which several electrodes are connected through resistors joined to a common point, a high electrode resistance is incompatible with the low value of averaging resistors presently in use (5000 ohms). He further illustrated his point by making recordings with low-and high-resistance electrodes. Although such a condition may obtain when high-resistance electrodes are used in this situation, provision could easily be made to electronically add the voltage from each individual electrode and thereby remove all restrictions on the resistance of electrodes employed in procedures in which averaging techniques are involved.

It is important therefore to note that electrodes and the electrolytes used for electrical contact should not be considered as independent from the recording equipment to which the electrodes are connected. Presented elsewhere in this chapter are additional studies relative to the type of distortion encountered when small-area electrodes are employed with amplifiers having input impedances that are not sufficiently high.

Although most of the commercially available electrode pastes are satisfactory for recording a variety of bioelectric events, various authors have presented their own recipes. Among these are Jenks and Graybiel (1935), Bell et al. (1939), Marchant and Jones (1940), Thompson and Patterson (1958), Shackel (1958), Lykken (1959), Edelberg and Burch (1962), Asa et al. (1964), and Fascenelli et al. (1966).

11-6. TISSUE RESPONSE TO ELECTROLYTES

When recording bioelectric events with surface electrodes, attention should be given to the choice of the metal and electrolyte employed, since each may produce its own physiological effects. The constituents of some electrode pastes can cause allergic reactions, erythema, or discoloration of the skin. Some species of ions stimulate cells; others are toxic. For example, a high concentration of calcium chloride, such as was used in the older electrode jellies and pastes, causes sloughing of the skin. Seelig (1925) showed by subcutaneous injections of calcium chloride that solutions with concentrations greater than 1% produced sloughing.

When recording the GSR, the ionic composition of electrolytes merits special consideration. For example, Edelberg and Burch (1962) conducted a series of ingenious experiments in which the responses at test and control sites were compared and found that solutions of 1 molar ($1.0 M$) calcium chloride, ammonium chloride, and potassium sulfate potentiated the GSR by 100 to 300%. Aluminum chloride potentiated by 1000%, and zinc chloride ($0.5 M$) approximately doubled the response. Very dilute acids, alkalis, and detergents decreased the response. A solution of $0.05 M$ sodium chloride had negligible effect on the GSR, and Edelberg recommended its use for this purpose. Thus, in the routine recording of a bioelectric event from skin surfaces containing sweat glands, what may appear as an artifact may actually be an enhanced GSR. On the other hand, if one is attempting to record the GSR, the electrolyte may enhance or diminish the response. Scarification of the region under the electrode can produce unwanted voltages. Edelberg and Burch (1962) reported that, while cuts or skin punctures lower skin resistance, they also reduce the GSR.

11-7. TISSUE RESPONSE TO ELECTRODE METALS

In many recording situations electrodes must remain in direct contact with body tissues and fluids for prolonged periods. For example, electrodes have been implanted in muscle and brain tissue to record the bioelectric signals of these structures for periods of months. Under such circumstances special consideration must be given to the type of metal employed. There have been a few studies of the relative toxicity of the various species of metallic ions. In the early days of depth electrode recording in the human brain, Dodge et al. (1955) had the opportunity to study the tissue response to two electrodes, each consisting of 6 strands of Formvar-insulated copper wire (97.5 microns in diameter), which had been *in situ* for 6 days. Nineteen months later the brain was examined histologically. Tissue changes were seen at the points of entry of the electrodes. Minimal tissue changes were found along the tracks of the electrodes.

Faced with the problem of recording the electrical activity of structures deep within the brains of human and animal subjects, Fischer et al. (1957) studied the responses of the brains of cats to 1-cm lengths of 24-gauge wires left *in situ* for periods up to 4 weeks. The wires employed were of chlorided silver, bare copper and stainless steel. Both bare and insulated[15] wires were employed. After 1 week histological studies showed tissue responses to all of the materials used. The responses were dependent on the types of metals employed; the insulating compounds were virtually without tissue response. Silver and copper wires proved to be the most toxic to brain tissue. After 3 weeks a narrow ring of necrotic tissue surrounded the silver wire. Around this ring was a circular edematous region 2mm in diameter. The reaction to the copper wire at the same time was similar except that an increase in vascularity had also occurred. The copper wire was encircled by necrotic tissue and an edematous region. The diameter of the lesion varied between 1.5 and 7 mm. With the stainless steel wire the size of the lesion was determined by the extent of the mechanical trauma produced by its introduction into the brain. Only minimal edema was found. Fischer and his co-workers concluded therefore that the electrode material of choice for such studies is stainless steel.

Another study, carried out by Collias and Manuelidis (1957), in which bundles of six stainless steel electrodes (125 microns in diameter) were inserted into the brains of cats, described the histological changes that occurred over periods extending up to 6 months. They found that an orderly sequence of changes took place in the tissue surrounding the electrode track. At the end of 24 hours there was a zone of hemorrhage, necrosis, and edema extending to about 1 mm from the electrode. After 3 days there was less hemorrhage and necrotic debris, and by the seventh day a 0.1-mm layer of capillaries occupied the necrotic zone. By the fifteenth day the capillaries had almost completely replaced the necrotic region and connective tissue had started to form. After the passage of 1

[15]Tygon, Formvar, Thermobond M472, and polyethylene.

month the necrotic debris had disappeared, and a well defined capsule surrounded the electrode track. Capsule formation was virtually complete after 4 months, at which time a thick, dense capsule completely encircled the electrode.

Robinson and Johnson (1961) carried out studies similar to those reported above. Into cat brains they implanted wires (125 microns in diameter) of gold, platinum, silver, stainless steel, tantalum, and tungsten and studied the tissue responses at different times over a period extending to 6 months. Responses similar to those previously described were observed. After about 1 week the differences between the metals in regard to the reaction produced began to be detectable. Gold and stainless steel evoked the least tissue response; tantalum, platinum, and tungsten produced more. Silver precipitated a vigorous tissue reaction. Encapsulation of all electrodes was evident at 15 days, with thicker capsules around the metals that provoked the greatest tissue response.

The authors hasten to emphasize that these tissue changes were studied in cat brains with electrodes which carried no current. Studies on the responses of other tissues to other electrode materials and on tissue responses to current-carrying electrodes have yet to be made. It is anticipated that the tissue response to current-carrying electrodes will be quite different in view of the many electrolytic reactions that can occur.

11–8. EQUIVALENT CIRCUIT FOR EXTRACELLULAR ELECTRODES

When extracellular electrodes, such as those just described, are employed to measure a bioelectric event, an approximate equivalent circuit which relates the bioelectric generator and electrode impedance to the impedance measured between the electrode terminals is as shown in Fig. 11–16. The voltage of a typical bioelectric generator is designated by E_t which in most cases is the summation of propagated action potentials of the cells between the electrodes. Sometimes E_t consists of slow variations in membrane potential. R and r are voltage-divider impedances which account for the attenuaton of the bioelectric event by the volume conductor action of body tissues and fluids. R_{pa}, R_{pb} and C_{pa}, C_{pb} are the resistive and capacitive components of the polarization impedances of electrodes a and b. E_a and E_b simulate the half-cell potentials of the electrodes. The magnitude and polarity of these voltages and the values for the resistive and capacitive components depend on the electrode metal and electrolyte.

Looking toward the event from the terminals of the electrodes, the impedance-frequency characteristic of this circuit resembles those shown in Figs. 11–9 and 11–13. Looking outward, the bioelectric generator sees impedances r, R, which attenuate the amplitude of the signal. The

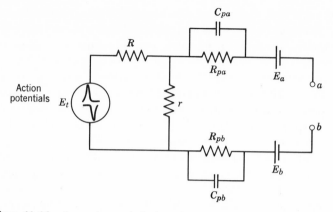

Figure 11–16. Approximate equivalent circuit for extracellular electrodes.

attenuated event is coupled to the bioelectric recorder through the electrode impedances (due to R_{pa}, C_{pa}, R_{pb}, C_{pb}), and if the input impedance of the bioelectric recorder is not high enough, frequency-dependent distortion can occur. This subject will be discussed in detail in the next section.

11–9. INPUT IMPEDANCE OF THE BIOELECTRIC RECORDER

When recording bioelectric events, it is customary to make the input impedance of the bioelectric recorder many times larger than the electrode impedance. When this technique is employed, only a small current flows through the electrode impedance and there is a minimal loss of voltage at the electrode-electrolyte interface. However, if the bioelectric recorder has an input impedance which is not high with respect to the electrode polarization impedance, there can occur a distortion in the waveform of the bioelectric event. Because of the resistive and reactive components of the electrode polarization impedance, the various components of the bioelectric event will not be presented to the input stage with the same relative amplitudes that they initially possessed. Moreover, phase distortion accompanies such amplitude-frequency distortion and the time relations between the various frequency components will be altered. In addition, it has been shown by Schwan (1963, 1965) that the resistive and reactive components of the electrode polarization impedance of platinum-iridium electrodes change when high current densities are encountered. Similar investigations carried out by Weinman and Mahler (1964), who studied electrodes of various metals, verify the nonlinear characteristic of electrode polarization impedance at high current densities. If the input impedance of the bioelectric recorder is so low that high current densities result, it is possible for the electrode impedance to become dependent on the amplitude of the bioelectric event. If this occurs, small and large-amplitude signals will be injected differently into the input of the bioelectric recorder. It is thus apparent that the use of an input stage which does not have an impedance very high with respect to the electrode impedance virtually guarantees that the bioelectric event will be distorted. A high electrode current density can occur when the electrode area is small (as it is with metal microelectrodes), and a conventional amplifier is employed.

It has already been demonstrated that waveform distortion of clinical significance occurs when high-resistance electrodes are employed with recorders having a low-resistive input impedance. In the early days of electrocardiography, when string galvanometers with their relatively low resistance (5 to 20 kilohms) were used, Lewis (1915) showed that a normal ECG was distorted when recorded with polarizable platinum electrodes. In such cases attenuated P and T waves and enhanced S waves were obtained. Similarly Pardee (1917), using a string galvanometer and German silver electrodes applied to a bandage soaked in saline, showed that the rectangular wave calibration signal was distorted when the area of each electrode was decreased from 300 to 8 cm². With the smaller electrodes, the calibration signal, instead of rising rapidly and exhibiting a flat top, showed a sharp overshoot and an *R-C* decay to a sustained plateau. On turning off the calibrate signal, there was an undershoot and *R-C* decay to the baseline. Pardee (1917) observed a similar type of distortion when electrodes were applied to patients with thick, dry skin or when the blood vessels under the electrodes were constricted. The distortion disappeared when an electrolyte was rubbed into the skin. It often disappeared as time passed and the electrolyte penetrated the dry, horny layers of the skin. Although Pardee did not investigate the phenomenon thoroughly, his observations were in agreement with those of previous and later workers, notably Einthoven (1928), who showed that the electrode-subject interface impedance introduced a time constant into the circuit which electrically differentiated the P and T waves.

The practical importance of these facts in recording the ECG was again demonstrated by Sutter (1944) and Roman and Lamb (1962). These investigators applied small-area electrodes to the chest of a human subject and used them first with an amplifier having a high input impedance to obtain control records. They then lowered the input impedance of the amplifier by connecting different resistances across it. The distortions in the ECG were what would be called clinically significant, consisting of a displacement of the S-T segment and a slight depression in the latter part of the T wave.

Recent studies which focused attention on the relationship between recorder input impedance and electrode impedance were those of Maxwell (1957–1958) and Lewes (1965), mentioned previously. Geddes and Baker investigated the relationship between resistive input impedance and electrode area in recording the ECG (1966) and the EMG (1967). By using electrodes of differing areas and shunting the amplifier input with various resistors, the effect of electrode interface impedance was made to manifest itself.

Figure 11–17 illustrates the type of distortion encountered when this technique was employed. This illustration shows a lead II ECG in an anesthetized dog. Stainless steel needle electrodes such as those shown in Fig. 11–12a were employed. The needles were insulated to within 1 mm of the tip. The geometric area in contact with the body tissues and fluids was approximately 1 mm². To illustrate the nature of the distortion, a square pulse was inserted in series with the electrodes.

Figure 11–17 a shows the control ECG and square pulse recorded with an amplifier having a 4.4-megohm resistive input impedance. Figures 11–17 b-e illustrate the changes produced by placing resistors of successively lower values across the input of the amplifier. During the various trials the electrodes were not disturbed. In Figs. 11–17a-d inclusive, the recording sensitivity was the same. In Fig. 11–17e the recording sensitivity was doubled for clearer comparison with Fig. 11–17a.

The outstanding changes seen in these records are those expected in a system which is deficient in low-frequency response. Such a situation could be predicted on the basis of the general nature of the impedance-frequency curves of electrodes. With 300 kilohms across the input terminals, there were recognizable P- and T-wave changes and a noticeable tilt appeared on the square pulse. With 100 kilohms and especially with 30 kilohms across the input terminals, the P and T waves and the square pulse were dramatically changed, all becoming diphasic. As loading was increased, there was a continued loss of overall amplitude, and in Figs. 11–17d, e the resemblance to the control record was all but lost. In Fig. 11–17e, recorded with twice the amplification, the ECG is seen to be vastly different from that shown in Fig. 11–17a. The outstanding differences are the loss of P- and T-wave amplitudes and the addition of diphasic components to each. The QRS complex has similarly been changed by exaggeration of the S wave.

The manner in which this type of distortion is related to electrode area is shown in Fig. 11–18. In this illustration the ECG's of anesthetized dogs were recorded with various pairs of needle electrodes connected in lead II configuration. The control records, shown along the top of the illustration, were all obtained with an input impedance of 4.4 megohms. The changes

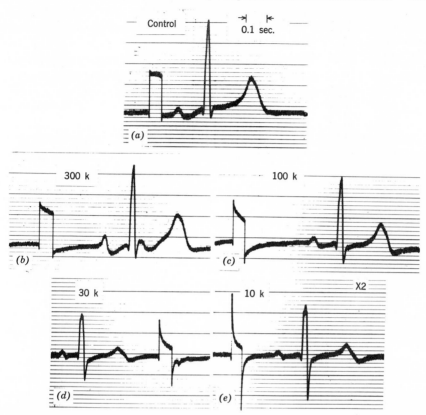

Figure 11–17. Distortion in the ECG produced by lowering input impedance. [From L. A. Geddes and L. E. Baker, *Med. Biol. Eng.* (1966). By permission.]

that occurred as the input impedance of the amplifier was lowered can be appreciated by reading from top to bottom of any column; for example, for the 1-mm^2 electrodes noticeable distortion occurred when the input impedance was reduced to 100 kilohms. For the 10-mm^2 electrodes detectable distortion occurred when the input impedance was 20 kilohms. Clearly evident in this illustration is the inverse relationship between distortion, amplifier input impedance, and electrode area.

The relationship between amplifier input impedance and electrode area is not the same for all metals. Cooper (1963) compared the distortions encountered when silver-silver chloride, platinum, silver, copper, gold, and stainless steel electrodes, all of the same area (0.1 mm^2), were connected to an amplifier with a 750-kilohm input impedance. The test consisted of passing a square wave of current through a saline bath in which the electrode pairs were immersed. The types of waveforms detected by the various

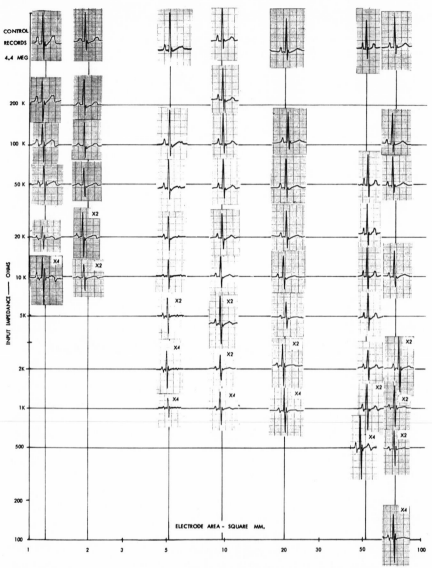

Figure 11–18. The relationship between input impedance and electrode area. [From L. A. Geddes and L. E. Baker, *Med. Biol. Eng.* **4**:439–450 (1966). By permission.]

electrode pairs are shown in Fig. 11–19. Clearly evident is the same kind of distortion as that shown in Figs. 11–17 and 11–18, namely, electrical differentiation or, stated differently, a loss of low-frequency response. Interestingly enough under these circumstances, the silver-silver chloride

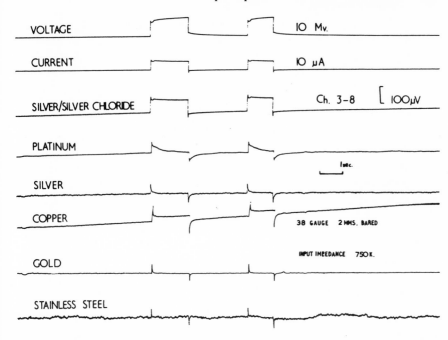

Figure 11–19. The relationship between surface area and input impedance for electrodes of various metals [From R. Cooper, Am. J. EEG Technol. 3:91–101 (1963). By permission.]

electrodes reproduced the waveform most accurately and the stainless steel electrodes provided the poorest reproduction of the test signal. The authors hasten to point out that this does not mean that stainless steel electrodes cannot be used with success; it does indicate that an amplifier having high input impedance is required with stainless steel electrodes of small surface area.

These results, which are consistently reproducible, are in agreement with those described by other investigators. They call attention to the need to use an input stage with an input impedance many times larger than that of the bioelectric generator-electrode system.

The distortion illustrated in Figs. 11–17 to 11–19 is caused primarily by two factors. First, with loading (i.e., the use of an amplifier input circuit in which the input impedance is not high with respect to the electrode-bioelectric generator system) the electrode polarization impedance becomes a dominant part of the input circuit, and the voltage across the input terminals of the bioelectric recorder is reduced. Second, the amount of phase shift is different for the various frequency components of the bioelectric event. With loading, the electrode current density is increased and the resistive and reactive components of the electrode polarization impedance become nonlinear, resulting in the magnitude of the electrode polarization impedance becoming a function of the amplitude of the bioelectric event. Thus, small- and large-amplitude signals will encounter different impedances. The exact contribution of each of the two sources of distortion is as yet unknown for the various electrodes employed in recording bioelectric events.

Not only does an increase in current density alter the electrode impedance, it also changes the half-cell potential. Even with such a relatively nonpolarizable electrode as the calomel cell, current flow alters the half-cell potential. Rothschild (1938) showed that the maximum current density for this type of electrode was $15\mu a/cm^2$ before the half-cell potential was changed. The exact limits of current densities permissible for the various types of electrodes have not as yet been investigated adequately.

11–10. MICROELECTRODES

When it is necessary to investigate the characteristics of the fundamental bioelectric generator (i.e., the single cell), microelectrodes are employed. For an electrode to be classed as a microelectrode, it need only be small enough with respect to the size of the cell in which it is inserted so that penetration by the electrode will not damage the cell.

Electrodes described as micro in dimensions are of two general types, metallic and nonmetallic. Metallic electrodes consist of a slender needle of a suitable metal sharpened to a fine point or formed by electrolytic etching; nonmetallic electrodes consist of a glass micropipette filled with an electrolyte.

Grundfest and Campbell (1942) described the method of grinding fine wires to produce 5 to 10-micron points. Grundfest (1950) gave complete details for making 1-micron stainless steel electrodes by electrolytic etching. His technique has become known as "electropointing." Hubel (1957) described a similar method for pointing tungsten wire to obtain electrodes with a tip diameter of 0.4 micron. A most useful and simple automatic electropointing machine for making stainless steel microelectrodes was developed by Mills (1962). With multiple needles mounted radially on a turning rod that dips them into and out of the etching solution 5 times per minute, the electrodes were pointed to have tip diameters in the range of 1 to 6 microns in 6 hours.

Before use, metal microelectrodes are coated almost to the micro tip with an insulating material which often requires baking in an oven. Guld (1964) described a technique for insulating platinum microelectrodes with a glass covering. When an insulating coating is applied to metal microelectrodes constructed by any of these techniques, it is often difficult to measure the exposed area of the tip, which is rarely if ever covered because of the action of the surface tension of the insulating material. The layer of insulating coating is usually so thin near the tip that microscopic examination frequently fails to uncover the true extent of the insulation regardless of its color. Under such circumstances the tip area can often be determined by using a method developed by McGoodwin working with the authors (1967). A drop of saline is placed on a glass slide and viewed with a microscope. A small wire is then placed in the drop and connected to one pole of a battery; the other pole is connected to the metal microelectrode, which is advanced into the drop and viewed in the microscope. The active area can be estimated by observation of the region from which bubbles are evolved.

As early as 1925 Taylor described the technique of drawing a 35-gauge platinum wire in heated glass tubing. By cutting or breaking the drawn section, an electrode with a tip diameter of less than 1 micron was produced. This method was revived by Svaetichin (1951), who heat-pulled silver solder in a glass tube to produce electrodes with tip diameters of 0.5 to 1 micron. The electrode tip was then covered with electrolytically deposited platinum to lower the electrode resistance. Dowben and Rose (1953) used a mixture of gallium and indium for the metal and heat-pulled the alloy in a glass tube to a tip 2 to 4 microns in diameter, which was gold plated to lower the electrical resistance. They pointed out that this particular alloy "wetted" the surface of the glass and produced electrodes having a high degree of uniformity.

It is possible to reduce the impedance of metal microelectrodes by electrolytic processing of the tip. Because some metals, notably platinum and silver, can be laid down in a spongy deposit, electrodeposition of these substances produces a substantial increase in surface area, and a reduction in impedance can be attained without much increase in diameter. A similar technique was described by Marmont (1949), who made an electrode of silver (13 mm long × 100 microns in diameter) that was first chlorided and then "developed" by a photographic developer. The procedure resulted in decreasing the electrode impedance from one-twentieth to one-thirtieth of its "undeveloped" value.

The nonmetallic microelectrode consists of a glass micropipette filled with an electrolyte compatible with the fluid inside the cell being studied. Connection to the electrolyte is made by means of a larger wire inserted into the electrolyte which fills the shank of the micropipette. The microelectrode thus resembles the larger wick electrode made from a medicine dropper (Fig. 11–11). There are numerous descriptions of this technique in the literature, and many microelectrode-fabricating machines are available commercially. Excellent reviews of the fabrication techniques have been presented by Kennard (1958) and Frank and Becker (1964).

When micropipette electrodes are to be applied to tissue which moves, breakage of the tip often occurs. An ingenious method of solving this problem was offered by Woodbury and Brady (1956), who introduced the floating micropipette. In their electrode the shaft was made of glass tubing 1 to 2 mm in diameter. After filling the micropipette with 3 M KCl, they introduced a thin, flexible tungsten wire into the stem. The friction between the wire and the stem of the micropipette and fluid surface tension held the micropipette on the wire. The tungsten wire was mounted to a rigid support, and its flexibility permitted the micropipette to follow contracting cardiac muscle.

In the search for precise knowledge of the mechanisms underlying bioelectric phenomena, the microelectrode has made it possible to measure the magnitude of the resting membrane potential and the action potential of an intact single cell and even of separate parts of a cell. Previously, attempts to measure the membrane and monophasic action potential relied on killing or damaging the cells under one electrode and placing the other electrode on uninjured cells. This resulted in much ambiguity concerning the conditions at the site of injury. However, with the advent of electrodes small enough to be inserted into single cells without excessive damage, it became possible to measure membrane and action potentials with accuracy and thereby discover the true nature of fundamental bioelectric generators.

When a microelectrode is employed to measure membrane and action potentials, it is located within the cell. The reference (indifferent) electrode is situated outside the cell. The size of an intracellular microelectrode is dictated by the size of the cell and the ability of its enveloping membrane to tolerate penetration by the microelectrode tip. Because single living cells are rarely larger than 0.5 mm (500 microns) and are usually less than one-tenth of this size, typical microelectrodes have tip dimensions ranging from 0.5 to 5 microns. When the tip of either a metal or glass micropipette electrode penetrates the cell membrane, the membrane potential suddenly appears between the intracellular and reference electrodes. The nature of the electrical circuits in these two situations of measurement will now be analyzed.

11–11. METAL MICROELECTRODES

When a metal microelectrode is advanced into a cell surrounded by other cells or by tissue fluids, as shown in Fig. 11–20, the potential appearing between terminals connected to the microelectrode and the indifferent electrode is the sum of three potentials: the metal-electrolyte junction potential at the microelectrode tip E_e, the cell membrane potential MP,

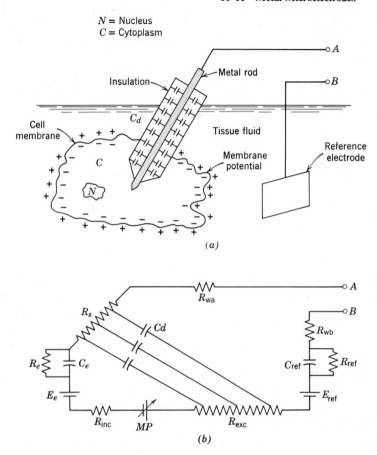

N = Nucleus
C = Cytoplasm

(a)

(b)

Figure 11–20. Intracellular metal microelectrode: (a) inserted into cell; (b) equivalent circuit.

and the reference electrode-electrolyte junction potential E_{ref}. When measuring the membrane potential, it is assumed that the sum of the first and the third potentials is known and constant.

In addition to the three sources of potential, several impedances are of special importance when action potentials are to be measured. If we neglect for the moment the potentials in the circuit and trace out the circuit from the active electrode terminal A to the terminal of the reference electrode B, there are encountered the resistance of the connecting wire R_{wa} (negligible), the resistance R_s of the shank of the microelectrode, the microelectrode tip-intracellular fluid interface impedance $R_e C_e$, the resistance of the intracellular fluid R_{inc}, the resistance of the extracellular

fluid R_{exc}, and the reference electrode-extracellular fluid interface impedance $R_{ref}C_{ref}$. The resistance of the wire connected to the reference electrode
R_{wb} is negligible.

In addition to the obvious impedances identified above, there is another
of some importance. It is the capacitive reactance of the distributed
capacitance C_d between the insulated shank of the microelectrode and the
extracellular fluid. Although the insulated shank extends into the cell, the
capacitance between it and the intracellular fluid can be neglected because
the potential difference across it does not change.

An approximate circuit that identifies these components is shown
in Fig. 11–20b. Although this circuit is relatively simple in appearance,
it cannot be analyzed because the component values cannot be specified.
Fortunately the values of some of the components are such that they
can be neglected, and in many instances it is possible to collect them and
to synthesize a simple electrical circuit which mimics the electrical behavior of the actual circuit. For example, in comparison to the junctional
impedance of the microelectrode tip $R_e C_e$, the resistance of the shank of
the metal microelectrode R_s can be neglected, as can the resistances of the
intracellular and extracellular fluids, R_{inc} and R_{exc}, respectively. Because
the area of the reference electrode is many times greater than that of the
microelectrode tip, its junctional impedance $R_{ref}C_{ref}$ can be neglected.
The distributed capacitance C_d between the shank and the extracellular
environment can be collected to form a single capacitance C_d'; its magnitude is small and hence its reactance is large with respect to the impedance
of the combination R_e and C_e, and in many cases can be neglected.

The electrochemical potentials of nonbioelectric origin (E_e, E_{ref}) can
likewise be collected to form E', and the equivalent circuit reduces to that
shown in Fig. 11–21. In practice C_d' is small and can often be neglected.
The impedance of the microelectrode tip, constituted by R_e and C_e is

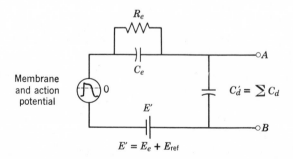

Figure 11–21. Approximate equivalent circuit for a metal microelectrode used to measure
the potential of a cell membrane.

inversely dependent on the area of the tip and the frequency. Thus the bioelectric event, i.e., the membrane potential and its excursions, is coupled to the amplifying device by a circuit which has a decreasing impedance with increasing frequency. The effect of such a circuit on the waveform of an action potential is determined by the input impedance of the amplifier to which it is connected. If the input impedance is not high enough, the low-frequency components of the bioelectric event will be attenuated as shown in Figs. 11–17 and 11–18. The relationship between electrode area and input impedance is also discussed in Section 11–9.

11–12.   THE MICROPIPETTE

Figure 11–22a diagrams a micropipette electrode inserted into a cell for the measurement of the membrane potential. The electrolyte filling the micropipette is frequently 3 M KCl, and the electrode wire in the stem is

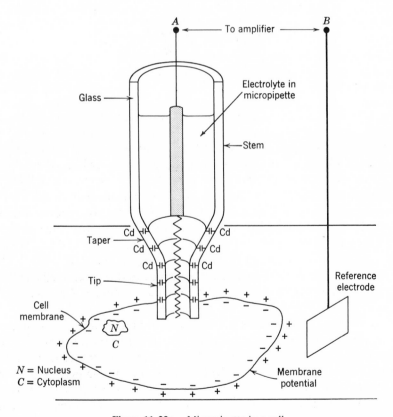

Figure 11–22a. Micropipette in a cell.

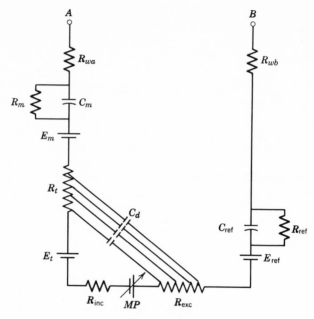

Figure 11–22b.

often chlorided silver, stainless steel or tungsten. Thus, in the circuit between the microelectrode and the indifferent electrode, there are actually four potentials, as shown in Fig. 11–22b. If we start from terminal A and trace out the circuit, the first potential encountered is E_m, the junctional potential between the electrode metal and the electrolyte filling the micropipette. If the fluid in the cell is different from that in the microelectrode tip, there will be a potential E_t at the tip. In practice the tip potential is larger than accountable for on the basis of ionic concentration differences (Nastuk, 1953; del Castillo and Katz, 1955; Adrian, 1956). Next to appear in the circuit is the membrane potential MP, followed by the potential between the indifferent electrode and the extracellular fluid E_{ref}. Thus the potential between the electrode terminals A,B consists of the sum of four potentials: E_m, E_t, MP and E_{ref}.

If we neglect the potentials for the moment and examine the impedances, in traversing the circuit there are encountered the resistance of the connecting wire R_{wa}, which is negligible, then the impedance of the electrode-electrolyte junction in the stem of the micropipette R_mC_m, the resistance R_t of the electrolyte filling the tip of the micropipette, the resistance of the electrolyte inside the cell R_{inc}, the resistance of the electrolyte outside the cell R_{exc}, the impedance of the reference electrode-electrolyte interface $R_{ref}C_{ref}$, and finally the resistance of the wire R_{wb} connecting the reference electrode to terminal B. All of these impedances form a series circuit in conjunction with the four potentials previously identified. In addition a distributed capacitance C_d exists between the fluid in the micropipette and the extracellular fluid. The magnitude of this important capacitance largely determines the response time of the microelectrode.

It is possible to assemble the components identified in Fig. 11–22b in an approximate equivalent circuit for the situation in which a micropipette is used to measure the membrane potential. In many measurement situations the relative magnitudes of the various impedances are known and it is therefore possible to simplify the circuit. For example, the resistance of the connecting wires R_{wa}, R_{wb} amounts to a fraction of an ohm and can be neglected. In the whole circuit, the resistance of the tip of the micropipette is by far the largest, amounting to about 10 to 200 megohms for typical microelectrodes filled with $3M$ KCl (Frank and Becker 1964). The area of the electrode-electrolyte interface in the stem is usually large or can be made large, resulting in the impedance of R_m C_m being negligible with respect to the 10- to 200-megohm resistance that exists at the tip. Likewise the resistance of the intracellular fluid R_{inc}, the resistance of the extracellular fluid R_{exc}, and the reference electrode-electrolyte impedance R_{ref}, C_{ref} can also be neglected. The distributed capacitance C_d cannot be neglected. Hence with reasonable accuracy the circuit can be reduced to that shown in Fig. 11–23a. This first simplification shows that the membrane potential MP is

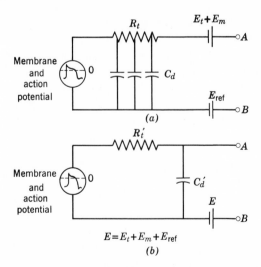

Figure 11–23. Equivalent circuits for a micropipette used to measure membrane and action potentials: (a) simplified circuit; (b) circuit with lumped parameters.

connected to the amplifier input terminals A, B via the 10- to 200-megohm resistance (R_t) of the tip of the micropipette, which is shunted by the distributed capacitance (C_d), amounting to about 0.5 $\mu\mu f$ per millimeter of tip length. Across the terminals a voltage appears which is the sum of the membrane potential, the potential of the electrode-electrolyte interface in the stem E_m, the tip potential E_t, and the potential of the reference electrode-electrolyte junction E_{ref}.

In many circumstances E_m, E_t, and E_{ref} are stable and can be corrected for in determining the membrane potential. Therefore they can be summed to form E. In addition, the distributed capacitance C_d and tip resistance R_t can be represented as shown in Fig. 11–23b, in which R_t' and C_d' are the single resistance and capacitance values which approximate the same electrical behavior as R_t with its distributed capacitance C_d.

Inspection of Fig. 11–23b shows that the membrane potential is coupled to the amplifier terminals A,B via a high series resistance and a moderate shunt capacitance. The effect of this particular combination of circuit elements is to place a limit on the response time of the circuit and hence restrict the faithful presentation of the rapidly changing portions of the action potential to the electrode terminals A,B.

In summary, therefore, the electrical characteristics of metal microelectrodes and of fluid-filled micropipettes are quite different. In the former, the metal electrode-electrolyte area is small and accounts for almost all of the impedance of the electrode; in the latter, the high impedance is constituted largely by the electrolyte-filled microtip. Both types require the use of an amplifying system having an input impedance many times higher than that of the microelectrode. Failure to use a high enough input impedance with the metal microelectrode causes it to behave as a high-pass filter. The micropipette behaves as a low-pass filter even when connected to an amplifier with a high input impedance. This limitation can be removed by the use of a "negative input capacity" amplifier (see Chapter 13). Under the conditions just described, the statement, attributed to Svaetichin by Gesteland et al. (1959), that metal microelectrodes resemble high-pass filters and micropipettes resemble low pass-filters is seen to be valid.

11–13. OHMIC NOISE

Another important characteristic of electrodes derives from the ohmic component of the electrode impedance. All resistors are generators of spurious voltages of all frequencies. This unwanted voltage, called Johnson noise after its discoverer (1928), results from the random motion of the charge carriers in the material making up the conductor. Johnson showed that the actual voltage measured is dependent on the magnitude of the resistance, the absolute temperature, and the bandwidth of the recording system. This voltage varies as the square root of these three quantities, and increasing any or all of them raises the noise voltage displayed by the recording system. For example, Terman (1943) stated that the thermal agitation voltage developed across a 500,000-ohm resistor at 27°C operating into a system with a bandwidth of 0 to 5000 cps is 6.4 μv rms. Although ohmic noise may not be an important factor when bioelectric recordings are made with large low-resistance electrodes, when the electrode resistance is high, as it is with microelectrodes, and the bandwidth of the recording equipment wide, resistive noise places a limit on the minimum signal detectable. For this reason it is advisable not to use a bandwidth in excess of that required for faithful reproduction of the waveform under investigation (see Chapter 14).

11–14. CONCLUSION

Although many penetrating studies of the electrochemistry of electrodes have been made, many factors remain to be investigated before there is an adequate description of the electrical nature of the circuit between a pair of electrodes from which a bioelectric event is recorded. Only when this is accomplished will it be possible to ascribe a proper magnitude to the type of distortion to be expected with the various electrodes and recording systems. The following statement, made by Curtis and Cole in 1938, retains much validity: "Unexplained effects, analogous to polarization impedance are found at metal-electrolyte interfaces, in imperfect dielectrics and internal viscosity of solids, but the equation which describes them all is purely empirical and the use of the term polarization impedance is an admission of our ignorance."

In summary, it is obvious that electrodes can produce their own distortions. To minimize galvanic potentials, the electrodes should be of the same metal and each should contact the same type of electrolyte. Although a steady electrode potential may not be bothersome, it nonetheless causes current to flow through the input resistance of the bioelectric recorder. Often this is not objectionable, but if electrodes are moved, the resistance of the circuit will alter and result in a change in current flowing through the input circuit. The use of electrodes with equal half-cell potentials and of a recording apparatus having high input impedance will minimize this type of artifact. Disturbance of the double layer at either electrode will also alter the half-cell potential. Stabilization can be attained by protecting the double layer by moving it away from the source of the movement. This is one of the reasons for the superiority of floating electrodes. Maintenance of a low current density at the electrode interface will reduce the tendency for the electrode impedance to distort the waveform of a bioelectric event. With large-area electrodes and a bioelectric recorder of high input impedance, the risk of encountering this type of distortion is minimized.

REFERENCES

Adrian, E. D., and D. W. Bronk, 1929. Impulses in motor nerve fibers, Part II. *J. Physiol.* **67**:119–151.

Adrain, R. H. 1956. The effect of internal and external potassium concentration on the membrane potential of frog muscle. *J. Physiol.* **133**:631–658.

Asa, M. M., A. H. Crews, E. L. Rothfield, E. S. Lewis, I. R. Zucker, and A. Berstein. 1964. High fidelity radioelectrocardiography. *Am. J. Cardiol.* **14**:530–532.

Atkins, A. R. 1961. Measuring heart rate of an active athlete. *Electron. Eng.* **33**:457.

Barnett, A. 1937. The basic factors involved in proposed electrical methods for measuring thyroid function. *Western J. Surg. Obs. Gyn.* **45**:540–554.

Basmajian, J. V. and G. Stecko. 1962. A new bipolar electrode for electromyography. *J. Appl. Physiol.* **17**:849.

Bell, G. H., J. A. C. Knox, and A. J. Small, 1939. Electrocardiography electrolytes. *Brit. Heart J.* **1**:229–236.

Blank, I. H., and I. G. Finesinger. 1946. Electrical resistance of the skin. *Arch. Neurol. Psychiat.* **54**:544–557.

Boter, J., A. den Hertog, and J. Kuiper 1966. Disturbance-free skin electrodes for persons during exercise. *Med. Biol. Eng.* **4**:91–95.

Burns, R. C. 1950. Study of skin impedance. *Electronics* **23**:190 and 196.

Burr, H. S., 1944, 1950. In O. Glasser (ed.), *Medical Physics*, 1944, Vol. 1; 1950, Vol. 2. Chicago, Yearbook Publishers.

Carbery, W. J., W. E. Tolles, and A. H. Freiman. 1960. A system for monitoring the ECG under dynamic conditions. *Aerospace Med.* **31**:131–137.

del Castillo, J., and B. Katz. 1955. Local activity at a depolarized nerve-muscle junction. *J. Physiol.* **128**:396–411.

Clark, L. C., and R. J. Lacey. 1950. An improved skin electrode. *J. Lab. Clin. Med.* **35**:786–787.

Cohn, A. E. 1920. A new method for use in clinical electrocardiography. *Arch. Int. Med.* **26**: 105–113.

Collias, J. C., and E. E. Manuelidis. 1957. Histopathological changes produced by implanted electrodes in cat brains. *J. Neurosurg.* **14**:302–328.

Cooper, R. 1956. Storage of silver chloride electrodes. *EEG. Clin. Neurophysiol.* **8**:692.

Cooper, R. 1963 Electrodes. *Am. J. EEG Technol.* **3**:91–101.

Curtis, H. J., and K. S. Cole. 1938. Transverse electric impedance of the squid giant axon. *J. Gen. Physiol.* **21**:757–765.

Davis, D. A., and W. E. Thornton, 1965. *Radiotelemetry in anesthesia and surgery.* International Anesthesiology Clinics. Boston, Mass., Little, Brown & Co., 586 pp.

Day, J., and M. Lippitt. 1964. A long term electrode system for electrocardiography and impedance pneumography. *Psychophysiology* **1**:174–182.

Delgado, J. M. R. 1952. Permanent implantation of multilead electrodes in the brain. *Yale J. Biol. Med.* **24**:351–358.

Delgado, J. M. R. 1955. Evaluation of permanent implantation of electrodes within the brain. *EEG Clin Neurophysiol.* 7:637–644.

Delgado, J. M. R. 1964. Electrodes for extracellular recording and stimulation. Chap. 3 in W. L. Nastuk (ed.), *Physical Techniques in Biological Research.* New York, Academic Press, 460 pp.

Dodge, H. W., C. Petersen, C. W. Sem-Jacobsen, G. P. Sayre, and R. G. Bickford. 1955. The paucity of demonstrable brain damage following intracerebral electrography: report of a case. *Proc. Staff Mtgs. Mayo Clinic* 30:215–221.

Dowben, R. M., and J. E. Rose. 1953. A metal-filled microelectrode. *Science* 118:22–24.

Dower, G. E., J. A. Osborne, and A. D. Moore. 1959. Measurement of the error in Wilson's central terminal. *Brit. Heart J.* 21:352–360.

Edelberg, R. 1963. Personal communication.

Edelberg, R., and N. R. Burch. 1962. Skin resistance and galvanic skin response. *Arch. Gen. Psychiat.* 7:163–169.

Einthoven, W. 1928. Die Aktionsstrome des Herzens. *Handbuch der Normalen und Pathologischen Physiologie.* Berlin, Julian Springer, pp. 758–862.

Fascenelli, F. W., C. Cordova, D. G. Simons, J. Johnson, L. Pratt, and L. E. Lamb, 1966. Biomedical monitoring during dynamic stress testing; 1. *Aerospace Med:* 37:911–922.

Fischer, G., G. P. Sayre, and R. G. Bickford 1957. Histologic changes in the cat's brain after introduction of metallic and plastic coated wire used in electroencephalography. *Proc. Staff Mtgs. Mayo Clinic* 32:14–22.

Forbes, A., S. Cobb, and McK. Cattell. 1921. An electrocardiogram and an electromyogram in an elephant. *Am. J. Physiol.* 55:385–389.

Forbes, T. W. 1934. An improved electrode for the measurement of potentials on the human body. *J. Lab. Clin. Med.* 19:1234–1238.

Frank, K., and M. Becker. 1964. Microelectrodes for recording and stimulation, in *Physical Techniques in Biological Research,* Vol. V, part A. New York and London, Academic Press, 460 pp.

Geddes, L. A. 1948–1949. Cortical electrodes. *EEG Clin. Neurophysiol.* 1:523. Illustrated on cover of *Sci. Amer.* 1948, 179, No. 4.

Geddes, L. A., and L. E. Baker 1966. The relationship between input impedance and electrode area in recording the ECG. *Med. Electr. Biol. Eng.* 4:439–450.

Geddes, L. A., and L. E. Baker 1967. Chlorided silver electrodes. *Med. Res. Eng.* 6: 33–34.

Geddes, L. A., L. E. Baker, and McGoodwin. 1967. The relationship between electrode area and amplifier input impedance in recording muscle action potentials. *Med. Biol. Eng.* 5:561–568.

Geddes, L. A., J. D. McCrady, H. E. Hoff, and A. Moore. 1964. Electrodes for large animals. *Southwestern Vet.* 18:56–57.

Geddes, L. A., M. Partridge, and H. E. Hoff. 1960. An EKG lead for exercising subjects. *J. Appl. Physiol.* 15:311–312.

Gesteland, R. C., B. Howland, J. Y. Lettvin, and W. H. Pitts. 1959. Comments on microelectrodes. *Proc. IRE.* 47:1856–1862.

Gibson, T. C., W. E. Thornton, W. P. Algary, and E. Craige. 1962. Telecardiography and the use of simple computers. *New Engl. J. Med.* 267:1218–1224.

Goldstein, A. G., W. Sloboda, and J. B. Jennings. 1962. Spontaneous electrical activity of three types of silver EEG electrodes. *Psychophysiol. Newsletter* 8:10–16.

Grahame, D. C. 1941. Properties of the electrical double layer at a mercury surface. *J. Am. Chem. Soc.* 63:1207–1214.

Grahame, D. C. 1952. Mathematical theory of the faradic admittance. *J. Electrochem. Soc.* **99**:370C–385C.

Gray, J. A. G., and G. Svaetichin. 1951–1952. Electrical properties of platinum tipped microelectrodes. *Acta Physiol. Scand.* **24**:278–284.

Greenwald, D. U. 1936. Electrodes used in measuring electrodermal responses. *Am. J. Psychol.* **48**:658–662.

Grundfest, H., and B. Campbell. 1942. Origin, conduction and termination of impulses in dorsal spino-cerebellar tracts of cats. *J. Neurophysiol.* **5**:275–294.

Grundfest, H., R. W. Sengstaken, and W. H. Oettinger. 1950. Stainless steel microneedle made by electro-pointing. *Rev. Sci. Instrs.* **21**:360–361.

Guld, C. 1964. A glass-covered platinum microelectrode. *Med. Electr. Biol. Eng.* **2**:317–327.

Haggard, E. A., and R. Gerbrands. 1947. An apparatus for the measurement of continuous changes in palmar skin resistance. *J. Exp. Psychol.* **37**:92–98.

Hendler, E., and L. J. Santa Maria. 1961. Response of subjects to some conditions of a simulated orbital flight pattern. *Aerospace. Med.* **32**:126–133.

Henry, F. 1938. Dependable electrodes for the galvanic skin response. *J. Gen. Psychol.* **18**: 209–211.

Hill, D. 1967. In Hales, Marey, and Chauveau, Report on 1966 course "Classical Physiology with Modern Instrumentation." NIH Grant Report HE 05125.

Hubel, D. H. 1957. Tungsten microelectrode for recording from single units. *Science* **125**: 549–550.

James, W. B., and H. B. Williams. 1910. The electrocardiogram in clinical medicine. *Am. J. Med. Sci.* **140**:408–421.

Janz, G. J., and F. J. Kelly. 1964. Reference electrodes. In C. A, Hampel (ed.), *Encyclopedia of Electrochemistry.* New York, Reinhold Pub. Co., 1206 pp.

Janz, G. J., and H. Taniguchi. 1953. The silver-silver halide electrodes. *Chem. Rev.* **53**: 397–437.

Jasper, H. H., R. T. Johnson, and L. A. Geddes. 1945. The RCAMC electromyograph. Can. Amy. Med. Report C6174.

Jenks, J. L., and A. Graybiel. 1935. A new simple method of avoiding high resistance and overshooting in taking standardized electrocardiograms. *Am. Heart J.* **10**:683–695.

Johnson, J. B. 1928. Thermal agitation of electricity in conductors. *Phys. Rev.* **32**:97–109.

Kado, R. T. 1965. Personal communication.

Kado, R. T., W. R. Adey, and J. R. Zweizig. 1964. Electrode system for recording EEG from physically active subjects. *Proc. 17th Ann. Conf. Eng. Med. Biol.*, Cleveland, Ohio. Washington, McGregor and Werner, 129 pp.

Kahn A. 1964. Fundamentals of biopotentials and their measurement. Biomedical Sciences Instrumentation, 1964, Dallas, Texas. *Am. J. Pharm. Educ.* **28**:805–814.

Kahn, A. 1965. Motion artifacts and streaming potentials in relation to biological electrodes. *Digest 6th Int. Conf. Med. Electr. Biol. Eng.*, Tokyo, Japan, pp. 562–563.

Kennard, D. W. 1958. Glass microcapillary electrodes. Chap. 35 in P.E.K. Donaldson (ed.), *Electronic Apparatus for Biological Research*, London, Butterworth's Scientific Publication's 718 pp.

King, E. E. 1964. Errors in voltage in multichannel ECG recordings using newer electrode materials. *Am. Heart J.* **18**:295–297.

Lewes, D. 1965a. Electrode jelly in electrocardiography. *Brit. Heart J.* **27**:105–115.

Lewes, D. 1965b. Multipoint electrocardiography without skin preparation. *Lancet* **2**: 17–18. U.K. Patent application 52253/64.

Lewes, D., and D. Hill. 1966. Personal communication.

Lewis, T. 1914–1915. Polarisable as against non-polarisable electrodes. *J. Physiol.* **49**:L-Lii.

Lucchina, G. G., and C. G. Phipps. 1962. A vectorcardiographic lead system and physiologic electrode configuration for dynamic readout. *Aerospace Med.* 33:722–729.

Lucchina, G. G., and C. G. Phipps. 1963. An improved electrode for physiological recording. Aerospace Med. 34:230:231.

Lykken, D. T. 1959. Properties of electrodes used in electrodermal measurement. *J. Comp. Physiol. Psychol.* 52:629–634.

Marchant, E. W., and E. W. Jones. 1940. The effect of electrodes of different metals on the skin current. *Brit. Heart J.* 2:97–100.

Marmont, G. 1949. Studies on the axon membrane. *J. Cell. Comp. Physiol.* 34:351–382.

Mason, R. E., and I. Likar. 1966. A new system of multiple lead electrocardiography. *Am. Heart J.* 71:196–205.

Maxwell, J. 1957 and 1958. Preparation of the skin for electrocardiography. *Brit. Med. J.* 1957, 2:942; 1958, 1:41.

Mills, L. W. 1962. A fast inexpensive method of producing large quantities of metallic microelectrodes. *EEG Clin. Neurophysiol.* 14:278–279.

Nastuk, W. 1953. The electrical activity of the muscle cell membrane at the neuromuscular junction. *J. Cell. Comp. Physiol.* 42:249–283.

O'Connell, D. N., and B. Tursky. Special modifications of the silver-silver chloride sponge electrode for skin recording. U.S. Air Force Office of Scientific Research. Contact AF 49 (638)-728, 37 pp.

O'Connell, D. N., B. Tursky, and M. T. Orne. 1960. Electrodes for recording skin potential. *Arch. Gen. Psychiat.* 3:252–258.

Offner, F. F. 1942. Electrical properties of tissues in shock therapy. *Proc. Soc. Exp. Biol. Med.* 49:571–575.

Pardee, H. E. B. 1917a. Concerning the electrodes used in electrocardiography. *Am. J. Physiol.* 44:80–83.

Pardee, H. E. B. 1917b. An error in the electrocardiogram arising in the application of the electrodes. *Arch. Int. Med.* 20:161–166.

Parker, T. G. 1966. Personal communication. V. A. Hospital, Houston, Texas.

Parsons, R. 1964. Electrode double layer. In C. A. Hampel (ed.), In *The Encyclopedia of Electrochemistry*. New York, Reinhold Pub. Co., 1206 pp.

Patten, C. W., F. B. Ramme, and J. Roman. 1966. Dry electrodes for physiological monitoring. NASA Technical Note NASA TN D-3414. National Aeronautics and Space Administration, Washington, D.C., 32 pp.

Plutchik, R., and H. R. Hirsch. 1963. Skin impedance and phase angle as a function of frequency and current. *Science* 141:927–928.

Rappaport, M. B., C. Williams, and P. D. White, 1949. An analysis of the relative accuracies of the Wilson and Goldberger methods for registering unipolar and augmented unipolar electrocardiographic leads. *Am. Heart J.* 37:892–917.

Ray, C. D. 1966. A new-multipurpose human brain probe. *J. Neurosurg.* 24:911–921.

Robinson, F. R., and M. T. Johnson. 1961. Histopathological studies of tissue reactions to various metals planted in cat brains. ASD Tech. Rep. 61–397, 13 pp. USAF Wright-Patterson AFB, Ohio.

Roman, J. 1966. Flight research program—III. High impedance electrode techniques. *Aerospace Med.* 37:790–795.

Roman, J., and L. Lamb. 1962. Electrocardiography in flight. *Aerospace Med.* 33:527–544.

Rose, K. D. 1963. Telemetering physiologic data from athletes. *Proc. Intern at. Telemetering Conf.* 1:225–241.

Roth, I. 1933–1934. A self-retaining skin contact electrode for chest leads in electrocardiography. *Am. Heart J.* 9:526–529.

Rothschild, Lord, 1938. The polarization of a calomel electrode. *Proc. Roy. Soc (London)* *Ser. B.* **125**:283–290.

Rowland, V. 1961. Simple non-polarizable electrode for chronic implantation. *EEG Clin. Neurophysiol.* **13**:290–291.

Rowley, D. A., S. Glagov, and P. Stoner. 1961. Fluid electrodes for monitoring the electro-cardiogram during activity and for prolonged periods of time. *Am. Heart J.* **62**:263–269.

Schmitt, O. H., M. Okajima, and M. Blaug. 1961. Skin preparation and electrocardiographic lead impedance. *Digest IRE Internat. Conf. Med. Electron.* New York. Washington, D.C., McGregor and Werner, 288 pp.

Schwan, H. P. 1963. Determination of biological impedances. In W. Nastuk (ed.),*Physical Techniques in Biological Research*, Vol. VI, part B. New York and London, Academic Press, 425 pp.

Schwan, H. P., and J. G. Maczuk. 1965. Electrode polarization impedance; limits of linearity. *Proc. 18th Ann. Conf. Eng. Biol. Med.* Philadelphia, Pa. Washington, D. C., McGregor and Werner, 270 pp.

Schwarzchild, M. M., I. Hoffman, and M. Kissin. 1954. Errors in unipolar limb leads caused by unbalanced skin resistances, and a device for their elimination. *Am. Heart J.* **48**:235–248.

Scott, R. N. 1965. A method of inserting wire electrodes for electromyography. *IEEE Trans. Bio-Med. Eng.* BME–**12**:46–47.

Seelig, M. C. 1925. Localized gangrene following the hypodermic administration of calcium chloride. *J. Am. Med. Assoc.* **84**:1413–1414.

Shackel, B. 1958. A rubber suction cup surface electrode with high electrical stability. *J. Appl.* **13**:153–158.

Shackel, B. 1959. Skin drilling: a method for diminishing galvanic skin potentials. *Am. J. Psychol.* **72**:114–121.

Simons, D. G., W. Prather, and F. K. Coombs. 1965. Personalized telemetry medical monitoring and performance data-gathering for the 1962 SAM-MATS fatigue study. SAM-TR-65-17. USAF Brooks AFB, Texas.

Skov, E. R., and D. G. Simons. 1965. EEG electrodes for in-flight monitoring. SAM-TR-65-18. USAF Brooks AFB, Texas.

Sullivan, G. H., and G. Weltman. 1961. A low mass electrode for bioelectric recording. *J. Appl. Physiol.* **16**:939–940.

Sutter, von C. 1944. Ueber die Beeinfluss der Ekg-curve durch elektrische Eigenschaften der Aufnahmeanordrung. *Cardiologia*, **8**:246–262.

Svaetichin, G. 1951. Low resistance microelectrode. *Acta Physiol. Scand. Suppl. 86*, **24**:1–13.

Tasaki, I. 1952–1953. Properties of myelinated fibers in a frog sciatic nerve and in spinal cord as examined with microelectrodes. *Japan. J. Physiol.* **3**:73–94.

Taylor, C. V. 1925. Microelectrodes and micromagnets. *Proc. Soc. Exp. Biol. Med.* **23**: 147–150.

Telemedics, Inc. 1961. *Medical Electronics News.* **1**(4):9.

Terman, F. E. 1943. *Radio Engineers Handbook*, 1st ed. New York, McGraw-Hill, 1019. pp.

Thompson, N. P., and J. A. Patterson. 1958. Solid salt bridge contact electrodes—System for monitoring the ECG during body movement. Techn. Rep. 58–453. ASTIA Doc. AD215538. April.

Ungerleider, H. E. 1939. A new precordial electrode. *Am. Heart J.* **18**:94.

Weale, R. A. 1951. A new micro-electrode for electrophysiological work. *Nature* **167**:529.

Weinman, J., and J. Mahler. 1964. An analysis of electrical properties of metal electrodes. *Med. Elect. Biol. Eng.* **2**:299–310.

Whalen, R. E., C. F. Starmer, and D. H. McIntosh, 1964. Electrical hazards associated with cardiac pacemaking. *Annals N.Y. Acad. Sci.* **111**:922–931.

Wilson, F. N., F. C. Johnston, A. G. Macleod, and P. S. Baker. 1934. Electrocardiograms that represent the potential variations of a single electrode. *Am. Heart J.* **9**:447–458.

Woodbury, J. W., and A. J. Brady. 1956. Intracellular recording from moving tissues with a flexibly mounted ultramicroelectrode. *Science* **123**:100–101.

Woodbury, L. A., J. W. Woodbury, and H. Hecht. 1950. Membrane and resting action potentials of single cardiac fibers. *Circulation* **1**:264–266.

12

The Bioelectric Events

12–1 ORIGIN OF BIOELECTRIC EVENTS

Electrical potentials exist across the enveloping membranes of living cells, and many cells have the ability to propagate a change in these potentials. Nerve, muscle, and gland, as well as many plant cells, exhibit this phenomenon, which is related to the functioning of the cell. When such a cell responds to a stimulus, the membrane potential exhibits a series of reversible changes which are called the action potential. Action potentials, unlike many other physiological events, require no specialized transducers for their detection. Suitable electrodes, amplification, and appropriate display are the only requirements for their presentation.

Because each type of cell exhibits a characteristic electrical activity, measurement of this activity yields important information relating to cellular function. From this fact has developed the clinical study of bioelectric signals, which usually deals with the measurement of the electrical activity of large numbers of cells. Because dysfunction frequently reveals itself in the bioelectric signal, much diagnostic information can be obtained from such recordings. In this chapter are presented simplified explanations of the manner in which living cells develop action potentials and present them to electrodes.

Because many of the bioelectric signals can be detected at a distance from their source, the electrographic devices, by virtue of their ability to "peer" inside the body, can be likened to the x-ray, which reveals information hidden from view. In addition, the measurement of a bioelectric signal usually does not interfere with the event being measured, resulting in a true electrical representation of function. Moreover, because of the great practicality and ease of making electrographic recordings on human subjects, the techniques are ideally applicable to clinical medicine. There is little doubt that, because of these facts, the future will see a considerable expansion of electrographic techniques.

Although the bioelectric signals recorded from the various cells vary considerably in amplitude and form, they all have a common origin in the membrane potential, which is the potential difference that exists between the interior and exterior surfaces of the cell. The enveloping membrane serves as a semipermeable barrier to the passage of certain substances and ions. The resulting ionic gradient is maintained by virtue of metabolic energy expended by the cell. In mammalian nerve cells, for example, the concentration of potassium ion is in the vicinity of 30 times higher inside the cell than in the extracellular fluid. On the other hand, sodium ion is approximately 10 times more concentrated in the fluid bathing the outside of the cell than in the intracellular fluid; similar conditions obtain for other ions. The net result is a potential difference across the membrane with the inside negative with respect to the outside. Membrane potentials vary within wide limits, ranging from a few tens of millivolts to about 100 mv. Table 12–1 presents the resting membrane potentials of a variety of cells measured under the circumstances indicated.

In response to a stimulus of adequate intensity to cause local depolarization, many types of cells propagate this disturbance over their membranes. The process of depolarization, reverse polarization, and repolarization constitutes the action potential. In nerve the propagated disturbance travels at a rate governed by the nerve fiber diameter and the temperature. The speed of propagation in the fastest nerves is approximately 150 meters per second, which represents the highest rate of propagation in any tissue. In muscle propagation is much slower and contraction follows development of the action potential.

The genesis of the action potential can be understood by considering a single strip of irritable tissue (as shown in Fig. 12–1) forming whole or part of a cell in which the membrane is intact and an ionic gradient exists to produce a membrane potential of 70 mv. This potential is measured by placing an electrode A on the intact surface of the cell and inserting a microelectrode[1] B into the cell. In Fig. 12–1(2), at the arrow, the microelectrode has penetrated the cell membrane, revealing the resting membrane potential at electrode A.

Assume now that a stimulus intense enough to depolarize the membrane is applied elsewhere to the same cell. An ionic current will flow from the surrounding polarized region to the depolarized area. This current is adequate to depolarize the adjacent regions, and a wave of depolarization will travel in all directions over the membrane.

[1] A microelectrode must be small with respect to the size of the cell so that its insertion will not produce cellular damage.

Table 12-1 Resting Membrane Potentials

Type of Tissue	Type of Environment	Membrane* Potential (mv)	Investigator and Year
Frog: myelinated axon	Excised—Ringer's	67.6± 1.4	Huxley and Stampfli (1951)
Rabbit: superior cervical ganglion cell	Excised—physiological solutions	65–80	Eccles (1955)
Cat: spinal motoneuron soma	In vivo	70	Coombs, Eccles and Fatt (1955)
Cat: cortical pyramidal cell	In vivo	55	Phillips (1955)
Rat: skeletal muscle fiber	In vivo	99.8± 0.19	Bennett, Ware, Dunn, and McIntyre (1953)
Dog: papillary muscle	Excised	85	Hoffman and Suckling (1953)
Dog: auricle	Excised	85	Hoffmann and Suckling (1953)
Dog: Purkinje fiber	Excised—Tyrode's	90	Draper and Weidmann (1951)
Guinea pig: intestinal smooth muscle fiber	Excised—physiological solutions	51.5–70	Holman (1958)
Kid: Purkinje fiber	Excised	94	Draper and Weidmann (1951)
Frog: ventricle	In vivo—Ringer's	62	Woodbury et al., (1950)
Squid: giant axon	Excised—sea water	45	Hodgkin and Huxley (1939)
Frog: skeletal muscle	Excised—Ringer's	92.2	Adrian (1956)
Frog: myoneural junction	Excised—Ringer's	90	Natsuk (1953)

*Interior of the cell is negative with respect to the exterior.

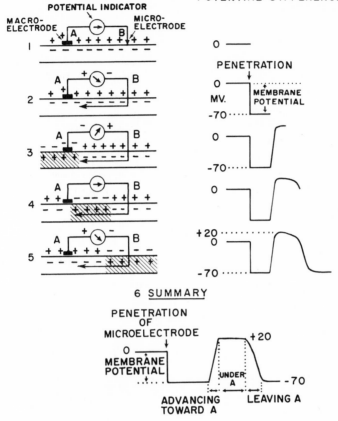

Figure 12–1.   Genesis of the monophasic action potential.

In most cells the process does not consist merely of depolarization; a slight reverse polarization also is found to occur, causing the outside of the portion of the cell which is active to be negative with respect to the inside. When this wave of depolarization-reverse polarization advances under electrode *A* [Fig. 12–1(3)], the potential indicator, which was previously indicating the membrane potential, shows a potential that drops to zero (depolarization of the membrane), and then a potential that is in the opposite direction to the membrane potential, indicating that the region of reverse polarization is under *A*. This sequence of events is shown on the right of Fig. 12–1(3).

As the wave of depolarization-reverse polarization advances, in its wake the metabolic activity of the cell causes recovery (re-establishment of the membrane potential) to occur. Thus, as the wave passes electrode *A* [Fig. 12–1(4)], the membrane potential is becoming restored, and when full repolarization has occurred the potential indicator reads the membrane potential again [Fig. 12–1(5)]. When the wave passes point B, the potential indicator shows no change because the electrode is inside the cell.

This sequence of events is summarized in Fig. 12–1(6), in which it is seen that the fundamental bioelectric event consists of a traveling wave of changing membrane polarity; first depolarization, then reverse polarization, followed by re-establishment of the membrane potential. Many cells exhibit a rapid depolarization and repolarization. Action potentials of such short duration are called spikes. In many cells during recovery the rate of repolarization slows, and there appears another component called the negative afterpotential. Some cells overshoot their repolarization to produce what is called a positive afterpotential. Some even produce a second negative afterpotential before stabilization of the membrane potential occurs. In pacemaker cells, before the propagated action potential there occurs a decay in membrane potential called the prepotential. The prepotential is respresentative of an unstable membrane potential, which upon reaching a critical value causes the cell to depolarize and a propagated action potential results. In summary, a bioelectric event derives its form from the manner in which a cell membrane depolarizes to produce a simple or complex action potential. Compilations of the various forms of action potentials have been presented by Grundfest (1947, 1966), Hodgkin (1951), and Durnstock et al. (1963).

A diagrammatic representation of the sequence of events that a hypothetical cell may display is shown in Fig. 12–2. Depolarization is rapid; repolarization is slower and follows a time course which is characteristic of the type of cell, resulting not in a flat-topped action potential, as sketched in Fig. 12–1, but in a smooth curve, as shown in Fig. 12–2. In this illustration are diagramed four of the types of potential changes exhibitable

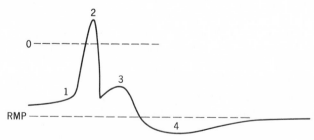

Figure 12–2. Changes in membrane potential for a hypothetical cell, showing prepotential (1), spike (2), negative (3), and positive (4) after potentials. RMP is the resting membrane potential.

by an irritable cell: (1) the prepotential, (2) the spike, (3) the negative afterpotential, and (4) the positive afterpotential.

During passage of the wave of depolarization, a small quantity of heat is liberated, the membrane impedance drops, and there is movement of ions across the cell membrane. Many of the extracellular ions enter the cell, and many of those in the cell move outward. During recovery there is a flow of the same ions in the opposite direction to re-establish the membrane potential; the inward and outward flows do not occur at the same rate. The rate of occurrence of this sequence of events and consequently the form of the action potential are characteristic of each type of cell.

The part of the cell that is occupied by the propagated wave of depolarization is unable to respond to a second stimlulus, and for this reason it is said to be refractory. However, during repolarization there is a cyclic variation in excitability, for a strong stimulus delivered early in the recovery phase will often produce another response. Later, during the phase of the negative afterpotential (if it occurs), when the membrane is almost fully repolarized, a weaker stimulus will often produce a response. During a positive afterpotential (if it occurs), an effective stimulus would need to be stronger. Thus the action potential, in addition to indicating that a cell is active, reveals the approximate time when it can be reactivated.

Figures 12–3 to 12–6 illustrate typical monophasic action potentials of various cells measured with microelectrodes. The monophasic action potential of a single nerve fiber of the squid is shown in Fig. 12–3. This fiber is so large (ca. 100 microns) that it is relatively easy to make a microelectrode to study the membrane and action potential. In addition the large size permits cannulation and replacement of the axoplasm with solutions of known ionic content. As illustrated, the membrane potential measured in sea water at 20°C was 45 mv, and during the spike the membrane potential became nearly +40 mv. Thus the total amplitude of the action potential was 85 mv. During the recovery phase a positive afterpotential was recorded.

The action potential of a single frog skeletal muscle fiber and its relationship to the twitch is shown in Fig. 12–4. In this experiment the resting membrane potential was −92 mv, and at the peak of the spike the potential difference was +30 mv. During recovery a negative afterpotential is clearly visible.

The membrane potential changes in frog cardiac muscle are shown in Fig. 12–5. Starting from a resting value of about −55 mv, during peak activity the membrane potential became about +25 mv. Because recovery is prolonged in cardiac muscle, a relatively flat-topped monophasic action potential is produced. Clearly evident in this illustration is a positive afterpotential.

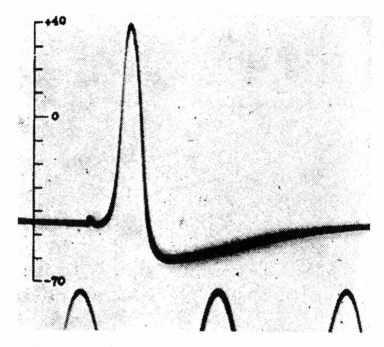

Figure 12–3. Membrane and action potential of giant axon of squid. Time pulses = 2 ms. [From Hodgkin and Huxley, *Nature* **144**:711 (1939). By permission.]

The electrical activity of smooth muscle of the guinea pig gut is shown in Fig. 12–6. During activity the membrane potential is seen to change from −46 mv to +10 mv. During recovery the afterpotentials previously mentioned can be seen.

In order to understand how a bioelectric event appears to a pair of distant electrodes, it is first necessary to analyze two situations in which

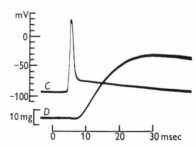

Figure 12–4. Action potential of a single skeletal muscle fibre in the frog (*C*) and the tension developed (*D*). [From Hodgkin and Horowicz, *J. Physiol.* **136**:18P (1957). By permission.]

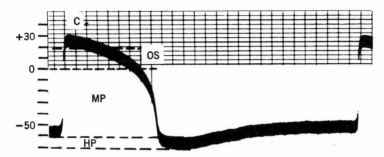

Figure 12–5. Membrane and action potential in a single cardiac muscle fiber in the frog. [From Woodbury et al., *Circulation* **1**:264–266 (1950). By permission of the American Heart Association.]

both electrodes are active, that is, both are on the intact surface of a strip of irritable tissue. The first is diagramed in Fig. 12–7. In this idealized situation it is assumed that the electrodes are small and widely separated. The dimensions were chosen so that the traveling wave of excitation and recovery in the tissue occupies a small fraction of the electrode spacing. In addition, the bioelectric event is considered as a simple monophasic action potential without prepotentials and after-potentials.

In Fig. 12–7(1), when the tissue is inactive, both electrodes are in regions of equal positivity and the potential difference seen by the indicator is zero. When the region under electrode A is excited, this electrode becomes negative with respect to electrode B and the indicator rises [Fig. 12–7(2)]. As the wave of excitation passes onward toward electrode B and occupies the region between the two electrodes, the region under A is recovered and that under B is not excited. Under these conditions no voltage is

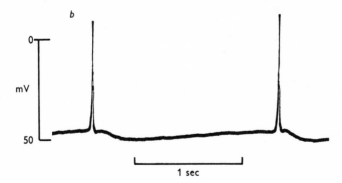

Figure 12–6. Membrane and action potential of single smooth muscle fibre of guinea pig gut. [From Holman, *J. Physiol.* **141**: 466 (1958). By permission.]

registered by the potential indicator [Fig. 12–7(3)] and the first (upward) phase of the monphasic action potential has been completed. As the wave of excitation occupies the region under electrode *B*, this electrode becomes negative with respect to *A* and hence the potential indicator falls [Fig. 12–7(4)]. As the wave of excitation passes *B*, recovery occurs; the membrane potential is re-established, the potential indicator reads zero, and the downward phase of the action potential is completed. Under these circumstances the time between the two phases of the action potential is determined by the speed of conduction in the tissue and the spacing of the electrodes. If the electrodes are appropriately spaced, the two monophasic action potentials will fuse to form a continuous and symmetrical biphasic action potential. If the temporal relations are such that the monophasic action potentials overlap, a smaller action potential will result. This situation is diagramed in Fig. 12–7(6).

In the situations analyzed thus far, the electrodes were placed along the direction of depolarization and repolarization. If they are placed opposite each other on either side of the uniform strip of irritable tissue, as shown in Fig. 12–8(1), the indicator will show no potential difference. When the wave of excitation arrives at the electrodes [Fig.12–8(2)],

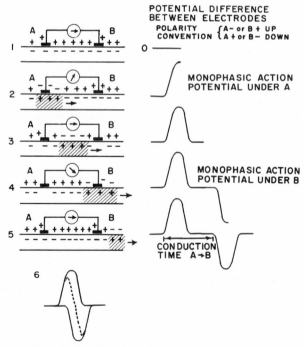

Figure 12–7. Genesis of the biphasic action potential.

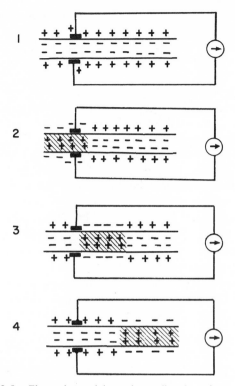

Figure 12–8.   Electrodes at right angles to direction of propagation.

depolarization and reverse polarization will occur simultaneously under both electrodes and the indicator will show no potential difference. As the wave of excitation passes onward and repolarization occurs, as shown in Fig. 12–8(3, 4), the indicator will continue to show no potential difference.

The second situation which must be examined before discussing the signals detected by distant electrodes is shown in Fig. 12–9. The foregoing examples considered uniform strips of irritable tissue in which the wave of excitation occupied a small portion of the tissue and was followed by recovery in a relatively short time. Although this situation is valid for nerve and skeletal muscle, it does not apply to cardiac muscle, in which the refractory period is long and the wave of excitation advances and occupies the whole of the tissue before recovery occurs. Moreover, in many circumstances recovery does not necessarily travel in the same direction as excitation. Therefore the action potentials developed under these conditions are expected to be different from those previously discussed.

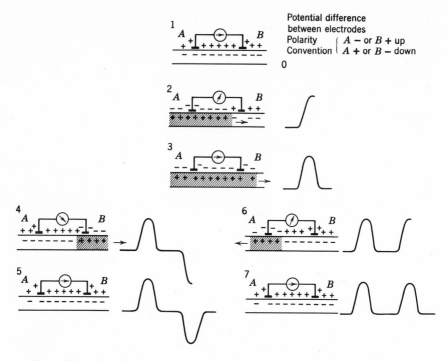

Figure 12–9. Genesis of an action potential in a tissue with a long refractory period.

Figure 12–9(1) diagrams a strip of irritable tissue in which the refractory period is long. Assume that the tissue has been stimulated and that a wave of excitation advances and occupies the region under electrode A [Fig. 12–9(2)]. Thus A is negative with respect to electrode B and the potential indicator rises. The wave of excitation continues to advance and ultimately occupies the region under electrode B. Because the refractory period is long, recovery will not have occurred under electrode A; hence both electrodes are over active tissue and the indicator shows no potential difference. Thus the first upward phase of the action potential will be described as shown in Fig. 12–9(3).

The sequence of events that follows depends upon the manner in which recovery takes place. If the strip of irritable tissue is uniform, recovery follows in the same direction as excitation. If this situation obtains [Fig. 12–9(4)], recovery will occur first under electrode A. Under this condition electrode B is negative, A is positive, and the potential indicator falls. When recovery occurs under electrode B, the potential indicator reads zero and the second (downward) phase of the action potential is completed as shown in Fig. 12–9(5).

In the sequence of events just described, the two monophasic action potentials have a special meaning. The peak of the first upward monophasic action potential indicates excitation under electrode A. The end of this action potential shows that the whole tissue is active. The beginning of the downward wave indicates that recovery is starting under electrode A, and recovery under this electrode becomes complete when the peak of the downward action potential is reached. Completion of the downward action potential shows full recovery of the tissue.

If the strip of irritable tissue is not uniform or a metabolic gradient exists, the sequence of events just described will not occur. If, when all of the tissue is active as shown in Fig. 12–9(3), recovery proceeds in the direction opposite to that of excitation, the second phase of the action potential will be different. In Fig. 12–9(6) recovery is shown to proceed from right to left, resulting in electrode B becoming positive with respect to A. Thus the potential indicator will rise, and the second phase of the monophasic action potential will be upward, that is, in the same direction as the first. As the tissue fully recovers, the second (upward) phase of the action potential is completed [Fig. 12–9(7)].

In the case just analyzed, the peak of the first upward phase described excitation under electrode A. At the end of the first monophasic action potential, when the indicator read zero, all of the tissue was active. The beginning of the second upward phase indicated the start of recovery under electrode B, which was complete when the second upward monophasic action potential was completed.

Thus in irritable tissue, in which the refractory period is long, if the two phases of the action potential are in opposite directions, excitation and recovery travel in the same direction. If the two phases are in the same direction, excitation and recovery travel in opposite directions.

The manner in which these fundamental facts can be shown to underlie the genesis of the ECG is shown in Fig. 12–10. In Fig. 12–10a the ECG was obtained with a macroelectrode and a microelectrode which, in the first part of the record, rested on the outside of a cardiac muscle cell. In the left of the illustration can be seen the familiar QRS-T complex of the ECG. In the middle of the record the microelectrode was pushed into a single cardiac muscle cell and the ECG was replaced by a monophasic action potential. Figure 12–10b shows the relationship between the ECG and the simultaneously recorded monophasic action potential.

In Fig. 12–11 are shown monophasic action potentials recorded from a frog ventricle. Because the recorder sees the algebraic temporal sum of the monophasic action potentials, the voltage recorded is the familiar R-T complex of the ECG. This situation is diagramed in Fig. 12–11c. The solid

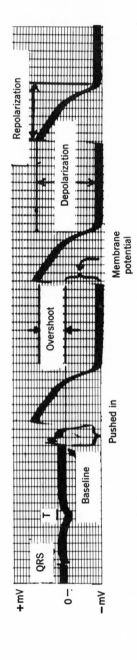

Figure 12–10a. Relationship of the electrocardiogram to the monophasic action potential. [From Hecht, *Ann. N.Y. Acad. Sci.* **65**: 7(1956–57). By permission.]

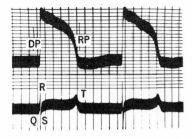

Figure 12–10b. Simultaneously recorded monophasic action potentials and the ECG, [From Hecht, *Ann. N. Y. Acad. Sci.* **65**: 7(1956–57). By permission.]

line represents the summated ECG developed when excitation and recovery travel in the same direction, that is, the monophasic action potentials are alike but displaced in time. The dotted line in Fig. 12–11*b* illustrates the situation when recovery occurs earlier at the last electrode to become active. The effect is to make the T wave upward, as shown dotted in Fig. 12–11*c*. That the ECG originated in this way was suggested by Burdon-Sanderson 1880, long before the action potentials of single cells were recordable.

The ECG, as conventionally recorded, reflects the potential difference between a pair of electrodes on the surface of the body. The origin of this time-dependent potential difference resides in the muscle fibers which make up the two masses of the heart, the atria and the ventricles, each fiber

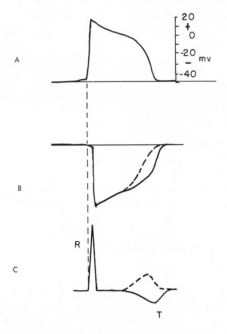

Figure 12–11. Summation of the monophasic action potentials to produce the ECG. (From Hoff and Geddes, Experimental Physiology, Baylor Medical College, Houston, Tex. By permission.)

producing its own action potential. Thus the ECG is the result of the temporal and spatial summation of the activities of all of the myocardial fibers. Notwithstanding the obvious complexity of the resultant potential difference, it is interesting to see how the nature of the fundamental bioelectric generator, the monophasic action potential, reveals itself in recordings made with appropriately placed surface electrodes.

The manner in which initial polarity indicates direction of propagation of the wave of excitation can be demonstrated easily. For example, in the normal mammalian heart, because excitation of the ventricles advances generally from base to apex and the polarity for recording the ECG is chosen so that in lead II negativity of the right arm electrode (and hence positivity of the left leg) causes the indicator to deflect upward, the monophasic action potentials summate to cause the R wave of the ECG to be upward, as shown in Fig. 12–11c. If excitation travels in the opposite direction (apex to base), the downward monophasic action potential will occur first and the R wave will be inverted.

In the experimental animal, if excitation is forced to travel in the normal direction from the base to the apex, by application of a stimulus to the base of the heart, the R wave is upward, as shown by R' in Fig. 12–12. If excitation is forced to travel from apex to base by delivery of a stimulus to the apex, the primary wave of excitation, QS in Fig. 12–12, will be downward. Note that in both instances the waves of excitation (R' and QS) are longer in duration than the normally conducted waves of excitation because the evoked extrasystoles traveled in myocardium, which has a slower conduction rate than the specialized conduction system of the heart (bundle of His and Purkinje fibers).

The situation of hastened recovery of the tissue under the electrode last to be excited can also be demonstrated experimentally. Figure 12–13 shows the ECG of a dog, recorded with one electrode on the right fore-limb and the other applied directly to the apex of the left ventricle. The ventricular electrode (thermode) was a hollow metallic chamber through which cold or warm water could be circulated.

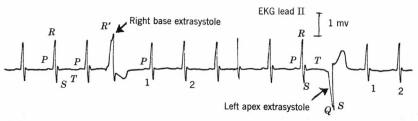

Figure 12–12. Normal canine ECG, showing induced ventricular basal (R') and apical (QS) systoles.

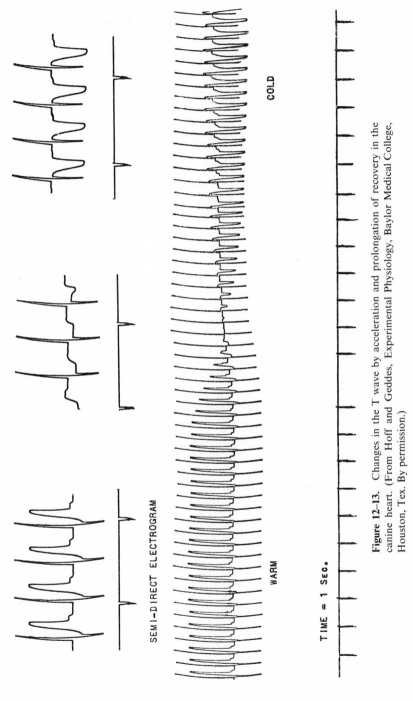

SEMI-DIRECT ELECTROGRAM

COLD

WARM

TIME = 1 SEC.

Figure 12-13. Changes in the T wave by acceleration and prolongation of recovery in the canine heart. (From Hoff and Geddes, Experimental Physiology, Baylor Medical College, Houston, Tex. By permission.)

When warm water was circulated through the thermode (Fig. 12–13, left), local metabolism was increased and recovery was hastened. Under these conditions the T wave became large and upright. By circulating cold water through the electrode recovery was prolonged, hence the T wave became inverted. This sequence of events is shown on the right in Fig. 12–13. In the center of the record it can be seen that at an intermediate temperature the T wave disappeared, indicating that the recovery occurred simultaneously in the regions of the ventricles seen by both electrodes.

Thus it is apparent that the form of an action potential, as detected by the pair of electrodes on the surface of a strip of homogeneous irritable tissue, is dependent on the time course of depolarization, reverse polarization, and repolarization, the speed with which it travels in the tissue, the amount of tissue occupied by the wave of excitation, and the orientation of the electrodes with respect to the direction of propagation of the wave of excitation, and recovery.

12–2.   LOCATION OF ELECTRODES

Because living tissues are reasonably good conductors, bioelectric generators send current through them and thereby establish potential distributions which make it possible to place electrodes distant from the generator and detect an attenuated version of the bioelectric signal. For example, in recordings of the ECG in man, the value of the voltage occurring at the peak of the R wave (lead II) is about 1.5 mv. On the other hand, the bioelectric generator, that is, the temporal and spatial summation of all of the fibers experiencing depolarization, produces a signal many times larger. The loss of amplitude is explainable on the basis of the asynchrony of depolarization, shunting by the conducting body tissues, and the orientation of the electrodes with respect to the spread of the wave of excitation.

By suitably orienting electrodes with respect to the bioelectric generator, it is possible to determine its location. The importance of this fact was brought to the attention of physiologists in 1889 by Waller, who was using the capillary electrometer[2] to investigate the magnitude of the electrocardiographic potentials picked up by electrodes placed on the body surface of a human subject. His studies, the first of their kind in man, revealed in a most dramatic way the fact that "favorable" and "unfavorable" locations for the electrodes existed, that is, there were some electrode locations where the deflection of the meniscus of the capillary electrometer was large and

---

[2] See Geddes and Hoff (1961).

others where the deflection was small. From a systematic study of the amplitudes recorded with different electrode locations, Waller deduced that the heart (in reality the ventricles) had a particular electrical orientation in the thorax. He characterized the orientation in terms of an equivalent dipole. These pioneering investigations not only laid the foundation for Einthoven's later studies, which initiated vectorcardiography, but also clearly demonstrated that the heart could be meaningfully represented as a dipole which could be located by multiple measurement of potentials appearing between distant electrodes on the surface of the body.

It is often assumed that a bioelectric generator can be represented as a dipole source embedded in a homogeneous conducting medium. Although this concept is useful, care must be exercised not to extend it beyond the point of physiological significance. In nearly every practical circumstance, bioelectric sources cannot be adequately represented by a single dipole embedded in an infinite volume conductor. More often a bioelectric source is better characterized by multiple dipoles representing islands of tissue which become simultaneously or sequentially active. Even with these restrictions in mind, equating the bioelectric generator to a simple dipole can provide a basis for understanding the importance of electrode orientation in the detection of bioelectric signals. In addition, study of such a simple situation not only serves to illustrate many important facts, but also permits an estimate of the distortions produced when the volume-conducting medium is inhomogeneous and not infinite in extent.

The relationship existing between the voltage picked up by a pair of electrodes and their distance and orientation with respect to the axis of a bioelectric generator can be appreciated by considering the generator to be a small dumbbell-shaped distribution of charge (dipole) placed in a conducting medium which extends to infinity in all directions. The potential distribution of such a dipole can be explored by means of two different electrode arrangements, which have their counterparts in the recording of a bioelectric event:

1. The potential distribution is explored with a single (monopolar) electrode, which is often designated the active electrode. The potential of the active electrode is measured with respect to a reference (indifferent) electrode located in a region of zero potential. This technique is called monopolar recording.

2. The potential distribution is explored with two similar and nearby electrodes, both of which are called active electrodes. This method is termed bipolar recording.

A typical biomedical application of monopolar recording is the V lead[3]

---

[3] See Wilson et al. (1934) and Rappaport et al. (1949).

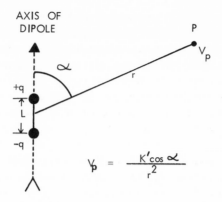

Figure 12–14. Potential at a point P at a distance r from a dipole $(+q, -q)$ of moment $M(=qL)$.

used in ECG. The indifferent lead is the V terminal; the active lead is on the chest. In electroencephalography (EEG) the ear lobes, nose, chin, and back of the neck are often used as sites for the indifferent electrode, the active electrode being placed on the scalp or cortex. In electromyography the active electrode is a needle inserted into the muscle, and the indifferent electrode is placed on the skin above the muscle. Bipolar as well as monopolar recording is employed routinely in the EEG laboratory. It is also apparent that the use of standard ECG limb leads is an example of bipolar recording.

Figure 12–14 diagrams a dipole embedded in a volume conductor. The potential at any point can be calculated by determining the work done in bringing a charge q_0 from infinity to point P, which is at a distance r from the dipole having a dipole moment M ($=qL$). Using Coulomb's law and carrying out the integration leads to the following expression[4] for V_p, the potential at the point P in a medium of dielectric constant K:

$$V_p = \frac{W}{q_0} = \frac{M}{K}\left(\frac{\cos \alpha}{r^2}\right).$$

Thus the potential varies inversely with the square of the distance and is dependent on the angle that the line from the dipole to the point P makes with respect to the axis of the dipole. Figure 12-15 diagrams the isopotential lines surrounding the dipole. It is important to note that in this situation three-dimensional symmetry exists.

---

[4] In deriving this expression it was assumed that point P was at a distance r many times greater than L, the length of the dipole.

Gross inspection of Fig. 12–15 reveals that the more distant an exploring electrode is from the dipole, the less the potential. In addition, in a plane perpendicular to the dipole axis and equidistant from the two poles of the dipole, no potential is measurable regardless of the location of the measuring electrode. Equally obvious is the fact that, if a pair of electrodes is used to explore the potentials surrounding the dipole, there are innumerable positions, near and far, where no potential difference will be measured between the electrodes. In these situations both electrodes are on the same equipotential line.

To analyze further the value of the information contained in Fig. 12–15, consider the measurement of a bioelectric event with a monopolar (active) electrode, the other (indifferent) electrode being located in a region of zero potential or at a great distance from the dipole. To illustrate the factors which determine the magnitude of the potential presented to the active electrode, it is instructive to bring the active electrode from a distant location toward the dipole, moving in a given plane containing both the electrodes and the dipole. In carrying out this procedure there are two important paths along which the active (exploring) electrode may be moved: (a) along a line at right angles to the axis of the dipole (Fig. 12–16), and (b) along a line parallel to the axis of the dipole (Fig. 12–17). These paths are of value in understanding monopolar measurement techniques.

In Fig. 12–16 is plotted the potential of the monopolar electrode V_p as it is moved along two lines perpendicular to the axis of the dipole. One is near ($d = 0.5$) the center of the dipole; the other is distant ($d = 1.5$). Clearly evident is the fact that for this specified movement of the active electrode the potential is maximum along the axis of the dipole (i.e., $D/d = 1.0$),[5] and that the potential at all points along the line nearer ($d = 0.5$) the dipole is greater than that at points on the distant line ($d = 1.5$).

Figure 12–17 diagrams the potential as the active electrode is moved along two lines parallel to the axis of the dipole. Clearly evident is the fact that, as the electrode is brought from a distance, the potential rises as the active electrode approaches the dipole and then decreases and drops to zero when the electrode is on a line perpendicular to the dipole axis at the center of the dipole ($D/d = 1.0$). As the movement of the electrode is continued in the same direction, the potential increases in the opposite direction, reaching a maximum and then decreasing as the electrode recedes from the dipole. The magnitude of potential is greater at all points along the line nearest the dipole ($d = 0.5$). Note

[5] D is the radial distance to the center of the dipole.

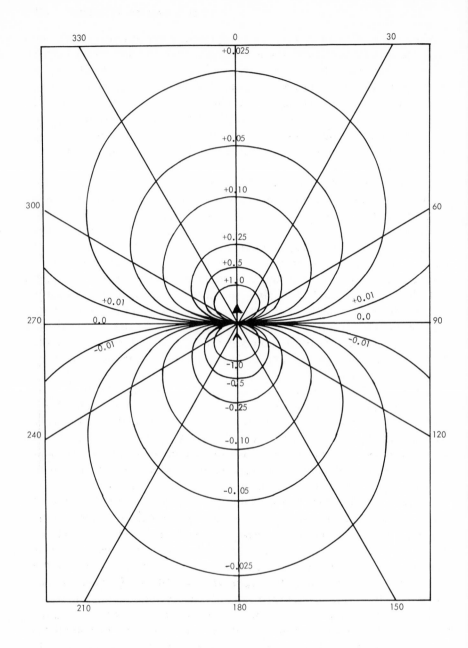

Figure 12–15. Isopotential lines around a dipole.

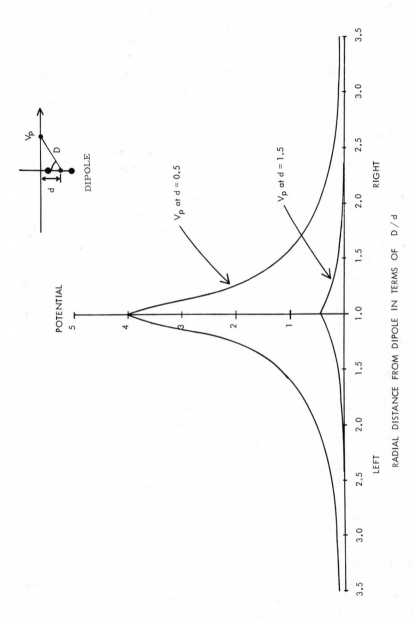

Figure 12–16. Potential of an electrode moved along lines perpendicular to the dipole axis.

that it is possible, as shown in Fig. 12–17, to have the active electrode very close to the dipole and yet detect no potential.

Figure 12–15 can also be employed to determine the potential presented to a pair of active electrodes, the use of which is described as bipolar recording. Bipolar recording introduces another variable: in addition to the distance and orientation with respect to the dipole, the spacing between the two electrodes must be considered. To display the relationship among these three quantities, it is convenient to consider bringing a pair of electrodes having a constant spacing (S) from a large distance toward the dipole, first along a line perpendicular to the axis of the dipole and then along a line parallel to it. The procedure will be repeated for different distances and electrode separations.

In Fig. 12–18 are plotted the potential differences measured between fixed separation electrodes as they are moved along lines perpendicular to the dipole axis. When the pair of electrodes is brought from afar toward the dipole, the potential difference is observed to increase, reach a maximum, and start to decrease. When the electrodes are symmetrical with respect to the dipole ($D/d = 1.0$), the potential difference is zero. With the continuation of movement in the same direction the electrodes pass over the axis of the dipole, and the potential difference starts to increase in the negative direction, reaches a maximum, and then decreases as the distance from the dipole becomes larger. This orderly sequence is repeated when closely ($S = 0.5$) or widely ($S = 1.5$) spaced electrodes are moved along a line near ($d = 0.5$) the dipole or distant ($d = 1.5$) from it. With constant spacing the farther the electrodes are away, the less the potential difference. When the electrodes are moved along either line, the effect of increasing the spacing is to increase the magnitude of the maximum.

Figure 12–19 illustrates the potential difference when electrodes with a constant spacing are brought from a distance toward the dipole along lines parallel to its axis. Although there are an infinite number of possible permutations of electrode spacing S and distance d, only a few values were chosen for presentation to illustrate the type of relationship to be expected. Perhaps of paramount importance is the fact that regardless of spacing and distance there is only one location on each side of the dipole where the potential is zero. These locations are complexly related to distance and spacing. Conspicuous also is the fact that, as the electrode pair is moved toward the dipole from the distant point, the potential rises, falls to zero, reverses, rises to a negative maximum, then falls to zero and reverses again to rise to a maximum, and decreases as the electrode pair is moved farther away.

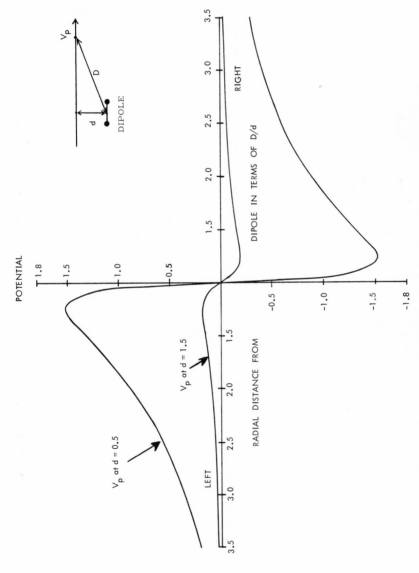

Figure 12-17. Potential of an electrode moved along lines parallel to the dipole axis.

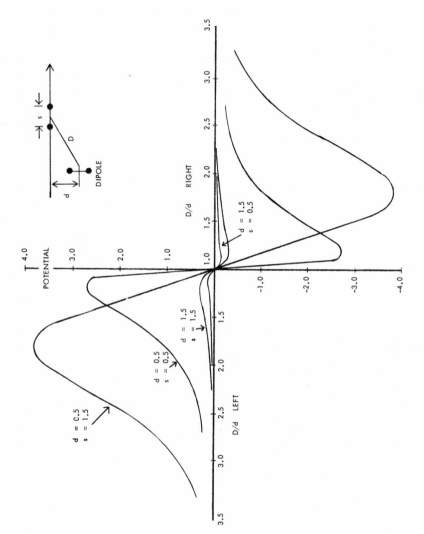

Figure 12-18. Potential between a pair of electrodes moved along lines perpendicular to the dipole axis.

In Fig. 12–19 it can be seen that, when the electrode pair is moved along a line at a constant distance d from the axis of the dipole, an increase in spacing between the electrodes raises the amplitude and distance D for the maximum potential. Also of interest is the fact that along each constant-distance (d) line there are two electrode separations that exhibit the same potential difference for different electrode spacings. Equal potential differences occur (1) at approximately $D/d = 2.0$ (for $d = 0.5$, $S = 1.5$ and $d = 0.5$, $S = 0.5$) and (2) at about $D/d = 1.4$ (for $d = 1.5$, $S = 0.5$ and $d = 1.5$, $S = 1.5$).

Thus, to understand the reason for a given potential difference appearing between a pair of electrodes in the vicinity of a dipole source, it is necessary to appreciate the relationship between the isopotential lines developed by the dipole source and the orentation, spacing, and distance of the electrode pair. The systematic measurement of the spatial distribution

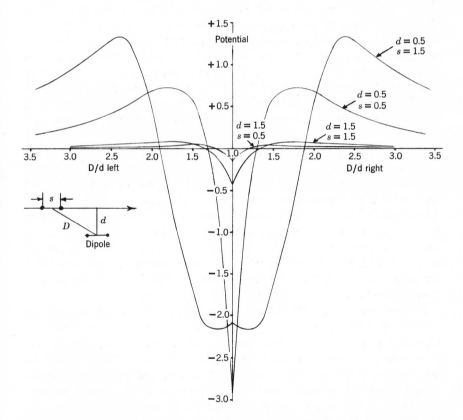

Figure 12–19. Potential between a pair of electrodes moved along lines parallel to the dipole axis.

of potentials existing at each instant in time permits speculation on the nature and location of the source. Although the theory is straightforward, its application often is accompanied by practical difficulties because bioelectric generators rarely exist as simple dipoles. It is important to recognize the fact that bioelectric generators usually present themselves to extracellular electrodes as regions of tissue which become active both simultaneously and sequentially.

12–3. POTENTIAL DISTRIBUTION AROUND BIOELECTRIC GENERATORS

After measuring the potential differences between leads placed on various points on the surface of the body, Waller (1889) postulated that the potential distribution at the peak of the R wave due to ventricular activity could be attributed to an equivalent dipole, as shown in Fig. 12–20. Since Waller's time many investigators have plotted the isopotential lines at various instants in the cycle of activity of bioelectric generators. Electrocardiographic isopotential lines appearing on the thorax at different instants during atrial and ventricular excitation and recovery were mapped in human subjects by Nahum et. al. (1951), Mauro et al. (1952), Nahum et al. (1952–1953), Simonson (1952), Frank (1955, 1956–1957), and Nelson (1956); in the dog by Mauro et al. (1952), Taccardi (1962), Horan et al. (1963), and Nelson et al. (1965); and in the monkey and lamb by Nelson et al. (1965).

It must be emphasized that such isopotential maps represent the potential distribution during one instant in the cardiac cycle. A complete display of the electrical activity for the whole cardiac cycle would require the plotting of instantaneous potential distributions at each instant in atrial and ventricular activity and recovery, that is, during the P, Tp, QRS, and T waves. Thus, it is apparent that the isopotential lines are time varying. Figure 12–21 illustrates the time-varying nature of the surface potential distribution during the ventricular depolarization process as described by the QRS wave of the ECG. The implications of these isopotential lines will be discussed in the next section.

Electroencephalographic isopotential lines have been plotted for various cerebral states. Two of the earliest to investigate this method of localizing active regions of the brain were Adrian and Matthews (1934). The study was continued by Brazier (1949), who presented a series of diagrams constructed from the EEG records of normal and abnormal subjects. Figure 12–22a,b present two of her diagrams from normal subjects. Figure 12–22a shows the scalp potential distribution during an instant in the development of the alpha rhythm, the normal background activity which characterizes the awake relaxed subject. Clearly evident is the

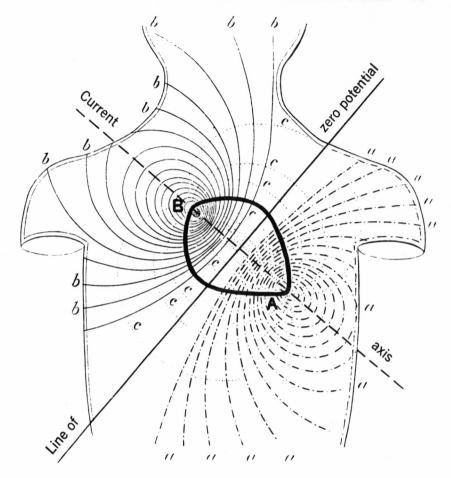

Figure 12–20. Waller's concept of the distribution of potential on the human thorax resulting from ventricular activity. [From A. C. Waller, *Phil. Trans. Roy. Soc.* **180B**: 169–194(1889). By permission of the Royal Society.]

focal location of this rhythm in the occipital region. Figure 12–22*b* shows the location of the origin of a low-frequency source in the sleeping subject.

Many penetrating theoretical studies have been carried out on the surface distributions of potentials for dipoles in irregularly shaped volume conductors. Those interested in this aspect of this field should consult the papers by Wilson and Bayley (1950), Frank (1953), Okada (1956, 1957), Geselowitz (1960), Brody et al. (1961), Hlavin and Plonsey (1963), and Plonsey (1963).

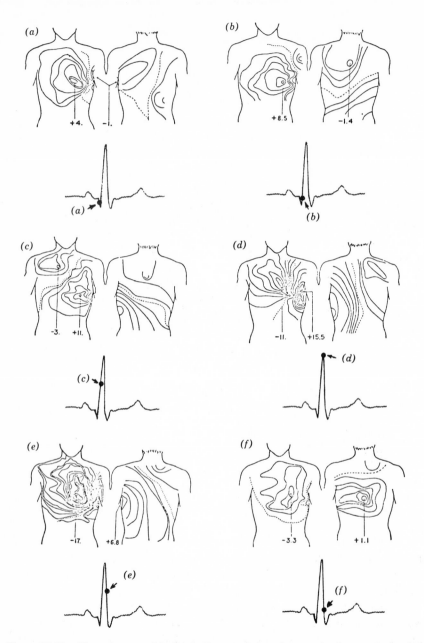

Figure 12–21. Thoracic potential distribution at various instants in the ventricular depolarization process. Lead I is shown for identification purposes. [From L. Nahum, in Fulton (Ed); *Textbook of Physiology*, 17th ed. Phila. Pa. W. B. Saunders Co, (1955). (By permission of the author and publisher).]

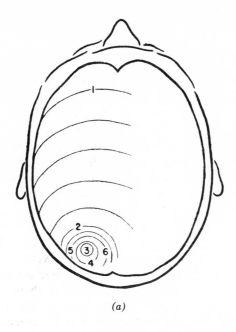

(a)

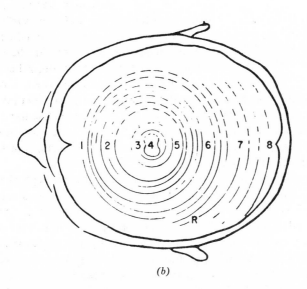

(b)

Figure 12–22. Potential distribution on the head due to electrical activity of the brain: (a) surface potential distribution of an alpha rhythm; (b) surface potential distribution at one instant during sleep. [From Brazier, *EEG Clin. Neurophysiol.* Supp. **2**:38–52 (1949). By permission of Masson & Cie, Publisher.]

12–4. VECTORCARDIOGRAPHY

The idea of locating the electrical axis of the ventricles by measuring potential differences appearing between limb electrodes was clearly demonstrated by Waller. Almost a quarter of a century later Einthoven postulated that in the human thorax the heart was almost in the center of an equilateral triangle in which the apices were the right and left arms (shoulders) and both feet (pubic area) (see Fig. 12–23). He stated:

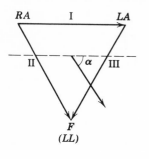

Figure 12–23. Einthoven's equilateral triangle. *RA* and *LA* are right and left-arm electrodes. *F* is the left leg (*LL*) electrode. [From Einthoven, trans. by Hoff and Sekelj, *Am. Heart J.*, **40**:163–211 (1950). By permission.]

"We now assume further that the ECG has been recorded from a subject that has in each of the three leads a simple form so that the summits of R_1, R_{11}, and R_{111} fall in the identical phases of a cardiac cycle. According to the well known formula, it can then be easily verified that $R_{11} - R_1 = R_{111}$. If we transfer the values found in the experimental subject over the schema (the triangle), we can determine in him the direction of the potential difference which was present in the heart during the registration of the R wave and thus was the cause of the formation of this wave."

Einthoven knew that he was recording only a component of ventricular depolarization in a plane parallel to the anterior surface of the body. In addition, on the triangle he plotted only a single line to represent the ventricular (manifest) vector of excitation, reflecting the R wave, although he knew that the R wave reached its peak at different times in the different leads. The notion that a series of instantaneous vectors could be drawn to describe the ventricular depolarization process was due to Williams (1914), who used the Einthoven triangle to plot the synchronous values of the amplitudes during the QRS wave derived from the limb leads.

It remained for Mann (1920) to introduce the concept of the vector loop by plotting the locus of the tips of the instantaneous values of the QRS and T vectors, as recorded by the three limb leads, to obtain loops which he called monocardiograms. He then proceeded in 1925 to build an instrument to record monocardiograms directly and demonstrated (1931) their value in the diagnosis of bundle-branch block, which was difficult to identify in the ECG at that time. A description of his instrument did not appear until 1938. Probably because no cathode-ray tubes were available, Mann constructed an ingenious galvanometer consisting of a single mirror which was deflected by three coils mounted with their axes

60 degrees apart, each axis corresponding to one of the leads as represented by the Einthoven triangle. A photographic record of the deflection of a light beam reflected from the mirror produced these early vectorcardiograms, although this name was not to be used until later.

The Braun cathode-ray tube was introduced to vectorcardiography by Schellong et al. (1937), who used a two-axis tube to obtain vector loops (vectordiagrams) in the frontal, horizontal, and sagittal planes (Fig. 12–24). Hollmann and Hollmann (1938) employed a cathode-ray tube with three pairs of deflection plates with 60-degree orientation and called the records that they obtained triograms (Fig. 12–25). Sulzer and Duchosal (1938) used the Braun tube to display what they called planograms derived from electrodes placed to record frontal, sagittal, and horizontal components of the ECG. Careful studies were carried out by Arrighi (1939) to locate the best electrode placement for the sagittal projection lead. His selection is shown in Fig. 12–26. At the same time Wilson and Johnston (1938) employed a cathode ray tube with the "central terminal" (Fig. 12–27) to make the Einthoven triangle method practical for clinical vectorcardiography. In this paper Wilson initiated the use of the word vectorcardiogram.

The manner in which the ventricular excitation vectorcardiogram (VCG) was developed from two limb leads and plotted on the Einthoven triangle is shown in Fig. 12–28. In this illustration the QRS waves recorded from leads I and III are mounted as shown. The loop is produced by joining the points formed by the intersections of the lines projected into the triangle from corresponding time points on the QRS waves. The major axis of the loop indicates the inclination of the electrical axis with the horizontal.

Because the electrocardiograph was in fairly widespread use and provided extremely valuable information on the condition of the heart, it was expected that the vectorcardiograph could provide more and different data about the functioning of the myocardium. With the availability of the

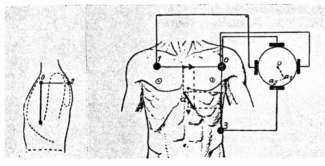

Figure 12–24. Schellong's method of producing vectordiagrams. [From Schellong et al., *Z. Kreislaufforsch.* **29**:497 (1937). By permission.]

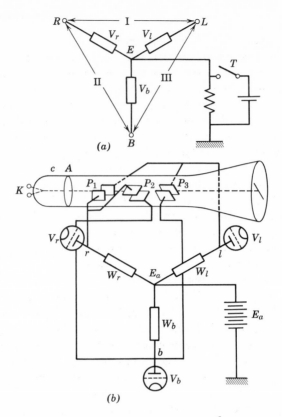

Figure 12–25. The Hollmann method of presenting triograms. [*From W. and H. E. Hollmann, Z. Krieslaufforsch.* **29**:546 (1937). By permission.]

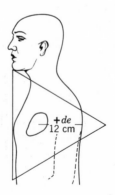

Figure 12–26. Arrighi's sagittal electrode placement. [From F. Arrighi, *Prensa Med. Arg.* **26**:253 (1939). By permission.]

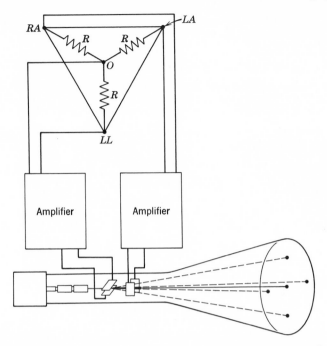

Figure 12–27. The vectorcardiogram derived from Wilson's central terminal. [From F. N. Wilson and F. D. Johnston, *Am. Heart J.* **16**:14 (1938). By permission.]

cathode-ray tube and high-fidelity voltage amplifiers after 1945, there arose a new interest in multiplane (spatial) vectorcardiography. To record such VCG's, many patterns of electrode location were proposed, most of which could be traced back to the reasoning behind the Einthoven triangle. However, before long it was realized that the basic assumptions in Einthoven's simple equilateral triangle were not entirely valid; for example, the heart is not at the center of an equilateral triangle with apices where the limbs join the trunk, nor is the resistivity of the tissues and fluids surrounding the heart uniform in all directions. Among the first to question the validity of Einthoven's concept were Burger and van Milaan (1947), who constructed a torso model, filled it with copper sulfate, and implanted a dipole generator in it in the position occupied by the heart as determined by x-ray studies on human subjects. Even in this homogeneously conducting model the potentials of the three limb leads were not those predicted on the basis of Einthoven's triangle. These investigators then altered their model by inserting masses of material to simulate the lungs (a bag of moist sand) and spinal column (cork), and showed that the potentials recorded by the limb leads were those represented by a scalene triangle having angles of

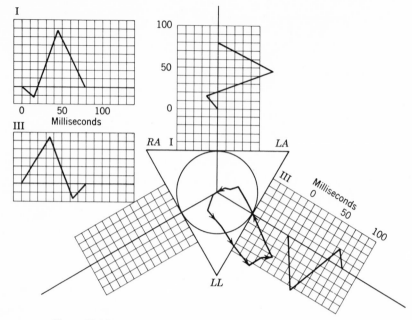

Figure 12–28. Development of the frontal plane vectorcardiogram.

96 degrees at the right arm, 56 degrees at the left arm, and 28 degrees at the left leg.

Despite knowledge that the torso is irregular in shape and anisotropic, many body-surface electrode arrangements were developed to obtain voltages from which the ventricular vector loop could be located spatially with reference to the electrode array. The electrode locations were usually chosen on the basis of equal distance from the "center" of the ventricles. The lines joining the electrodes formed the boundaries of a solid figure which was often used to identify the electrode array. Controversy over the ability of a particular electrode reference frame to locate the "cardiac vectors" has continued to the present time.

On the basis of considerable clinical experience with vectorcardiography, Sulzer and Duchosal (1945) advocated the two electrode schemes shown in Figs. 12–29a,b. Although both gave similar loops, they preferred system b, which became known as the double-cube system.

Wilson et al. (1947), after studying the potential distribution of an electrically driven dipole placed in a cadaver heart, introduced the equilateral tetrahedral reference frame (Fig. 12–30). With this system, limb electrodes and the central terminal were used to obtain the frontal plane projection. From a back electrode and the central terminal was derived

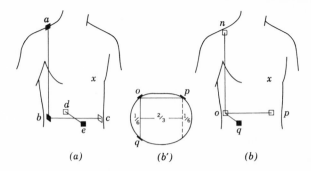

Figure 12–29. Sulzer and Duchosal's reference frames. [From R. Sulzer and P. W. Duchosal, *Cardiologia* 9:10–120 (1945). By permission.]

the sagittal projection. The relative voltages appearing between the various electrode pairs were in nearly all instances those predicted from the geometry of the torso. With such evidence the tetrahedral system gained considerable support.

Grishman et al. (1951), after obtaining clinical records with the Wilson tetrahedral, the Arrighi triangle, and the Duchosal reference frames, were led to develop the cubic electrode arrangement shown in Fig. 12–31. The no. 1 electrode was placed "near the right posterior axillary line at the level of the first and second lumbar vertebrae"; no. 2 in the left posterior

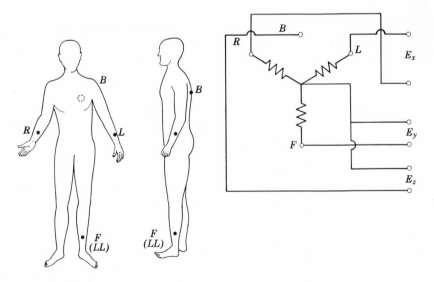

Figure 12–30. Wilson's tetrahedral reference frame. (Redrawn from G. Burch et al., *Spatial Vectorcardiography*, Lea and Febiger, Philadelphia, Pa.)

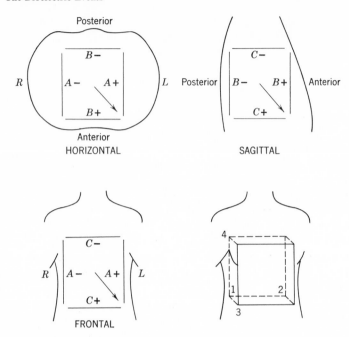

Figure 12–31. The cubic reference system employed by Grishman. [Adapted from Grishman et al., *Am. Heart J.* **41**:483–493 (1951). By permission.]

axillary line, no. 3 over the right anterior axillary line, and no. 4 over the left scapula. With this arrangement the authors claimed that the heart was as equidistant from the electrodes as the thorax allowed and that the electrodes were easily located anatomically.

Although all reference frames provided reasonable VCG's, the QRS and T loops derived from normal subjects exhibited a remarkably wide range of magnitudes and orientations even when the same vectorcardiographic reference frame was used. In addition, the data obtained with different reference frames were not easily comparable. It is not difficult to find possible reasons for this situation. At least two concerted attempts have been made to identify the variables by means of investigations in which electrically driven dipoles were implanted into electrolyte filled human torso models and the resulting body-surface potential distributions were studied. The investigations by Schmitt and Simonson (1955) and Frank (1956) are fine examples of this technique. From their studies both investigators developed orthogonal lead systems for spatial vectorcardiography. Schmitt's SVEC III system is shown in Fig. 12–32, and Frank's is sketched in Fig. 12–33. Both are used clinically.

In Schmitt's system fourteen active electrodes are employed. The voltage which represents the X component of the cardiac vector is derived from the right- and left-arm electrodes, along with components derived from chest and back electrodes placed at the level of the fifth intercostal space. The Y component is obtained from the head and left-leg electrodes, and the Z component from eight electrodes located on the chest and back at the third and sixth interspace.

Seven active electrodes are used with Frank's system (Fig. 12–33). The X component is derived from an array of electrodes that surround the heart approximately at the level of the fifth interspace. The Y component is obtained from the neck and left-leg electrodes, and the Z component from

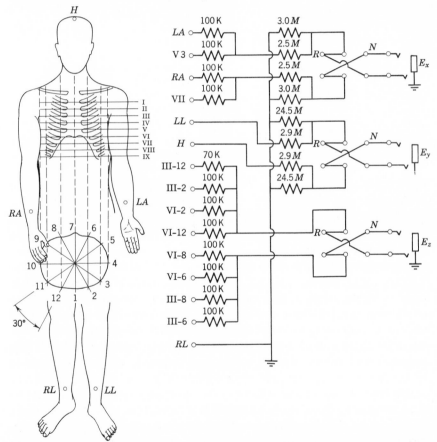

Figure 12–32. Schmitt's SVEC III orthogonal lead system. [Redrawn from O. H. Schmitt and E. Simonson. A.M.A. *Arch. Internal Med.* **96**:574–590 (1955), and as reported by Pipberger and Wood, *Circ. Res.* **6**:239–24 (1958). The resistor values shown are for an input impedance of 10 megohms to ground. By permission of the American Heart Association, Inc.]

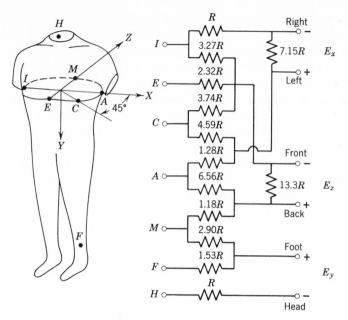

Figure 12–33. Frank's vectorcardiographic lead system. [From E. Frank, Circulation **13**: 737–749 (1956). By permission of the American Heart Association.]

the voltage appearing between an array of three electrodes on the anterior of the chest and one electrode in the back and one on the midaxillary line. To provide more accurate location of the level for the chest and back electrodes, Frank developed a three-electrode exploring tool and presented instructions for its use.

There have been several comparisons of the data obtained with the various vectorcardiographic reference frames. Frank (1954) presented one of the earliest studies, which examined the validity of the assumptions underlying the Duchosal double cube, the Wilson tetrahedron, and the Grishman cube arrays. Using human torso models filled with an electrolyte and containing a fixed dipole, he measured the potentials at 200 electrode positions and calculated the voltages presented to electrodes placed in the locations specified by the three reference frames. He found that "the scalar lead shapes of the Wilson tetrahedron deviate, on the average, by approximately 15% from the torso dipole variations, but the scalar lead shapes of the systems of Duchosal and Grishman show significantly larger discrepancies." He also found that the standardization factors employed in the Wilson system were too large, particularly with respect to the head-to-foot dipole component (by a factor of 2.3), and added, "Certain fortuitous features of the Wilson system enable a modification of the standardization factors which leads to results that are fairly satisfactory for a dipole located in the center of the heart. This system which possesses certain other advantages would appear to deserve further study."

The practical value of Wilson's system was also investigated by Abildskov and Pence (1956), who compared data obtained by means of Wilson's tetrahedron with those obtained with the corrected tetrahedron as advocated by McFee and Johnson (1954). In 75 subjects they found that, although the data were similar with both methods, the scatter was less with the corrected tetrahedron. Brody (1957) carried out another study on a series of human subjects, using the scalene tetrahedron and Wilson's equilateral tetrahedron, to find that, although the scalene tetrahedron was based on sound experimentally determined data, "the mean spatial QRS- and T-vector loci exhibited slightly less scatter and better coefficients of correlation within the uncorrected frame of reference," and that "the corrected frame of reference does not appear to possess sufficient merit to warrant its routine application to the analysis of mean QRS-and T-vector orientation." In another investigation of Wilson's tetrahedral system, Burger et al. (1956) applied their scalene triangle correction and compared data collected on a series of 96 patients with their own reference frame. They found good agreement between the two methods, using the electrode locations advocated by Wilson only when their correction was applied. It is probably because of such studies in which deviations from the "ideal" value turn out to be clinically unimportant that the Wilson method still enjoys considerable support.

The Schmitt, Frank, Helm, and McFee (corrected Einthoven triangle) systems have also been exposed to close scrutiny by Langner et al. (1958). The importance of the differences depends on how critical the reader may be. Langner found that for the Z lead the systems were interchangeable in over 90% of the cases for the QRS and T loops in regard to shape and orientation. For the X lead the systems were interchangeable in all cases for the QRS loop and in 90% for the T loop. In another study involving 4 normal and 182 elderly subjects, Simonson et al. (1959) compared the QRS and T loops obtained with eight popular orthogonal-lead systems to find large differences between these systems. However, they stated, "Most types of pathology can be recognized in any of the lead systems." Although their extensive study was carefully carried out, they were reluctant to advocate the superiority of one system over another.

Nonogawa (1966) called attention to the important fact that many of the popular electrode reference frames were derived from torso models of Caucasian adults. He wondered whether these frames were applicable to the Oriental torso. Therefore he constructed Caucasian and Oriental torso models into which he placed electrically excited dipoles and obtained VCG data with the Frank, Schmitt SVEC III, McFee, Polygraph III, and Grishman lead systems. He concluded that in each of the X, Y, and Z-axis leads the Schmitt and Frank systems were similar. The other lead systems showed larger differences. However, he also concluded that "these VCG systems, in their original networks, can be applied to the Japanese without appreciable error."

With such variety of reference frames and the lack of clear-cut clinical evidence to indicate the superiority of one reference system over another to identify specific myocardial diseases, it is difficult to set forth criteria which would lead to the adoption of a single method. Information on this interesting field can be found in the monographs by Grant and Estes (1951), Grishman (1952), Goldberger (1953), Burch et al. (1953), Grant (1957), Kowarzykowic (1961), Pozzi (1961), Uhley (1962), Guntheroth (1965), and Lamb (1965). In Pozzi's (1961) monograph there is an excellent bibliography of the original papers which describe the various vectorcardiographic lead systems and potential distributions around the heart of the human subject and in models of the human torso. The bibliography also lists studies in which field mapping was carried out with various dipole models.

In considering the merits of one reference frame over another, it is useful to remember that most of the carefully examined reference frames were derived from human torso models in which electrically driven dipoles were implanted. Although this is a good starting point, the situation in the actual human subject is quite different. Not only do human torsos come in a wide range of shapes and sizes, but also the tissues between the heart and body-surface electrodes have quite different electrical properties. Even within a single tissue the resistivity is not the same in all directions. Therefore there still remains the need to conduct more cadaver experiments such as those carried out by Wilson et al. (1947) to evaluate the magnitude of the distortions produced by the intrathoracic contents.

Traditionally the VCG is displayed in Cartesian coordinates on a two-axis cathode ray tube. Usually a single photograph is taken of each cardiac cycle. From such pictures the magnitude and orientation of the P-, QRS-, and T-vector loops are determined. Timing of the vector loops is accomplished by blanking the beam with a triangular pulse to indicate the direction of development of the loop. Continuous moving picture records of the same presentation produce figures that are grossly distorted.

With the conventional cathode-ray tube presentation, an adequate display for the large, rapidly developing QRS loop requires the use of a high-intensity beam. When this situation obtains, there is a bright halo around the P and T loops. Between heart beats the bright stationary spot soon damages the cathode-ray tube screen. To overcome this defect, Briller et al. (1950) described a method of obtaining a triggering signal from the P wave of the ECG to turn on the cathode ray tube beam only for the duration of the QRS or the T wave. Becking et al. (1950) described a most practical method of brightening the cathode-ray tube trace in proportion to the velocity of the excursion of the beam. This technique not only protects the screen between heart beats but also provides a means of obtaining photographs with high contrast. Isaacs (1964) described a method similar to Briller's in which the R wave was used to trigger delay generators that could be manually set to turn on the cathode-ray tube beam for all or part of the next heart beat. A combination of the techniques described by these investigators would undoubtedly improve display of the loops.

An interesting three-dimensional display system was described by Ishitoya et al. (1965). With this method the X, Y, and Z signals derived by using the Frank system were applied to three galvanometers with their deflection axes mutually perpendicular. A light beam was reflected from the first galvanometer to the second and to a screen on the third beside which was a half-silvered mirror used to view the screen. Three illuminated mutually perpendicular axes were placed behind the half-silvered mirror, and the whole assembly was mounted in a lightproof box. By looking into a viewing hole, the spatial orientation of the vector loops with respect to the three axes was clearly seen.

The use of polar coordinates for presentation of the VCG was described by Dower et al. (1965). Instead of a conventional cathode-ray tube display, they employed an analog computer which continuously calculated the spherical coordinates (R, Θ, ϕ) and presented them on a graphic record. Although such a presentation is not easy to comprehend, it does retain the important PR, QRS, and QT time intervals, which are lost in the conventional Cartesian coordinate presentations.

There is no doubt that the cathode-ray tube presentation of the spatial VCG provides an intellectually pleasing display and clearly illustrates the phase differences between the voltages in the various leads from which it is derived. The major piece of information that it presents is the direction of depolarization and repolarization of the atria and the ventricles. The most prominent feature, the QRS loop, is usually so large that it is difficult to see the P and T loops. Beam brightness-controlling techniques offer some solution to this problem.

At present there is not unanimity of opinion regarding the best location for body-surface electrodes and choice of weighting networks. A reference frame designed to give orthogonal components for ventricular depolarization (QRS) may not indicate repolarization (T) with the same accuracy. Moreover, the same reference frame may be quite inappropriate for atrial depolarization and repolarization. From these loops, as they are displayed on the conventional two-axis cathode-ray tube, it is impossible to determine the important time durations and intervals (PR, QRS, and QT), which contain a considerable amount of diagnostic information. Although conduction disturbances and ectopic beats identify themselves clearly in the VCG, they are equally well indicated by the ECG. Injury to the myocardium, as shown by S-T segment deviations, are better displayed in the ECG by precordial leads.

The preceding discussion appears to indicate that the VCG has limited clinical value and will not replace the ECG in routine electrocardiography. As a teaching device the VCG has much to offer. Its ability to display the rate of depolarization and repolarization is far superior to that of the ECG. Especially well displayed by the VCG are the small beat-by-beat changes in these quantities. Expanded clinical use of the VCG will depend on the clinical value of the information it produces. The fact that so many reference frames are employed will probably delay the time when the full usefulness of the VCG will be established.

12–5. HISTORICAL POSTSCRIPT

The electrical activity of nerve and that preceding the contraction of skeletal and cardiac muscle were known long before there were instruments adequate for their accurate reproduction. Galvani's three important experiments (ca. 1800) have been recounted frequently (Fulton and Cushing 1936; Hoff, 1936; Walker, 1937) because they led directly and immediately to the development of current electricity and to an intense interest in bioelectricity, despite the fact that Galvani's explanation for them was incorrect. Of the three experiments, only the third, which described contraction of the gastrocnemius muscle without the use of metals, need concern us here, for it was the only one which demonstrated the existence of a true bioelectric potential. This experiment, sketched in Fig. 12-34a, consisted of observing a twitch in a rheoscopic[6] frog preparation when the sciatic nerve was laid over a cut muscle so that contact was made between the intact and cut surfaces. Between the cut (injured) and the intact surface appeared the membrane potential, which was of sufficient magnitude to stimulate (on contact) the sciatic nerve of the rheoscope and produce a

---

[6]"Current-seeing" preparation, consisting of an isolated sciatic nerve-gastrocnemius muscle used before invention of the galvanometer to demonstrate the existence of an electric potential.

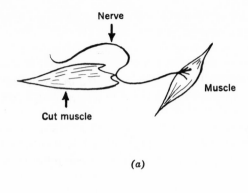

(a)

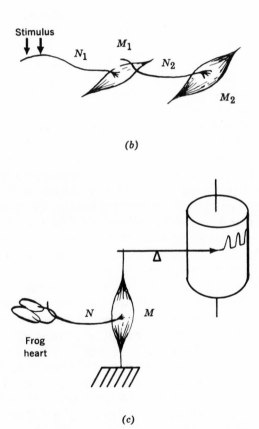

(b)

(c)

Figure 12–34. The beginnings of bioelectricity: (a) Galvani: (b) Matteucci: (c) Kolliker and Mueller, and Donders.

twitch in the muscle. In a primitive way this experiment demonstrated the existence of the membrane potential.

Carlo Matteucci (1842) used the rheoscopic frog to first demonstrate the existence of an action potential accompanying muscular contraction. His experiment, sketched in Fig. 12–34b, consisted of laying the sciatic nerve N_2 of a rheoscopic frog over the surface of a muscle M_1 in which the nerve N_1 was intact. Repetitive stimulation of nerve N_1 caused muscle M_1 to develop action potentials and twitches. The muscle action potentials stimulated nerve N_2 of the rheoscopic frog, causing twitches in its muscle M_2. Thus was demonstrated the first electromyographic signal.

The electrical activity accompanying the heart beat was also discovered with the rheoscopic frog by Kolliker and Mueller (1856) in the manner shown in Fig. 12–34c. When these investigators laid the nerve N over the beating ventricle of a frog heart, the muscle M twitched once and sometimes twice. Stimulation of the nerve obviously occurred with depolarization and repolarization of the ventricles. Because at that time there were no rapidly responding galvanometers, Donders (1872) recorded the twitches of the rheoscope to provide a graphic demonstration of the existence of an electrocardiographic signal.

The first measurements of bioelectric potentials by means of a physical instrument were those of Nobili (1828), who measured the injury current by connecting his astatic galvanometer to electrodes on the cut and intact surfaces of a pile of frog muscles. The next to measure myoelectric potentials was du Bois Reymond (1843), who postulated that a difference of potential existed between the interior and the exterior of muscle, another prediction of the existence of a membrane potential. Connecting a galvanometer to electrodes on the fingers of the two hands, he noted a deflection when the muscles of one arm were contracted; this was probably the first demonstration of the human electromyogram.

True voltage-time graphs of the bioelectric signals were made long before rapidly responding indicators were available. The actual waveform of the nerve action potential was determined by Bernstein (1868), using the rheotome;[7] this was perhaps one of the earliest applications of the sampling method. In this technique developed by the Russian physicist Lenz (1849, 1854), a commutator, for a brief time, connected a slowly responding galvanometer which averaged the voltage at different instants after a tissue had been stimulated by completion of a circuit, using a second pair of contacts on the commutator. A graph of the average values of voltage and time after the stimulus permitted Bernstein to plot the true voltage-time curve of the nerve action potential, which lasted 0.6759

---

[7] See Hoff and Geddes (1957).

ms. Figure 12–35 illustrates Bernstein's rheotome and the nerve action potential he obtained with it.

Using the rheotome, Marchand (1877), Englemann (1878), and Burdon-Sanderson and Page (1878) plotted accurate representations of the waveform of the ventricular component of the electrocardiogram. The record obtained by Burdon-Sanderson, which clearly reveals the R and T waves, is shown in Fig. 12-36. From this study came the proposal that the ventricular electrogram is the sum of two monophasic action potentials. This theory, now well substantiated by microelectrode measurements on single cardiac muscle cells, provided an understanding of the relationship of the T wave to recovery of the ventricles.

The first instrument to provide a continuous record of a rapidly changing bioelectric event was the capillary electrometer[8] developed by Marey (1876). This device, shown in Fig. 12–37a, consisted of a mercury-sulfuric acid interface enclosed in a capillary tube. Current, obtained from electrodes on an irritable tissue, altered the contour of the mercury meniscus. By the use of a high-intensity light and an optical system, the variations in the contour of the meniscus were photographed to display the first spontaneously occurring bioelectric signals, the tortoise and frog cardiac electrograms shown in Fig. 12–37b, c.

The capillary electrometer was the first instrument to display the ECG's of animals and man as they arose spontaneously. It was also the first instrument to record nerve and muscle action potentials as they occurred spontaneously. The first nerve action potentials were recorded by Gotch and Horsley. Figure 12–38 illustrates the records that they obtained. Because they wanted to be sure that the signals recorded by the capillary electrometer were not artifacts from the induction coil stimulator, they made a separate record of the stimulus to show that the make (m) and break (b) shocks moved the mercury meniscus in opposite directions. The nerve action potentials evoked by both make and break shocks always moved the mercury meniscus in the same direction, thereby proving the physiological origin of the waves recorded in Fig. 12–38.

Although the capillary electrometer was used to record muscle action potentials, great difficulty was encountered because of the long response time and the need to apply the correction technique described by Burch (1892). Moreover, it was difficult practically to excite skeletal muscle electrically and eliminate stimulus artifact. In addition, the waveforms of muscle action potentials had been determined previously with the rheotome. Because of these facts and because better bioelectric recorders were soon to appear, there are few good records of muscle action potentials

---

[8] See Geddes and Hoff (1961).

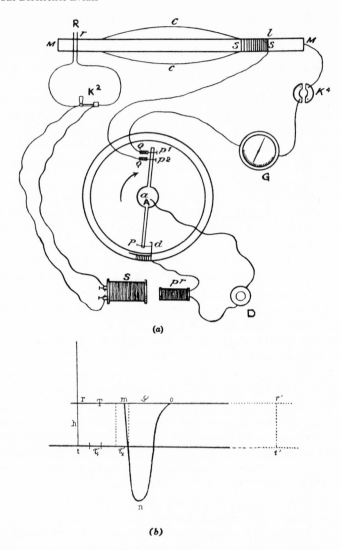

(a)

(b)

Figure 12–35. Bernstein's rheotome (a) 1876, and the nerve action potential (b). [From H. E. Hoff and L. A. Geddes, *Bull. Hist. Med.* **31**(3):212–347 (1957). By permission.]

taken with the capillary electrometer. Although the records obtained by the capillary electrometer could be corrected to provide true voltage-time graphs, this unnecessary inconvenience, along with the erratic behavior of the electrometer, so infuriated Einthoven that he set himself to the task of developing a rapidly responding recording instrument. Using as a starting point the telegraphic recorder of Ader (1897), he soon developed

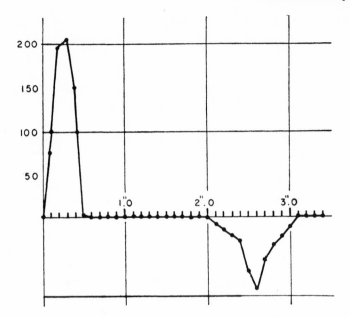

Figure 12–36. Burdon-Sanderson's record of the ECG, made by using the rheotome. [From H. E. Hoff, and L. A. Geddes, *Bull. Hist. Med.* **31**(3):212–347 (1957).]

his well known string galvanometer (1903). There is no doubt that this instrument (Fig. 12–39) ushered in clinical electrocardiography.

Although amplifier-type electrocardiographs with mirror galvanometers were demonstrated in the early 1930's[9], they did not gain popularity because of their excessively short time constants. These records, when compared with those of the string galvanometer, consequently exhibited distortions having clinical implications. Introduction of the hot stylus recorder by Haynes (1936) and its use with an amplifier having a long time constant resulted in the appearance of practical direct-writing electrocardiographs, which, since 1945, have displaced the Einthoven string galvanometer.

Although the electrical activity of the brain of a rabbit had been recorded by Caton in 1875 with a Thomson reflecting galvanometer,[10] it was not until 1929 that the first human electroencephalogram was recorded by Berger, using the Einthoven string galvanometer. By the early 1940's electroencephalography had become a clinical tool, and from the beginning

[9] See Pardee (1929–30), Ernstence and Levine (1928–29), Caldwell et al. (1932), Mann (1931–1932), and D'Zuma (1931).

[10] A moving-magnet instrument used for receiving telegraphic signals. British Patent 329 (1858).

multichannel direct-inking instruments were employed. For further information on electroencephalography relative to the techniques of recording, the types of waveforms obtained, and their physiological and clinical meanings, the reader should consult Cohn (1949), Gibbs and Gibbs (1950, 1964), Hill and Parr (1950, 1963), Straus (1952), Faulconer (1960), Hughes (1961), Stewart (1961), Brechner (1962), and Kiegler (1964).

The need for a rapidly responding recorder for transient bioelectric events led Gasser and Erlanger (1922) to introduce physiologists to the Braun tube, one of the first cathode ray tubes. In their pioneering study they built their own amplifiers and circuitry to operate the Braun tube, and with it they faithfully recorded nerve action potentials. This study paved the way for later investigations of Weddell et al, (1943, 1944) which developed the basic information on which clinical electromyography is based. The reader who is interested in obtaining detailed information on the amplitudes and waveforms of the EMG signals when recorded with a variety of electrodes in normal and pathological conditions should consulted the following original papers: Weddell et al. (1944), Kugelberg (1947), Jasper and Ballem (1949), Denny-Brown (1949), Petersen and Kugelberg (1949), Landau (1951), Lundervold and Li (1953), Buchtal et al. (1954), and Liberson (1962). Among the useful clinical text books on electromyography are those by Pearson (1961), Licht (1961), Norris (1963), and Marinacci (1965).

Despite successes in obtaining faithful records of many bioelectric events, only three have attained a prominent position in clinical medicine: the electrocardiogram, the electroencephalogram, and the electromyogram. Although these three events can be recorded with many different kinds of instruments, clinical use has imposed standards on techniques of recording and display. Such standards are necessary to guarantee not only that recordings made in one laboratory will be identical with those made of the same event in another, but that all will be obtained with instruments known to be capable of faithful reproduction of these events. In the United States minimum

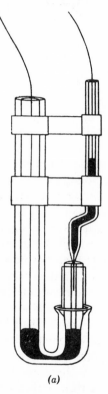

(a)

Figure 12–37. The capillary electrometer *a*, and the first electrocardiograms *b, c*. [From L. A. Geddes and H. E. *Hoff, Arch. Intern. Hist. Sci.* **56–57**:275–290 (1961).]

T

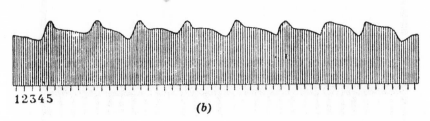

12345

(b)

G

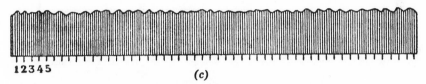

12345 *(c)*

(b) — *Marey and Lippmann's tortoise electrocardiogram. It is difficult to be certain of the identity of the waves because the authors did not provide enough information on the location of the electrodes. Quite probably the waves shown here are the R and T waves.*

(c) — *Marey and Lippmann's frog auricular electrogram. If as the authors say, the time divisions are 1/25 second, the auricular rate was 5 per second or 300 per minute, which is excessively fast for a frog heart. Very possibly the auricles were in a state of fibrillation, and if so, this is one of the earliest records of auricular fibrillation.*

Figure 12–37. (*continued*)

standards for many devices have been set by various professional societies in consultation with scientists who are considered leaders in their particular fields. These standards are usually published in reports of the Council on Physical Medicine of the American Medical Association in its journal. Those who want ECG and EEG recordings to have clinical value and who desire to make such records with instruments other than those which have been approved should check the specifications in these reports.

For faithful reproduction of the ECG[11] minimum requirements have been set to guarantee adequate low- and high-frequency responses and to standardize the speed of the recording chart and the sensitivity of the recording device. Interestingly enough the chart speed is that which Einthoven used (25 mm/second) and was derived from Marey's studies. The sensitivity,

[11]See Council on Physical Medicine (1950).

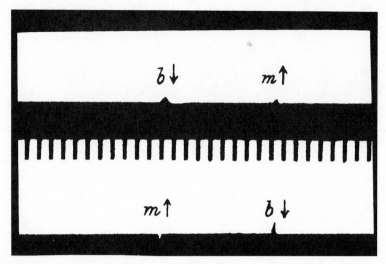

Figure 12–38. Nerve action potentials recorded with the capillary electrometer. (See text for explanation.) [From Gotch and Horsley, *Proc. Roy. Soc.* **45**: 18–26 (1888). By permission.]

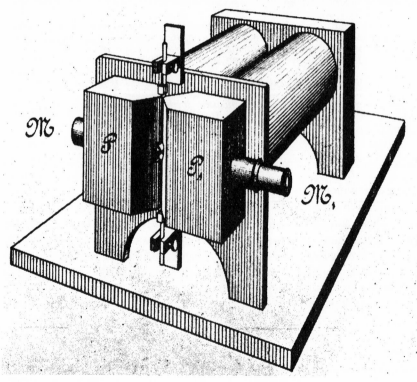

Figure 12–39. Einthoven's string galvanometer. [From W. Einthoven (1906), *Arch. Internat. Physiol.* **4**:132–164.]

1 mv per centimeter of deflection of the recording device, was adopted by Einthoven.

The minimum high- and low-frequency responses necessary for faithful reproduction of all of the various waveforms were not established without difficulty. Taking heed of precedent and of instances in which the ECG was known to be undistorted, the Council on Physical Medicine recommended as follows:

"3. One centimeter response to one millivolt peak sinusoidal voltage variation up to 15 cycles per second shall not fall below 90 percent and up to 40 cycles per second shall not fall below 80 percent of the square wave response to equivalent voltage variation. The amplitude response of the instrument to 1 millivolt peak sinusoidal voltage variation up to 300 cycles per second shall not exceed 100 percent of the square [wave] response to equivalent voltage variations."

The report defined the low-frequency response in the following manner:

"4. The response of the instrument at 0.2 second after the application of a direct current of 1.0 millivolt shall not deviate more than plus or minus 10 percent from the response at 0.04 second. The test voltage of 1 millivolt should be applied to the leads of the instrument through a series resistance of 2000 ohms."

The report of the Council concluded by defining other operating and safety features of an acceptable ECG.

A later report of the Committee on Electrocardiography of the American Heart Association (1954) specified lead configurations and terminology, and reviewed previous recommendations relating to standards for ECG instruments and only slightly altered the manner in which the frequency response was specified by stating, "When the instrument is adjusted for a maximum deflection of 1 cm in response to a direct voltage of 1 millivolt, the deflection resulting from a sinusoidal voltage of the same magnitude varying in frequency from 1 cycle to 15 cycles per second shall not be less than 0.9 cm from 15 to 40 cycles per second shall not be less than 0.8 cm, from 5 to 300 cycles per second shall not be more than 1 cm, and from 1 to 5 cycles per second shall not be more than 1.1 cm." In a footnote it was recommended that: "For a precise study of wave forms, the instrument used should display a flat frequency response from 0.5 to 100 cycles per second as a minimum characteristic." The same report continued with a description of electrodes, leads, voltage calibration, and nomenclature.

In January 1967 the recommendations for electrocardiographs and lead systems were updated by the Subcommittee on Instrumentation of the American Heart Association. Of particular importance is the revised frequency response characteristic, which was given as follows:

"(a) From 0.14 to 50 Hz, the response shall be flat to within ± 6 percent (± 0.5 dB). The response down to 0.05 Hz shall not be reduced by more than 30 percent (-3 dB) from the response at 0.14 Hz. This requirement corresponds to a "time constant" of at least 3.2 seconds, where "time constant" refers to the time required for a direct current step input (such as the calibration voltage) to decay to 36.8 percent of its original magnitude.

"(b) With an amplitude response of 5 mm peak-to-peak at 50 Hz, the response to constant amplitude sinusoidal input signals up to 100 Hz shall not be reduced by more than 30 percent (-3 dB), leaving an amplitude of at least 3.5 mm at 100 Hz.

"(c) The response shall at no frequency exceed the restraints specified for the 0.14 to 50 Hz range."

There is no doubt that there is some interest in recording the ECG with equipment having a higher frequency response. In the few studies carried out to date, no clinically useful information has been forthcoming. However, in the study reported by Langner (1952), which compared limb and precordial ECG's taken with a conventional direct writer and a system having a high-frequency response extending to 300 cps, the precordial leads exhibited notched R waves which were not detectable in the tracings taken by the direct recorder. In general the differences were greater between the precordial leads than between the limb leads. A study by Kerwin (1953) developed substantially the same information. Specifically he reported that, if the high-frequency half-power (70%) point was less than 73 cps, ECG records were distorted. With a frequency response extending to 135 cps satisfactory records were obtained. When high-speed tracings were made with a frequency response extending to 760 cps, notching of the QRS waves was observed. Whether or not the notched R waves are indicative of serious disturbances in intraventricular conduction cannot be established until further clinical studies are carried out.

In 1948 the Council on Physical Medicine of the AMA reported on the minimum requirements for acceptable direct-reading electroencephalographs. The report was based on earlier recommendations of the American Electroencephalographic Society. In addition to the obvious requirement of amplitude linearity within the operating range, the maximum sensitivity standard stated, "An input voltage change of 5 microvolts (5 μv) shall give a deflection of not less than 2 mm." For frequency response the recommendation was as follows:

"3(a) The overall frequency response of the system shall be such that between 1 and 60 cycles per second the deflections at all frequencies [presumably sinusoidal][12] shall be within 10 percent of the average of the maximum and the minimum deflections within this range.

"3(b) Overall time constant (*RC*) without low frequency cut-off filters should not be less than 0.2 second. This implies a square wave response which declines to 0.37 of its peak value in 0.2 second."

Because multichannel instruments were recommended, the permissible interchannel cross-talk was specified. In addition, because the EEG signals are small and require the use of differential amplifiers,[13] the minimum acceptable discrimination [common mode rejection][13] ratio was clearly specified as follows:

"7. 'Discrimination' here refers to the ratio of a potential difference applied between ground and the input terminals connected together (for a given deflection) to the potential difference applied between the input terminals for the same deflection. The discrimination of the instrument shall be at least 1000 to 1. The American Electroencephalographic Society recommends even more discrimination, particularly in portable apparatus."

To date there appear to be no minimum requirements for acceptable electromyographs, although there is considerable agreement on the need for such standards[14] At the 1954 meeting of the Committee on Instrumentation and Technique of the American Association for Electromyography and Electrodiagnosis, there was composed a document entitled "Information Concerning the Formulation of Minimal Requirements for Electromyographs for Clinical Use." This document listed several specifications which probably reflected the characteristics of good-quality electromyographs of that time.

The Committee recognized the difficulty in setting up standards in a new field in which techniques were varied. Nonetheless it recommended that when needle electrodes were employed the following criteria were to be satisfied. The maximum overall recording sensitivity should be 5 μv per millimeter of deflection of the indicating device. Recognizing that, although a frequency response uniform over the range of 2 to 10,000 cps would be ideal, difficulties encountered during the taking of routine EMG's dictated that a somewhat narrower frequency response would be adequate. The Committee stated:

"3(a). The overall frequency response of the system shall be such that between 40 and 3000 cps the deflections at all frequencies shall be within

[12] Authors' comments in brackets.
[13] See Chapter 13.
[14] See Lambert (1954), in Committee on Instrumentation and Techniques.

Bioelectric Event	Electrode Arrangement	Usual Calibration	Time Constant (seconds)	Rise Time (seconds)	Sine Wave Frequency Response		Usual Recorder
					Low	High (cps)	
ECG	Limb leads	1 mv/cm	3.2*	0.02†	0.08 (70%)	40 (80%)	Hot stylus
	Chest leads	0.5 mv/cm	3.2*	0.02†	0.08 (70%)	40 (80%)	Hot stylus
	Myocardial leads	10 mv/cm	2*	0.02†	0.08 (70%)	40 (80%)	Hot stylus
EEG	Scalp leads	2.5 μv/mm,‡	0.2		1.0 (90%)	60 (90%)	Ink
	Cortical leads						
EMG	Needles	5 μv/mm,‡	0.005§		40 (90%)	3000 (90%)	CRT

*Special low-frequency compensation used.
† Approximate values.
‡ Maximum recording sensitivity.
§ A range of 5 to 300 ms has been used. Authors prefer 50ms.

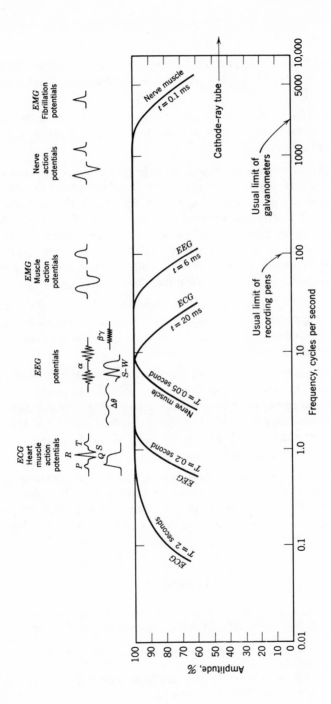

10 per cent of the average of the maximal and minimal deflections within this range.

"3(b). Overall time constant (RC) should be not less than 5 milliseconds. This implies a square wave response which declines to 0.37 of its peak value in 0.005 second."

The Committee recognized the importance of a high input impedance in view of the small-area needle electrodes ordinarily used. It therefore recommended as follows:

"8. The impedance between each input lead and the ground connection of the preamplifier, without the input cable, shall be at least 500,000 ohms in parallel with not more than 25 $\mu\mu$F. The input cable shall not add more than 250 $\mu\mu$F. These values are minimal requirements for use with needle electrodes having an exposed tip of not less than 0.1 millimeter in diameter; for needles having a smaller tip area and a relatively high impedance, the input impedance of the preamplifier should be greater. Micro-electrodes require a cathode follower input for undistorted recording."

Because the EMG signals are low in amplitude a differential input stage is required to provide the necessary amplification. In recognition of this fact, the Committee recommended that a high discrimination ratio (common mode rejection ratio) be provided:

"7. Discrimination ratio refers to the ratio of the deflection produced by a signal applied between the two input terminals to that produced by the same signal applied between ground and the two input terminals connected together. The discrimination ratio of the instrument shall be at least 2000 to 1. A greater ratio is desirable, particularly when the instrument is recommended for use in unshielded rooms."

A summary of the specifications for the instruments just described, along with other pertinent data, is presented in Fig. 12–40. The values in this illustration should be considered only as minimum requirements. Whenever possible, better lower and higher frequency response should be provided.

REFERENCES

Abildskov, J. A., and E. D. Pence. 1956. Comparative study of spatial vectorcardiograms with the equilateral tetrahedron and a corrected system of electrode placement. *Circulation* **13**:263–269.

Ader, M. 1897. Sur un nouvel appareil enregistreur pour cables sous-marins. *Comptes Rendus* **124**:1440–1442.

Adrian, E. D., and B. H. C. Matthews. 1934. The Berger rhythm: potential changes from the occipital lobes in man. *Brain* **57**:355–385.

Arrighi, F. P. 1939. El eje electrico del corazon en el espacio. *Prensa Med. Arg.* **26**:253–283.

Becking, A. G. T., H. C. Burger, and J. B. van Milaan. 1950. A universal vector cardiograph. *Brit. Heart J.* **12**:339–342.

Bennett, A. L., F. Ware, A. L. Dunn, and A. R. McIntyre. 1953. The normal membrane resting potential of mammalian skeletal muscle measured in vivo. *J. Cell. Comp. Physiol.* **42**:343–357.

Berger, H. 1929. Über das Elektronkephalogramn des Menschen. *Arch. Psychiat. Nervenkr.* **87**:527–570.

Bernstein, J. 1868. Ueber den zeitlichen Verlauf der negativen Schwankung des Nervenstroms. *Arch. Ges. Physiol.* **1**:173–207.

Brazier, M. A. B. 1949. A study of the electric fields at the surface of the head. *EEG Clin. Neurophysiol. Suppl.* **2**: 38–52.

Brechner, V. L. 1962. *Practical Electroencephalography for the Anesthesiologist.* Springfield, Ill., Charles C. Thomas, 107 pp.

Briller, S. A., N. Marchand, and C. E. Kossman. 1950. A differential vectorcardiograph. *Rev. Sci. Instr.* **21**:805–811.

Brody, D. A. 1957. An analysis of the planes and spatial electrocardiographic indices of normal subjects as referred to an orthogonalized lead system. *Am. Heart J.* **53**:125–131.

Brody, D. A., J. C. Bradshaw, and J. W. Evans. 1961. A basis for determining heart lead relations of the equivalent cardiac multipole. *IRE Trans. Bio-Med. Electron.* **BME-8**: 139–143.

Buchtal, F., C. Guld, and P. Rosenflack. 1954. Action potential parameters in normal human muscle and their dependence on physical variables. *Acta Physiol. Scand.* **32**:200–229.

Burch, G. J. 1892. On the time-relations of the excursions of the capillary electrometer, with a description of the method of using it for the investigations of electrical changes. *Phil. Trans. Roy. Soc. London,* **183**:81–106.

Burch, G., J. A. Abildskov, and J. A. Cronvitch, 1953. *Spatial Vectorcardiography.* Philadelphia, Pa., Lea and Febiger, 173 pp.

Burdon-Sanderson, J., and F. J. M. Page, 1878. Experimental results relating to the rhythmical and excitatory motions of the ventricle of the heart of the frog and the electrical phenomena which accompany them. *Proc. Roy. Soc. (London)* **27**:410.

Burdon-Sanderson, J., and F. J. M. Page. 1880. On the time relations of the excitatory process in the ventricle of the heart of the frog. *J. Physiol.* **2**:384–435.

Burger, H. C., and J. B. van Milaan. 1946. Heart vector and leads. *Brit. Heart J.* **8**: 157–161.

Burger, H. C., and J. B. van Milaan. 1947. Heart vector and leads. Part II. *Brit. Heart J.* **9**: 154–160.

Burger, H. C., J. B. van Milaan, and W. Klip. 1956. Comparison of two systems of vector-cardiography with an electrode to the frontal and dorsal sides of the trunk respectively. *Am. Heart J.* **51**:26–33.

Caldwell, S. H., C. B. Oler, and J. C. Peters. 1932. An improved form of electrocardiograph. *Rev. Sci. Instr.* **3**:277–286.

Caton, R. 1875. The electric currents of the brain. *Brit. Med. J.* **2**:278.

Caton, R. 1887. Researches on the electrical phenomena of cerebral gray matter. *Trans IX Internat. Med. Cong.* **3**:247–249.

Cohn, R. 1949. *Clinical Electroencephalography.* New York, McGraw-Hill. 639 pp.

Committee on Electrocardiography. 1954. American Heart Association. Recommendations for standardization of electrocardiographic and vectorcardiographic leads. *Circulation* **10**:564–573

Committee on Instrumentation and Technique of the American Association for Electromyography and Electrodiagnosis. 1954. Chairman E. H. Lambert. 11 pp. (Personal communication.)

Coombs, J. S., J. C. Eccles, and P. Fatt. 1955. The electrical properties of the moto-neurone membrane. *J. Physiol.* **130**:291–325.

Council on Physical Medicine. 1948. Tentative minimum requirements for acceptable direct reading electroencephalographs. *J. Am. Med. Assoc.* **138**:958–959.

Council on Physical Medicine and Rehabilitation. 1950. Minimum requirements for acceptable electrocardiographs. *J. Am. Med. Assoc.* **143**:654–655.

Denny-Brown, D. 1949. Interpretation of the electromyogram. *Arch. Neurol. Psychiat.* **61**: 99–128.

Donders, F. C. 1872. De secondaire contracties onder den involed der systolen van het hart, met en zonder vagus-prikkfung. *Utrecht Rijksuniv. Phys. Lab. Onder Zoekinjen,* **1,** Suppl. **3**:246–255.

Dower, G. E., H. E. Horn, and W. G. Ziegler. 1965. The Polarcardiograph. *Am. Heart J.* **69**:355–381.

Draper, M. H., and S. Weidmann. 1951. Cardiac resting and action potentials recorded with an intracellular electrode. *J. Physiol.* **115**:74–94.

du Bois-Reymond, E. 1843. Vorläufiger Abriss einer Untersuchung über dem sogenannten Froschstrom und über die electromotorische Fische. *Ann. Phys. Chem.* **58**:1–30.

duBois-Reymond, E. 1849. Intelligence and misc. articles (translation of duBois Reymond's article). Deflection of the magnetic needle by volition. *Phil. Mag.* **34**:543–545.

Duchosal, P., and J. R. Grosgurin. 1952. The spatial vectorcardiogram obtained by use of a trihedron and its scalar comparisons. *Circulation* **5**:237–248.

Duchosal, P. W., and R. Sulzer. 1949. *La Vectorcardiographie.* Bale, Switzerland, and New York, S. Karger, 172 pp.

Durnstock, G., M. E. Holman, and C. L. Prosser. 1963. Electrophysiology of smooth muscle. *Physiol. Rev.* **43**:482–528.

D'Zuma, A. P. 1931. A new electrocardiograph . *J. Am. Med. Assoc.* **96**:439–440.

Eccles, R. M. 1955. Intracellular potentials recorded from a mammalian sympathetic ganglion. *J. Physiol.* **130**:572–584.

Einthoven, W. G. Fahr, and A. de Waart. 1950. On the direction and manifest size of the variations of potential in the human heart and on the influence of the position of the heart on the form of the electrocardiogram. Translated by H. E. Hoff, and P. Sekelj. *Am. Heart J.* **40**:163–211.

Einthoven, W. 1903. Ein neues Galvanometer. *Ann. Physik 12,* Suppl. **4**:1059–1071.

Englemann, T. W. 1878. Ueber das electrische Verhalten des thätigen Herzens. *Arch. Ges. Physiol,* **17**:68.

Ernstence, A. E., and S. A. Levine. 1928–1929. A comparison of records taken with the Einthoven string galvanometer and the amplifier type electrocardiograph. *Am. Heart J.* **4**:725–731.

Faulconer, A. 1960. *Electroencephalography in Anesthesiology.* Springfield, Ill., Charles C. Thomas, 90 pp.

Frank, E. 1953a. Theoretical analysis of the influence of heart dipole eccentricity on limb leads, Wilson central-terminal voltage and the frontal plane vectorcardiogram. *Circ. Res.* **1**:380–388.

Frank, E. 1953b. A comparative analysis of the eccentric double-layer presentation of the human heart. *Am. Heart J.* **46**:364–378.

Frank, E. 1954. A direct experimental study of three systems of spatial vectorcardiography *Circulation* **10**:101–113.

Frank, E. 1955. Absolute quantitative comparison of instantaneous QRS equipotentials on a normal subject with dipole potentials on a homogeneous torso model. *Circ. Res.* **3**:243–251.

Frank, E. 1956. An accurate, clinically practical system for spatial vectorcardiography. *Circulation* **13**:737–749.

Frank, E. 1956–1957. Spread of current in volume conductors of finite extent. *Ann. NY. Acad. Sci.* **65**:980–1002.

Fulton, J. F., and H. Cushing. 1936. A bibliographical study of the Galvani and the Aldini writings on animal electricity. *Ann. Sci.* **1**:239–268.

Gasser, H. S., and J. Erlanger. 1922. A study of action currents of nerve with the cathode ray oscillograph. *Am J. Physiol.* **62**:496–524.

Geddes, L. A., and H. E. Hoff. 1961. The capillary electrometer. *Arch. Internat. Hist. Sci.* **56–57**:275–290.

Geselowitz, D. B. 1960. Multipole representation for an equivalent cardiac generator. *Proc IRE* **48**:75–79.

Gibbs, F. A., and E. L. Gibbs. 1950, and 1964. *Atlas of Electroencephalography.* Cambridge, Mass., Wesley Press, 3 vols.

Goldberger, E. 1953. *Unipolar Lead Electrocardiography and Vectorcardiography.* Philadelphia Pa., Lea and Febiger, 601 pp.

Grant, R. P. 1957. *Clinical Electrocardiography—The Spatial Vector Approach.* New York, McGraw-Hill, 225 pp.

Grant, R. P., and E. H. Estes. 1951, *Spatial Vector Electrocardiography*, Philadelphia, Pa., Blakiston Co., 145 pp.

Grishman, A. 1952. *Spatial Vectorcardiography.* Philadelphia, Pa., W. B. Saunders, 217 pp.

Grishman, A., E. R. Borun, and H. L. Jaffe. 1951. Spatial vectorcardiography. *Am. Heart J.* **41**:483–493.

Grundfest, H. 1947. Bioelectric potentials in the nervous system and in muscle. *Ann. Rev. Physiol.* **9**:477–506.

Grundfest, H. 1966a. Comparative electrobiology of excitable membranes. *Advan. Comp. Physiol. Biochem.* **2**:1–116.

Grundfest, H. 1966b. Heterogeneity of excitable membranes; electrophysiological and pharmacological evidence and some consequences. *Ann. N.Y. Acad. Sci.* **137**:901–949.

Guntheroth, W. G. 1965. *Pediatric Electrocardiography.* Philadelphia, Pa., W. B. Saunders, 150 pp.

Haynes, J. R. 1936. A heated stylus for use with waxed recording paper. *Rev. Sci. Instr.* **7**: 108.

Hecht, H. H. 1956–1957. Normal and abnormal transmembrane potentials of the spontaneously beating heart. *Ann. N.Y. Acad. Sci.* **65**:700–740.

Helm, R. A. 1957. An accurate lead system for spatial vectorcardiography. *Am. Heart J.* **53**: 415–424.

Hill, D., and G. Parr. 1950. *Electroencephalography: A Symposium on Its Various Aspects.* London, Macdonald & Co., 438 pp.

Hill, D., and G. Parr, 1963. *Electroencephalography: A Symposium on Its Various Aspects.* New York, Macmillan and Co., 509 pp.

Hlavin, J. M., and R. Plonsey 1963. An experimental determination of a multipole representation of a turtle heart. *IEEE Trans. Bio-Med. Electron.* **BME-10**:98–105.

Hodgkin, A. L. 1951. The ionic basis of electrical activity in nerve and muscle. *Biol. Rev. Cambridge Phil. Soc.* **26**:339–409.

Hodgkin, A. L., and P. Horowicz. 1957. The differential action of hypertonic solutions on the twitch and action potential of a muscle fiber. *J. Physiol.* **136**:17P-18P.

Hodgkin, A. L., and A. F. Huxley. 1939. Action potentials recorded from inside a nerve fiber. *Nature* **144**:710–711.

Hoff, H. E. 1936. Galvani and the pre-Galvani electrophysiologists. *Ann. Sci.* **1**: 157–172.

Hoff, H. E., and L. A. Geddes. 1957. The rheotome and its prehistory: A study in the historical interrelation of electrophysiology and electromechanics, *Bull. Hist. Med.* **31**:212–347.

Hoff, H. E., and L. A. Geddes. *Experimental Physiology*, (2nd ed.). Houston, Texas, Baylor University College of Medicine.

Hoffmann, B. F., and E. E. Suckling. Cardiac cellular potentials: effect of vagal stimulation and acetylcholine. *Am. J. Physiol.* **173**:312–320.

Hollmann, H. E., and W. Hollmann. 1938. Das Einthovensche Druckschema als Grudlage neuer elektrokardiograpischen Registriermethoden. *Z. für Klinik. Med.* **134**:732–753.

Holman, M. E. 1958. Membrane potentials recorded with high resistance micro-electrodes. *J. Physiol.* **141**:464–488.

Horan, L. G., N. C. Flowers, and D. A. Brody. 1963. Body surface potential distribution. *Circ. Res.* **13**:373–387.

Hughes, R. R. 1961. *An Introduction to Electroencephalography*. Bristol, J. Wright, 118 pp.

Huxley, A. F., and R. Stampfli. 1951. Direct determination of membrane resting potential and action potential in single myelinated nerve fibers. *J. Physiol.* **112**: 476–495.

Isaacs, J. H. 1964. A study of electrical fields. The differential vectorscope. *Am. J. Med. Electron.* **2**: 34–40.

Ishitoya, J. T. Sakurai, I. Aita, and K. Sasaki. 1965. A new type of spatial vectorcardiograph *Tohoku J. Exp. Med.* **85**:1–8.

Jasper, H. H., and G. Ballem, 1949. Unipolar electromyograms of normal and denervated human muscle. *J. Neurophysiol.* **12**:231–244.

Kerwin, A. J. 1953. The effect of frequency response of electrocardiographs on the form of electrocardiograms and vectorcardiograms. *Circulation* **8**: 98–110.

Kiegler, J. 1964. *Electroencephalography in Hospital and General Consulting Practice*. Amsterdam, Elsevier Publ. Co., 180 pp.

Kölliker, R. A., and J. Müller. 1856. Nachweis der negativen Schwankung des Muskélstroms am natürlich sich contrahirenden Muskel. *Verhandl. Phys. med. Gesellsch. Wurzburg* **6**:528–533.

Kowarzykowic, H., and Z. Kowarzykowic. 1961. *Spatial Vectorcardiography*. Oxford, Pergamon Press, 254 pp.

Kugelberg, E. 1947. Electromyograms in muscular disorders. *J. Neurol. Neurosurg. Psychiat.* **10**:122–136.

Lamb, L. E. 1965. *Electrocardiography and Vectorcardiography*. Philadelphia, Pa., W. B. Saunders, 609 pp.

Landau, W. M. 1951. Comparison of different needle leads in EMG recording from a single site. *EEG Clin. Neurophysiol.* **3**:163–168.

Langner, P. H. 1952. The value of high fidelity electrocardiography using the cathode ray oscillograph and an expanded time scale. *Circulation* **5**: 249–256.

Langner, P. H., R. Okada, S. R. Moore, and H. C. Fies. 1958. Comparison of four orthogonal systems of vectorcardiography. *Circulation* **17**:46–54.

Lenz, E. 1849, 1854. Über den Einfluss der Geschwindigkeit des Drehens auf den durch magneto-electrische Machinen erzeugten Inductronsstrom. *Ann. Physik. Chem.* 1849, **152**:494–523; 1854, **92**:128–152.

Liberson, W. T. 1962. Report on the standardization of reporting and terminology in electromyography. *EEG Clin. Neurophysiol.* **22**:107–172.

Licht, S. H. 1961. *Electrodiagnosis and Electromyography*. New Haven, Conn., E. Licht, 470 pp.

Lundervold, A., and C-L. Li. 1953. Motor units and fibrillation potentials as recorded with different kinds of needle electrodes. *Acta Psychiat. Neurol. Scand.* **28**:201–212.

McFee, R., and F. D. Johnston. 1954. Electrocardiographic leads. III. Synthesis. *Circulation* **9**:868–880.

Mann, H. 1920. *A method of analyzing the electrocardiogram. Arch. Int. Med.* **25**:283–294.

Mann, H. 1931. Interpretation of bundle-branch block by means of the monocardiogram. *Am. Heart. J.* **6**:447–457.

Mann, H. 1931–1932. A light weight portable EKG. *Am Heart J.* 1931–1932, **7**: 796–797.

Mann, H. 1938. The monocardiograph. *Am. Heart J.* **15**:681–689.

Marchand, R. 1877. Beiträge zur Kentniss der Reizwelle und Contractionswelle des Herzmuskels. *Arch. Ges. Physiol.* **15**:511.

Marey, E. J. 1876. Des variations électriques des muscles du coeur en particulier étudiées au moyen de l'électromètre de M. Lippmann. *Comptes Rendus* **82**:975–977.

Marinacci, A. A. 1965. *Clinical Electromyography.* Los Angeles, Calif., San Lucas Press, 199 pp.

Matteucci, C. 1842a. Correspondence. *Comptes Rendus* **159**, Suppl. 2:797–798.

Matteucci, C. 1842b. Sur un phénomène physiologique produit par les muscles en contraction. *Ann. Chim. Phys.* **6**: Suppl. **3**: 339–343.

Mauro, A., L. H. Nahum, R. S. Sikand, and H. Chernoff. 1952. Equipotential distribution for the various instants of the cardiac cycle of the body surface of the dog. *Am. J. Physiol.* **168**:584–591.

Mauro, A., L. H. Nahum, and R. Sikand. 1952–1953. Instantaneous equipotential distribution on the thoracic surface of human subjects with cardiac pathology. *J. Appl. Physiol.* **5**:698–704.

Nahum, L. H., A. Mauro, H. M. Chernoff, and R. J. Sikand. 1951. Instantaneous equipotential distribution on surface of the human body for various instants in the cardiac cycle. *J. Appl. Physiol.* **3**:454–464.

Nahum, L. H., A. Mauro, H., Levine, and D.G. Abrahams. 1952–1953. Potential field during the S T segment. J. Appl. Physiol. **5**:693–697.

Nelson, C. V. 1956. Human thorax potentials. *Ann. N.Y. Acad. Sci.* **65** 1014–1050.

Nelson, C. V., E. T. Angelakos, and P. R. Gastonguay, 1965. Dipole moments of dog, monkey and lamb hearts. *Circ. Res.* **17**:168–177.

Nobili, C. L. 1828. Comparison entre deux galvanomètres les plus sensibles, la grenouille et le multiplicateur à deux agiulles suivi de quelques resultats nouveaux. *Ann. Chim. Phys.* **38**, Suppl. 2:225–245.

Nonogawa, A. 1966, Comparison of five different vectorcardiographic systems. *Japan. Circ. J.* **30**:1009–1016.

Norris, F. H. 1963. *The EMG.* New York, Grune and Stratton, 134 pp.

Okada, R. H. 1956. Potentials produced by an eccentric current dipole in a finite-length circular conducting cylinder. *IRE Trans. Bio-Med. Electron.* **7**: 14–19.

Okada, R. H. 1957. An experimental study of multiple dipole potentials and the effects of inhomogeneities in volume conductors. *Am. Heart J.* **54**: 567–571.

Pardee, H. E. B. 1929–1930. The distortion of the EKG by capacitance. *Am. Heart J.* **5**: 191–196.

Pearson, R. B. 1961. *Handbook of Clinical Electromyography.* El Monte, Calif., The Meditron Co., 72 pp.

Petersen, I., and E. Kugelberg. 1949. Duration and form of action potential in the normal human muscle. *J. Neurol. Neurosurg. Psychiat.* **12**:124–128.

Phillips, C. G. 1955. The dimensions of a cortical motor point. *J. Physiol.* **129**:20P–21P.

Plonsey, R. 1963a. Current dipole images and reference potentials. *IEEE Trans. Bio-Med. Electron.* **BME-10**:1–8.

Plonsey, R. 1963b. Reciprocity applied to volume conductors and the ECG. *IEEE Trans. Bio-Med. Electron.* **BME-10**:9–12.

Pozzi, L. 1961. *Basic Principles in Vector Electrocardiography.* Springfield, Ill., Charles. C. Thomas, 292 pp.

Rappaport, M. B., C. Williams, and P. D. White. 1949. An analysis of the relative accuracies of the Wilson and Goldberger methods for registering unipolar and augmented unipolar and augmented unipolar electrocardiographic leads. *Am. Heart J.* **37**: 892–917.

Report of the Committee on Electrocardiography, American Heart Association. 1954. *Circulation* **10**:564–573.

Schellong, F., S. Heller, and E. Schwingel. 1937. Das Vektordiagramm. 1. *Z. Kreislaufforsch.* **29**:497–509.

Schellong, F., and E. Schwingel. 1937. Das Vektordiagramm. II. *Z. Kreislaufforsch.* **29**: 596–607.

Schellong, F., E. Schwingel, and C. Hermann. 1937. Die praktisch-klinische Methode der Vektordiagraphie und des normale Vektordiagramm. *Arch. Kreislaufforsch.* **1**: 1.

Schmitt, O. H., and E. Simonson. 1955. The present status of vectorcardiography. *AMA Arch. Int. Med.* **96**:574–590.

Simonson, E. 1952. The distribution of cardiac potentials around the chest in one hundred and three normal men. *Circulation* **6**:201–211.

Simonson, E. 1961. *Differentiation between Normal and Abnormal in Electrocardiography.* St. Louis, Mo., C.V. Mosby Co., 328 pp.

Simonson, E., O. Schmitt, and H. Nakagawa. 1959. Quantitative comparison of eight vectorcardiographic lead systems. *Circ. Res.* **7**:296–302.

Stewart, L. 1961. *Introduction to the Principles of Electroencephalography.* Springfield, Ill., Charles C. Thomas, 55 pp.

Straus, H. 1952. *Diagnostic Electroencephalography.* New York, Grune and Stratton, 282 pp.

Subcommittee on Instrumentation. 1967. Recommendations for standardization in electrocardiography and vectorcardiography. *IEEE Trans. Bio-Med. Eng.* **BME-14**:60–68.

Sulzer, R., and P. W. Duchosal, 1938. Applications de la planographie. *Arch Mal. Coeur Vaisseaux.* **31**:682–685, 686–696.

Sulzer, R., and P. W. Duchosal. 1945. Principes de cardiovectorgraphie. *Cardiologia* **9**: 106–120.

Taccardi, B. 1962. Distribution of heart potentials on dog's thoracic surface. *Circ. Res.* **11**:862–869.

Uhley, H. N. 1962. *Vector Electrocardiography.* Philadelphia, Pa., J. B. Lippincott, 339 pp.

Walker, W. C. 1937. Animal electricity before Galvani. *Ann. Sci.* **2**: 83–113.

Waller, A. D. 1889. On the electromotive changes connected with the beat of the mammalian heart and of the human heart in particular. *Phil. Trans. Roy. Soc. London* **180B**:169–194.

Weddell, G., B. Feinstein, and R. E. Prattle. 1943. The clinical application of electromyography, *Lancet* **1**:236–239.

Weddell, G., B. Feinstein, and R. E. Prattle. 1944. The electrical activity of voluntary muscle in man under normal and pathological conditions. *Brain* **67**:178–257.

Williams, H. B. 1914. On the cause of the phase difference frequently observed between homonymous peaks of the electrocardiogram. *Am. J. Physiol.* **35**:292–300.

Wilson, F. W., and R. H. Bayley. 1950. The electric field of an eccentric dipole in a homogeneous spherical conducting medium. *Circulation* **1**: 84–92.

Wilson, F. N., and F. D. Johnston, 1938. The vectorcardiogram. *Am. Heart J.* **16**:14–28.

Wilson, F. N., F. D. Johnston, and C. E. Kossman. 1947. The substitution of a tetrahedron for the Einthoven triangle. *Am. Heart J.* **33**:594–603.

Wilson, F. N., F. D. Johnston, A. G., Macleod, and P. S. Barker. 1934 Electrocardiograms that represent the potential variations of a single electrode. *Am. Heart J.* **9**:447–458.

Woodbury, L. A., J. W. Woodbury, and H. H. Hecht. 1950. Membrane resting and action potentials of single cardiac muscle fibers. *Circulation* **1**: 264–266.

13

Amplifiers

13–1 INTRODUCTION

The signals produced by physiological transducers and bioelectric events are small and therefore require amplification to suitable levels for recording or display. The purpose of this chapter is to discuss the fundamental principles of various types of amplifiers and to point out the operating characteristics of each to indicate its suitability for amplification and energizing display devices.

Amplification is obtained by means of either vacuum tubes or transistors or a combination of the two, each device being used for its unique characteristics. Circuits employing vacuum tubes are generally easier to analyze and are more familiar to most investigators in the life sciences, although solid-state circuits possess distinct advantages and have, in many newer systems, entirely replaced vacuum tubes. It is therefore important at this time to have knowledge of the characteristics of both devices.

The vacuum tube came into existance in 1884 when Edison placed a metallic plate in one of his light bulbs while seeking a method of preventing the bulb from darkening. In experimenting with the device, he noticed that current would flow between the plate and the heated filament when a galvanometer was connected between these elements. Without knowing the explanation for the current, he patented[1] the device and the phenomenon became known as the Edison effect. Its explanation, of course, had to await the discovery of the electron by J. J. Thomson some 13 years later.

The Edison effect was put to useful service in 1904 by Fleming, who discovered the unidirectional conducting properties of Edison's device. With one wire of a galvanometer connected to the plate and the other connected to the positive pole of a battery, the negative pole of which was

---

[1]U.S. Patent 307, 031, Oct. 21, 1884.

connected to the heated filament, it was observed that the current flowing was proportional to the voltage of the battery. With the polarity of the battery reversed, no current was detectable. Fleming likened the action to that of a valve. This is probably the origin of the designation "valve" used in the United Kingdom for a vacuum tube.

Because Fleming's valve could conduct in one direction, it could be used as a detector, and in the early days of radio it saw considerable service in this role. According to Upton (1957), De Forest began studying methods of improving the Fleming valve and was led to incorporate a third electrode between the plate and the filament.[2] Although this device proved to be a superior detector, its potential as an amplifier was not recognized until 1912, when De Forest and Logwood build the first vacuum tube amplifier. Because of its ability to amplify audio frequencies, the triode became known as the audion.

Despite financial and legal difficulties, De Forest succeeded in expanding development of the triode. In a remarkably short time its possibilities became recognized because there were technological gaps in communications that it filled adequately. Within a few years, the triode was used as an amplifier for long-distance telephony and as an oscillator for generating radio-frequency waves, thereby giving birth to modern communications.

The first triodes were made by lamp manufacturers. By 1920 about one million had been manufactured, and a few soon found their way into electrophysiological investigations. In this field, in which the Einthoven string galvanometer reigned supreme, there was need of a device to record a variety of low-voltage bioelectric events. Although the string galvanometer was adequate for human ECG's, it lacked the sensitivity needed for ECG's of small animals and obviously did not offer the response time required for nerve and muscle action potentials. Although investigators knew that sensitivity could be increased by slackening the string, the response time was thereby lengthened. It was soon recognized that the needed sensitivity could be obtained by the use of a vacuum-tube amplifier connected between the subject and the string galvanometer. Those who had used the capillary electrometer also saw the value of increasing its sensitivity with a vacuum-tube amplifier. With the availability of the first cathode-ray (Braun) tubes and rapidly responding mirror oscillographs, many vacuum-tube amplifiers were constructed and put into service for the amplification of bioelectric events.

Among the first to report on the use of the vacuum-tube amplifier for electrophysiological investigation were Forbes and Thacher (1920) and Gasser and Newcomer (1921) in the United States and Daly and Shillshear (1920–1921) in England. Acting on a suggestion by Williams, the pioneer

[2]U.S. Patents 841, 387 (1907) and 879, 532 (1908).

electrocardiographer, Forbes and Thacher built a single-stage amplifier and capacitively coupled it to a string galvanometer. With this apparatus they recorded action potentials of frog and cat nerves and human muscles. The amplifier built by Daly and Shillshear employed a vacuum tube in one arm of a Wheatstone bridge. The string galvanometer was used as a detector, and with this apparatus frog ECG's were recorded.

Gasser and Newcomer desired to record the action potentials of the canine phrenic nerve during respiration. To accomplish this, they built a three-stage resistance-capacitance coupled amplifier and connected it to a string galvanometer which was operated with a tight string. High-quality records of volleys of actions potentials were recorded, using two stages of amplification. Gasser and Erlanger (1922) desired to record nerve action potentials more carefully, therefore they abandoned the string galvanometer as a reproducer and used the Braun cathode-ray tube with a three-stage resistance-capacitance coupled amplifier. With this apparatus they obtained an overall amplification of 7400 and a response time of slightly less than 1 μ s. Details of the Gasser-Erlanger circuit were sent to Adrian (1926) in England; he constructed his own amplifier for use with the capillary electrometer. He chose this device as a reproducer because of the low light output of the Braun tube. Noteworthy is the fact that, with these instruments, Gasser and Erlanger conducted their fundamental studies which demonstrated that in nerve the speed of conduction is related to fiber diameter, and Adrian showed that in the nervous system, intensity is signaled by the frequency of nerve impulses. Both studies earned Nobel prizes for the investigators.

Many of the subsequent studies which employed the vacuum-tube amplifier were directed toward the development of a suitable reproducer. Rosenberg (1927) demonstrated nerve action potentials, using a three-stage transformer-coupled amplifier connected to a Siemens high-frequency oscillograph which was commercially available at the time. The response time attained was 0.1 ms. Matthews (1928) developed his moving-vane (tongue) mirror oscillograph for use with the vacuum tube amplifier and attained a response time of about 0.2 ms. With Matthews' oscillograph connected to a five-stage direct-coupled amplifier, Adrian (1931) recorded the spontaneous electrical activity in the abdominal ganglia of the water beetle.

Perhaps the ultimate refinement of the string galvanometer as a rapidly responding reproducer was due to Forbes et al. (1931). Basing their work on experiments carried out by Williams (1926), they built their own string galvanometers, using quartz fibers 0.5 to 1 micron in diameter and 7 mm long, which were tightened to have a resonant frequency of more than 10,000 cps. With these instruments connected to a six-stage resistance-capacitance coupled amplifier, they recorded the action potentials of the frog sciatic nerve.

Even before the string galvanometer became widely used clinically for ECG's its fragility was recognized, and several attempts were made to replace it with a rugged, rapidly responding mirror oscillograph connected to a vacuum tube amplifier. According to Marvin (1953), C. P. Steinmetz and W. R. G. Baker of the General Electric Company started to develop a vacuum-tube electrocardiograph in 1917 on the suggestion of Dr. L. H. Neuman of Albany, but the project had to be abandoned because of other commitments during World War 1. The project was resumed in 1921, and three years later what is believed to be the first vacuum-tube ECG was demonstrated. Although subsequent vacuum-tube ECG instruments did not gain popularity,[3] use of the vacuum tube in electrophysiology continued.

An ingenious electronic cardiotachometer, using chest electrodes connected to a four-stage, tuned transformer-coupled amplifier, was developed for Boas in 1928 by A. N. Goldsmith, a pioneer in radio engineering. This device was not only the first vacuum tube cardiotachometer but was also one of the first to use tuned circuits to separate the R wave from the P and T waves to obtain a sharp noise-free spike to operate the cardiotachometer.

By the early 1930's the use of vacuum-tube amplifiers in electrophysiology had increased substantially. Some were connected to string galvanometers to increase their sensitivity and to obtain a high input impedance; others were connected to mirror galvanometers, cathode-ray tubes, and direct-recording pens. With careful shielding, most of the amplifiers operated satisfactorily when single-channel records were made. However, many channels of amplification could not be employed easily to record multiple bioelectric events from the same preparation because of the need to use a common reference electrode. In addition, elimination of ground-referred interference was always difficult. A solution to all of these problems was provided by the various types of differential amplifiers which appeared around 1937. A discussion of them is presented in this chapter.

13-2. VACUUM TUBES

The simplest vacuum tube used for amplification is the triode, which is a three-element device consisting of a cathode, grid, and plate in an evacuated glass bulb. It is shown schematically in Figure 13–1. The cathode is frequently a cylindrical metallic sleeve coated with a material which emits a large number of electrons when heated. The heat is obtained from an electrically

[3] See Chapter 12.

energized filament placed inside the cylindrical sleeve but insulated from it by a refractory material. Cathodes are usually operated at approximately 1000°K. The grid is an open screen surrounding the cathode and often concentric with it. Its function is to control the electric field in the vicinity of the cathode, which in turn determines the number of electrons permitted to pass through the grid structure. The grid is usually operated with a potential which is negative with respect to the cathode and thereby exerts a repulsive force on the electrons liberated by the cathode. The plate consists of a cylindrical metallic sleeve, concentric with the grid and cathode. Its operating potential is positive with respect to the cathode, and its function is to collect the electrons which have passed through the grid structure. Thus there is a competitive action on the electron stream; the positive anode attracts the electrons and the negatively charged grid repels them. Because the grid is in close proximity to the cathode, a very small change in grid voltage will produce a large change in the number of electrons traveling to the anode. Since the plate current is constituted by the electron flow, a small change in grid voltage produces a considerable charge in plate current. By allowing a change in plate current to flow through a resistance, a change in voltage can be developed: this technique forms the basis of the operation of the vacuum tube as a voltage amplifier. By using the plate current to produce to a magnetic field, electromagnetic devices such as relays, transformers, and deflection coils can be operated.

13–3.   VOLTAGE-CURRENT CHARACTERISTICS

The operation of the triode is completely specified in terms of the instantaneous potential differences existing between the three elements and the resulting currents which flow in them. It is customary to think of the vacuum tube (and more complex systems) in terms of two input terminals and two output terminals, that is, a four-terminal network. This concept is illustrated in Fig. 13–2. In order to place a three-element device in such an arrangement of four terminals, it is necessary that one element be common to two terminals. This concept is useful not only in examining the various possible circuit configurations for vacuum tubes

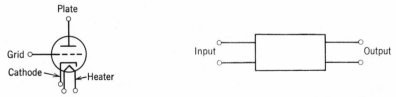

Figure 13–1.   The triode vacuum tube.   **Figure 13–2.**   The four-terminal network.

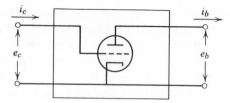

Figure 13-3. The triode represented as a four-terminal network with the cathode common.

but also applies equally well to transistors; for example, in Fig. 13-3 the cathode is common and the variables of interest are the input voltage and current e_c and i_c, respectively, and the output voltage and current e_b and i_b. A practical circuit for measuring these quantities is shown in Fig. 13-4. In this figure the currents and voltages are shown in capital letters to indicate that, once adjusted to specific values, they remain fixed until one or more is reset, that is, the values reflect static or no-signal conditions in the vacuum tube.

In determining the relationship between the voltages and currents, it is found that, if the voltage from grid to cathode is maintained negative, the grid current I_c is, in most practical applications, negligibly small. The operation of the triode is specified therefore by the simultaneous values of grid voltage E_c, plate voltage E_b, and plate current I_b. It is customary to assign fixed specific values to one of these quantities (in which case it is called a parameter) and to examine the relationship between the remaining two (called variables), which can be displayed by a conventional two-dimensional graph. The plate characteristic curve, which shows the plate current I_b as a function of the plate voltage E_b with the grid voltage E_c as the parameter, is the relationship between these quantities most frequently given in vacuum tube manuals. A typical triode plate characteristic curve is shown in Fig. 13-5. From the static characteristic can be derived other quantities, called the tube parameters, important in describing the dynamic operation of the tube: the plate resistance r_p, the amplification factor μ, and the transconductance g_m; their use in predicting the operation of the tube as an amplifier will be discussed subsequently.

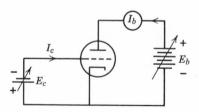

Figure 13-4. Circuit for the measurement of currents and voltages in the triode.

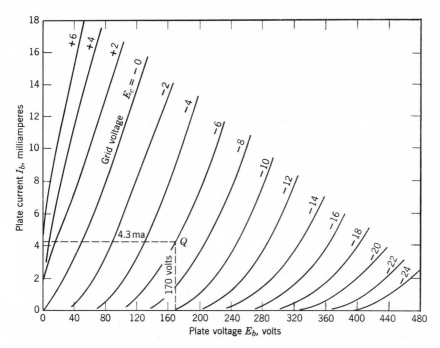

Figure 13–5. Plate characteristics of type 6J5 vacuum tube.

In analyzing the operation of the vacuum tube by means of the static characteristic curve it is important to note that the curve describes the behavior of the tube only with respect to the voltages actually appearing across the elements of the tube and the current(s) through the tube regardless of the circuitry to which the tube may be connected. Therefore, as shown in Fig. 13–5, if for any reason the voltage from plate to cathode is 170 volts and from grid to cathode is –6 volts, the current flowing from plate to cathode has the value 4.3 ma.

The circuit shown in Fig. 13–4 is useful for little else than applying the voltages E_c and E_b directly to the tube elements for the purpose of obtaining the static characteristics of the tube. The addition of a resistor R_L in the plate circuit, as shown in Fig. 13–6, permits the tube to function as a voltage amplifier. In order to understand how amplification is achieved it is necessary to introduce the concept of the load line.

13–4. THE LOAD LINE

The operation of a transistor or vacuum tube amplifier can be analyzed graphically by means of the load line. Its use will be demonstrated by applying Ohm's law to the plate circuit of Fig. 13–6, in which it is apparent that

$$E_B = e_r + e_b, \tag{A}$$

where E_B = the applied battery or power supply voltage,
$e_r = i_b R_L$, the voltage drop across R_L resulting from the plate current i_b flowing through R_L,
e_b = the plate-to-cathode voltage of the tube.

Equation (A) may be written as

$$E_B = i_b R_L + e_b, \tag{B}$$

whence

$$i_b = -\frac{1}{R_L} e_b + \frac{E_B}{R_L}, \tag{C}$$

which is the equation of straight line of the "slope-intercept" form:

$$y = m(x) + b$$

Thus the plate current i_b is a linear function of the plate-to-cathode voltage e_b. This function is completely described in terms of the slope $-1/R_L$ and intercept E_B/R_L. Equation C states that over the total range of possible values of e_b (from $e_b = 0$ to $e_b = E_B$) the corresponding values of plate current are constrained to the straight line, and that the values of I_b corresponding to $e_b = 0$ and $e_b = E_B$ are E_B/R_L and 0, respectively. A straight line is also described if i_b is made the independent variable:

From equation B

$$e_b = -R_L(i_b) + E_B, \tag{D}$$

from which it is seen that, over the possible range of values of i_b, e_b is constrained to the same straight line described above. Equation D perhaps allows better visualization of the tube operating path in that one can

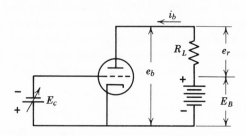

Figure 13–6.   The triode amplifier.

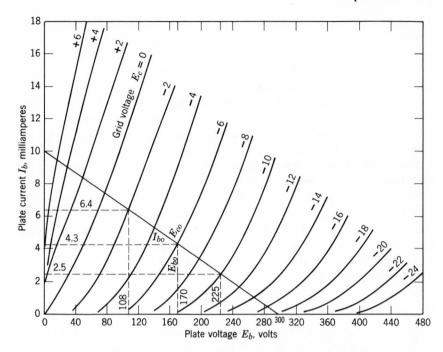

Figure 13-7. Use of the load line to determine amplification.

easily picture the grid potential controlling the number of electrons permitted to pass to the plate per second (i_b), which then determines the plate-to-cathode voltage e_b. This information may now be applied to a practical problem to demonstrate the construction and use of the load line to display the dynamic operation of the tube as an amplifier.

13-5. AMPLIFICATION

Assume that the tube in Fig. 13-6 has the characteristics shown in Fig. 13-7 and that the following values have been chosen: $R_L = 30,000$ ohms, $E_B = 300$ volts, $E_c = -6$ volts. Because the load line is a straight line, it is determined by any two points which satisfy equation C. Two convenient points can be found as follows: when

$$i_b = 0, \qquad e_b = E_B = 300,$$

$$e_b = 0, \qquad i_b = \frac{E_B}{R_L} = \frac{300}{30,000} = 10 \text{ ma.}$$

The load line has been drawn in Fig. 13–7. Observe that when the grid voltage E_c is set at -6 volts the plate current I_b is 4.3 ma and the plate-to-cathode voltage E_b is 170 volts. This arbitrarily selected set of conditions may be defined as the operating point, and these fixed voltage and current values designated as E_{c0}, I_{b0}, and E_{b0}.

If E_c is now changed from the operating point value $(-6$ volt) to a new value such as -2 volts, the plate circuit operation is constrained to move upward along the load line to the point where $E_b = 108$ volts and $I_b = 6.4$ma. Likewise, if E_c is given the value -10 volts, E_b and I_b become 225 volts and 2.5 ma, respectively. Suppose that conditions are then returned to the operating point by resetting E_c to -6 volts.

From these data it is seen that a total change in the grid voltage magnitude of 8 volts (from -2 to -10 volt) resulted in a corresponding change in the plate voltage magnitude of 117 volts (from 108 to 225 volts). The voltage amplification from grid to plate is therefore $117/8 = 14.6$, that is, a 1-volt change in grid-to-cathode voltage produced a plate-to-cathode voltage change of 14.6.

13–6. PHASE SHIFT

In the common-cathode circuit the output voltage e_b is opposite in phase to the input voltage. Thus, in the example above, when the grid-to-cathode voltage was increased (made less negative) from -6 to -2 volts, the plate-to-cathode voltage was decreased (made less positive) from 170 to 108 volts. Phase shift is of great importance when several stages of amplification are coupled together and feedback (either intentional or unintentional) is considered. Also, the relative phase of voltages is fundamental to the operation of differential amplifiers, which are especially prominent in electrophysiological studies.

13–7. DISTORTION

Although there are several ways of defining distortion, it exists in an amplifier when the waveform of the output differs from that of the input. How this can occur is shown by the following example.

Instead of manually causing the grid (bias) battery voltage E_c to move from the operating point in discrete steps, assume that a sinusoidal voltage source is connected in series with the bias battery as shown in Fig. 13–8. Let the sinusoidal voltage vary between $+4$ and -4 volts, that is, it is said to have a peak-to-peak value of 8 volts. Clearly then, if the bias battery is used to set the operating point to the value previously designated (-6 volts), the sinusoidal voltage will cause the tube operation to move up and down the load line between the grid voltage limits of -2 to -10 volts.

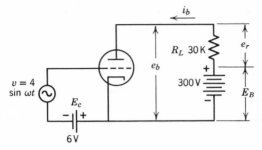

Figure 13–8.   The biased triode amplifier.

It is instructive to examine the degree of symmetry about the operating point. For example, referring to Fig. 13–7, when the grid voltage is changed from the operating point value of -6 to -2 volts, the plate voltage changes from 170 to 108 volts, resulting in a voltage amplification in this direction of $(108{-}170)/[-2{-}(-6)] = -15.5$; the negative sign denotes a phase shift of 180° between the input and output voltages. When the grid voltage is changed from the operating point (-6 volts) to -10 volts, the corresponding plate voltage change is from 170 to 225 volts and the voltage amplification is $(225{-}170)/[-10{-}(-6)] = -13.8$. Recall that the voltage amplification, considering the total grid voltage and plate voltage changes, was found to be 14.6. It is apparent that, for this particular set of tube characteristics and with operation in the manner described, a sinusoidal wave of 4 volts peak amplitude applied to the input will be amplified but somewhat distorted. This point is emphasized because the limitations of the vacuum tube as a linear device are clearly demonstrated in terms of the actual voltage and current values which characterize its behavior. It is important to keep this fact in mind because many analyses of vacuum tube (and transistor) circuits are based upon linear equivalent circuits for these devices which neglect the curvature and variations in spacing between the characteristic curves.

Published plate circuit characteristics, as shown in Fig. 13–7, are merely representative of the tube type. In this respect it is instructive to determine and compare the characteristics of a group of vacuum tubes of the same type with one another and with the published characteristics. The variation is often considerable.

13–8.   THE TUBE PARAMETERS μ, g_m AND r_p

The vacuum tube parameters μ, g_m, and r_p are characteristic quantities which describe the tube as a circuit element. They are often called constants and single specific values are assigned, although the actual values depend upon the operating point. In the data sheets describing the vacuum tube, these quantities are always given. They are defined as follows:

Amplification factor: $\qquad \mu = \dfrac{\Delta e_b}{\Delta e_c}\bigg|_{i_b = \text{constant}}$

Transconductance: $\qquad g_m = \dfrac{\Delta i_b}{\Delta e_c}\bigg|_{e_b = \text{constant}}$

Plate resistance $\qquad r_p = \dfrac{1}{g_p} = \dfrac{\Delta e_b}{\Delta i_b}\bigg|_{e_c = \text{constant}}$

where g_p is described as the plate conductance, and Δe_b, Δe_c, Δi_b represent small corresponding changes in the plate-to-cathode voltage, grid-to-cathode voltage, and plate current, respectively. If the voltage-current characteristics of the triode consisted of equally spaced, straight lines the parameters μ, g_m, and r_p would indeed have constant values. These conditions are met sufficiently in the "linear portion" of the characteristics to permit assigning values to the parameters and using them in linear equivalent circuits which closely approximate the behavior of the tube for operation confined to the linear portion of the characteristics.

13-9. THE LINEAR EQUIVALENT CIRCUIT

Because it is often impractical to employ a graphical method to determine the operating characteristics of a vacuum-tube circuit, the vacuum-tube is represented by an equivalent circuit. The linear-equivalent circuit makes possible the solution of a large number of vacuum-tube problems by means of the well-established techniques of linear-network theory. As implied in the designation linear-equivalent circuit, it will be assumed that the vacuum-tube characteristics are straight lines. It will be assumed further that the lines are parallel and equally spaced. Certainly for small-signal operation the approximation is close over a reasonable range of the tube characteristics. The assumption of straight, parallel, and equally spaced lines simplifies greatly the mathematical considerations in deriving the equivalent circuit. The derivation will not be presented here. The interested reader is referred to a textbook such as that of Alley and Atwood (1966) for complete details. Under the conditions just mentioned, it can be shown that the vacuum tube may be represented as either a constant-voltage source of magnitude μe_g in series with a resistance of r_p or a constant-current source of magnitude $g_m\, e_g$ shunted by the plate

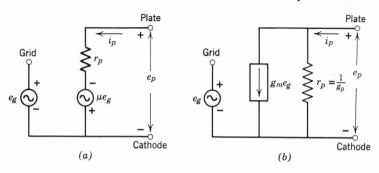

Figure 13–9. Linear equivalent circuits for the vacuum tube: (*a*) constant-voltage circuit; (*b*) constant-current circuit.

resistance r_p. The two circuits are of course equivalent, and either may be used. Mathematical convenience often indicates a preference.

The equation $\mu e_g = i_p r_p - e_p$ represents a constant-voltage equivalent and describes the circuit shown in Fig 13–9*a*. The constant-current equivalent is represented by

$$i_p = \frac{1}{r_p} e_p + g_m e_g$$

or since $\dfrac{1}{r_p} = g_p$

$$i_p = g_p e_p + g_m e_g$$

The circuit described by this equation is shown in Fig. 13–9*b*.

It is easily seen from the graphical analysis of the triode operation, or it can be shown analytically, that $e_p = -i_p R_L$, so that the a-c equivalent circuit for the triode connected to load R_L is as shown in Fig. 13–10. The advantage of this simplification can be demonstrated by using it to calculate the voltage gain and comparing it with the value found by graphical analysis. The voltage equation is

$$\mu e_g = i_p R_L + i_p r_p,$$

from which

$$i_p = \frac{\mu e_g}{r_p + R_L},$$

but

$$e_0 = -i_p R_L = -\frac{\mu e_g R_L}{r_p + R_L},$$

and

$$\text{amplification (gain)} = A = \frac{e_0}{e_g} = -\frac{\mu R_L}{r_p + R_L}.$$

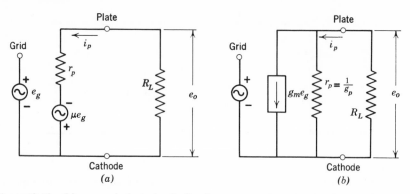

Figure 13–10. Linear equivalent circuits for the vacuum tube connected to a resistive load: (*a*) constant-voltage circuit; (*b*) constant-current circuit.

Substituting $R_L = 30$ K, as used in the graphical analysis, and $r_p = 11$ K, $\mu = 19.8$ (as determined from the plate characteristic curves):

$$A = -\frac{19.8 \times 30}{11 + 30} = -14.5,$$

which may be compared to the average value 14.6 obtained graphically.

The benefits derived from use of the a-c linear equivalent circuit are not fully demonstrated by this simple example. It is only for pure resistive loads that the load line is unambiguously defined, rendering use of the load line impractical for analysis of vacuum-tube operation with reactive loads. The equivalent circuit may be employed to predict performance when the tube is connected to such complex networks, although it must always be borne in mind that the linear-equivalent circuit is valid only for representing tube operation in a region in which the characteristic curves approximate straight, parallel, equally spaced lines. Within these limitations the equivalent circuit transforms a vacuum-tube problem into an a-c network problem, a field in which standardized and powerful techniques of problem solution have been developed for linear circuits and important beginnings have been made in nonlinear analysis.

13–10.   CATHODE BIAS

In the circuit shown in Fig. 13–8, the battery E_c was used to bias the grid negatively with respect to the cathode and thereby establish a fixed operating point. The use of a battery for this purpose is, in most cases, impractical and expensive, and may be obviated by placing a resistor R_K in the cathode as shown in Fig. 13–11.

For the purpose of more clearly illustrating this biasing technique, assume that the signal voltage source v_g has been temporarily removed from the input terminals A, B and replaced by a direct connection as shown. Note that both the grid and the bottom end of the cathode resistor are connected to the common point G. The current through the tube (plate current) flows through R_K, making the cathode end more positive than point G. Because the grid is connected to point G, the cathode is positive with respect to the grid. This condition can be described equally well by stating that the grid is negative with respect to the cathode. The value of R_K required to provide a specified bias voltage E_c can be determined by drawing the load line for R_L and noting the plate current I_{bo} which will flow for the desired value of grid bias voltage E_c. The required value of $R_K = E_c/I_{bo}$. Because the d-c load line is determined by $R_L + R_K$, if the load line is to remain the same after placing R_K in the cathode the value of R_L must be reduced by the amount R_K. It is shown in Section 13–22 that the voltage developed across R_K produces negative feedback which reduces the gain of the amplifier stage but offers benefits in the form of gain stabilization and increased bandwidth. A capacitor may be placed across R_K to maintain constant the voltage produced by the d-c component of the plate current, while "bypassing" the alternating components. The use of a capacitor eliminates the negative feedback at the frequencies for which it effectively provides a low-impedance bypass (i.e., the capacitive reactance is small with respect to R_K), and the stage gain is increased, but at the expense of gain stability and bandwidth. Both bypassed and unbypassed cathode resistors are encountered frequently in instrumentation circuitry.

13–11.   RESISTANCE-CAPACITANCE COUPLED AMPLIFIER

It is not always possible to obtain the desired voltage gain from a single stage of amplification. Therefore, to obtain higher voltage gain several

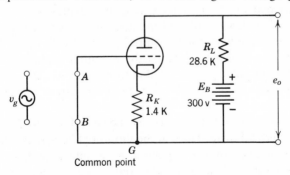

Figure 13–11.   Triode amplifier with cathode bias.

amplifier stages, with the output of one connected to the input of the next are required. In such an arrangement the stages are said to be connected in cascade, and the overall amplification is the product of the individual stage gains. The need for cascading raises the problem of coupling the stages together. A simple and inexpensive method uses a resistor and capacitor to couple the signal voltage from the output of one stage to the input of the next.

Because a capacitor blocks the d-c component of a waveform while passing the a-c components, it is useful in transferring a-c voltage variations between two points which are at different d-c potentials. For example, the signal variations at the plate of one amplifier operating at a relatively high d-c potential may be applied to the grid of a second stage which is biased negatively without disturbing the d-c operating potentials of either the plate or the grid. Because such a coupling capacitor effectively isolates the d-c levels of one stage from another, the stages may be individually designed for high, stable gain and may be operated more easily from a common power supply. Amplifiers containing stages coupled through such resistance-capacitance (*RC*) networks are termed a-c amplifiers because of their insensitivity to d-c (baseline) levels at the input. Direct-coupled amplifiers, which will amplify sustained d-c voltages introduced into the input, are designated as d-c amplifiers; they are discussed in Section 13–12. It is pertinent to mention that one very useful method of securing d-c amplification makes use of amplifiers that are *RC* coupled and respond only to a-c signals. This technique is described in Sections 13–46 and 13–38.

The behavior of two stages coupled together by an *RC* circuit is determined by the properties of the circuit. The responses of a simple *RC* network to various input voltage are shown in Figs. 13–12 *a,b,c*. Figure 13–12*a* shows the voltage V_R which appears across the resistor when the fixed voltage E is suddenly applied to a series *RC* circuit. Upon closing the switch, V_R jumps immediately to the value E and then decays to zero. The decay is described by the familiar exponential expression $V_R = Ee^{-(t/RC)}$. The product RC is defined as the time constant. It is measured in seconds and defines the length of time required for V_R to decay to $0.37E$. It is important to note that, with a steady d-c potential applied as an input to this circuit, the output V_R is modified in form as shown. It is apparent that this circuit possesses limitations as a coupling system for sustained d-c potentials.

If a sinusoidal voltage v is applied as shown in Fig. 13–12*b*, the voltage v_r is also sinusoidal. Furthermore, if the sinusoidal frequency is high enough so that the reactance of the capacitor X_c is much smaller than R, the voltage drop across C is insignificant, and v_r is essentially the same as v. For sinusoidal frequencies for which X_c is not small in comparison to R, the

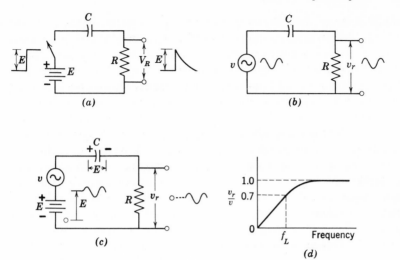

Figure 13–12. The response of a series RC circuit to a step function and a sinusoidal voltage.

voltage v_r will still be sinusoidal but will be of lesser magnitude than v and also will be shifted in phase.

Figure 13–12c shows the sinusoidal voltage source v and the battery E connected in series as input to the RC circuit. After a time lapse of approximately five time constants from the initial completion of the circuit, the capacitor C will be charged to the battery voltage E and only the sinusoidal voltage will appear across R. Because any d-c component of the input voltage is lost with RC coupling, no baseline information appears in the output which contains only the time-varying components of the input signal with periods $(T = 1/f)$ which are short compared with the time constant RC.

This simple illustration demonstrates the fundamental nature of the RC-coupling circuit—that is, varying voltages are coupled across it; a steady voltage is not. Therefore with RC-coupled amplifiers the output contains no information regarding the level about which an input signal is varying. The sinusoidal frequency response characteristic of the circuit in Fig. 13–12c is shown in Fig. 13–12d.

13–12.   DIRECT-COUPLED AMPLIFIER

Frequently it is desirable, and sometimes it is necessary, to amplify bio-electric or physiological signals which are referenced to a baseline, such as direct blood pressure or slow variations in membrane potential. The limitations in the use of RC coupling for such purposes have been discussed briefly. Figure 13–13 shows two triode stages, similar to the one analyzed in Figs. 13–6 and 13–7, connected together without using coupling capacitors. The only requirement to be met is that the potentials appearing across the elements of each tube be within the proper operating range of the tube regardless of the actual values of potential appearing elsewhere in the circuit. In Fig. 13–13, with the input terminals A, B connected together, tube V_1 is biased at the operating point shown in Fig. 13–7. The grid bias is -6 volts and the plate-to-cathode voltage is therefore 170 volts as shown. The operating point of V_2 can be set to the same operating point as V_1 by "bucking out" the plate voltage of V_1 with a battery of 176 volts connected as shown. This leaves the grid of V_2 biased 6 volts negatively with respect to its cathode. The 170 volts which appears from plate to cathode of V_2 can then be "bucked out" to produce zero volts of output to correspond to zero volts at the input. The short circuit may then be removed from the input terminals, and an input containing a d-c component may be connected.

Suppose that a signal consisting of a sinusoidal source of 0.02 volt peak-to-peak in series with a battery of 0.1 volt is connected to the input terminals A, B as indicated. This situation is similar to recording a membrane potential with superimposed oscillations. Each stage will amplify the input voltage presented to it by 14.6 (as calculated previously) so that the voltage from the grid to cathode of V_2 will be 0.292 peak-to-peak sinusoidal voltage super-imposed upon a steady voltage of 1.46 volts. Note that the phase of both of these voltages has been shifted 180 degrees. In a similar manner, tube V_2

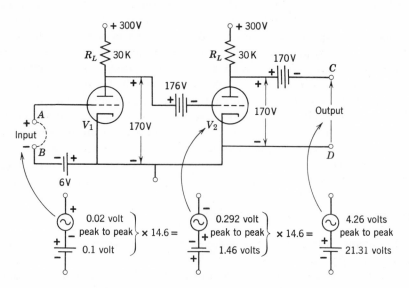

Figure 13–13.   The two-stage direct-coupled amplifier.

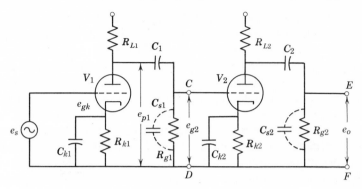

Figure 13–14.   The two-stage RC coupled amplifier.

increases the amplitude by 14.6 and shifts each voltage by 180 degrees. At the output terminals C, D, the sinusoidal and d-c components are 4.26 volts peak-to-peak and 21.31 volts, respectively. Because the total phase shift in the two stages of amplification is $180 + 180 = 360$ degrees, the output voltage is in phase with the input.

A direct coupled amplifier of the type described above has limited practicality. Its basic limitation results from the fact that a d-c level change anywhere in the circuit (for whatever reason) is indistinguishable from an input signal. Slight inherent d-c shifts due to thermal effects or voltage supply instabilities, especially in the input stage, must be small compared to the desired input signal because the system treats both in the same manner. As pointed out previously, the use of capacitor coupling between stages eliminates these problems, but at the expense of a loss of baseline information.

The cost and commercial availability of well designed, stable, and reliable direct-coupled amplifiers have become so attractive that it is hardly worthwhile for any investigator to build his own. The brief discussion just given will have served its purpose if it provides enough insight into the difficulties encountered with these amplifiers to discourage such an undertaking. An excellent review of the factors which conspire to limit the stability of direct-coupled amplifiers was presented by Harris and Bishop (1949). The reader interested in either designing such an amplifier or improving the performance of an existing one will obtain a wealth of practical information from this paper.

13–13.   FREQUENCY RESPONSE OF AN *RC*-COUPLED AMPLIFIER

Figure 13–14 shows two vacuum tube stages coupled by a resistance-capacitance network consisting of C_1 and R_{g1}. In a similar manner, the output of the second stage is coupled to the output terminals E, F by the network consisting of C_2 and R_{g2}; C_{s1} and C_{s2}, shown with dotted connections, are "stray" capacitances existing between circuit wires and metal chassis, from one wire to another, and between vacuum tube elements. Although the capacitances so formed are small and are minimized by good design and construction practice, they nevertheless exist and provide shunting reactance which decreases in magnitude with increasing frequency. It will be shown in a later section that the effective capacitance appearing between the input terminals of a vacuum tube stage operated in the common-cathode mode is dependent upon the voltage gain of the stage. This factor can be dominant in determining the shunting capacitance and, accordingly, the frequency response.

The frequency characteristics of the two-stage vacuum-tube amplifier of Fig. 13–14 can be determined from the general equivalent circuit shown in Fig. 13–15, which shows the voltage presented to the second stage e_{g2} after passing through the coupling network $C_1 R_{g1}$. The frequency characteristic of interest is the ratio of the output voltage of this network

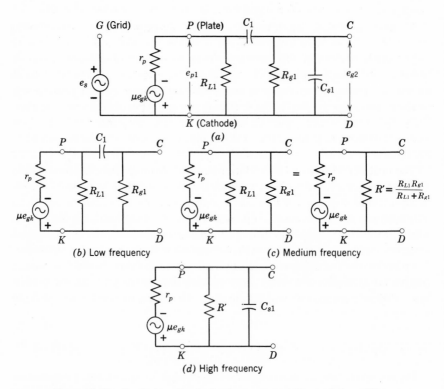

Figure 13–15.   Equivalent circuits for the two-stage RC-coupled amplifier.

e_{g2} to the input voltage e_{p1} over the sinusoidal frequency range from low to high values. The general circuit may be reduced to more simple equivalents through consideration of the effects of the reactances of C_1 and X_{s1} (X_{c1} and X_{cs1}) on the rest of the circuit, for example:

At low frequencies:	(a) X_{c1} is high and will influence the value of e_{g2}.
	(b) X_{cs1} is very high and can be considered an open circuit. It will have no effect on e_{g2}.
At medium frequencies:	(a) X_{c1} is low and may be considered a short circuit.
	(b) Although the value of X_{cs1} is not as high as at low frequencies, it is still too high to affect e_{g2}.
At high frequencies:	(a) X_{c1} is very low and acts even more as a short circuit than at medium frequencies.
	(b) X_{cs1} is low. It effectively shunts the terminals C-D and reduces the value of e_{g2}.

The low-, medium-, and high-frequency equivalent circuits are shown in Figs. 13–15 b,c,d, respectively. A plot of the network response (gain and phase) as a function of frequency is shown in Fig. 13–16, where f_L and f_H and the low and high frequencies for which the response is 0.707 of the mid-frequency value. These frequencies are designated the "half power" or "3 db down" points, and the range of frequencies between them is called the bandwidth. It can be shown that, in addition to the phase shift produced by the vacuum tube itself, which may be assumed to remain 180 degrees for all-frequency components, the network produces a phase shift of 45 degrees at the frequencies f_L and f_H. The consequences of this reduction in amplification and associated shift in phase will be examined in Chapter 14. Thus it can be seen that the RC-coupled amplifier exhibits both a low- and a high-frequency limit beyond which amplification begins to decrease. In addition, the foregoing analysis indicates the direction in which a change can be made to alter the frequency response. For example, if an increase in low-frequency response is desired, it is necessary to raise either R_{g1} or C_1 or both, that is, to increase the time constant. If attenuation of the low frequencies is desired, a reduction in either R_{g1} or C_1, or in both, will accomplish this end. Since the product $R_{g1} C_1$ is the time constant, a decrease in time constant reduces the low-frequency response.

To increase the high-frequency response it is necessary to decrease C_{s1}; if the high frequencies are to be excluded, C_{s1} should be increased.

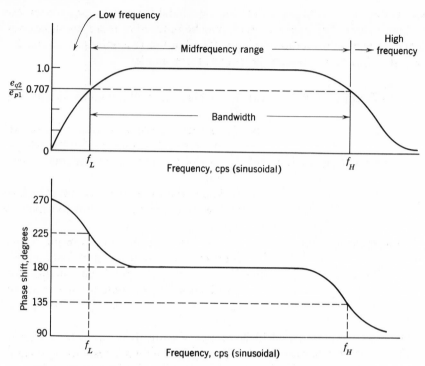

Figure 13–16. The frequency and phase response of an RC-coupled amplifier.

Of the three components, it is most difficult to decrease C_{s1}. This will become apparent from the following discussion.

13–14. INPUT IMPEDANCE

The necessity for making the input impedance of the bioelectric amplifier many times larger than the electrode impedance has been discussed in Chapter 11. In the preceeding analysis of the operation of a vacuum tube amplifier it has been assumed that with the grid biased negatively the input impedance of the triode is extremely high. The validity of this assumption for different sinusoidal frequencies will now be examined.

In Fig. 13–17 is shown the equivalent circuit for the triode amplifier, taking into consideration the interelectrode capacitances of the tube, which may be augmented in various amounts by stray capacitance contributed by circuit wiring. For simplification in analysis, assume that no grid resistor is present between grid and cathode so that the input impedance is governed entirely by the capacitive reactance appearing across the grid-to-cathode terminals. These terminals are shunted directly by the grid-to-cathode

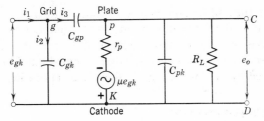

Figure 13–17.   Equivalent circuit for the input impedance of the triode amplifier.

capacitance C_{gk}, which is in the order of a few picofarads. Because of its small value C_{gk} offers a high-impedance path for low frequencies with the shunting effect increasing with rising frequency. It will be shown that it is the grid-to-plate capacitance C_{gp}, rather than C_{gk}, which reduces the input impedance of the common-cathode triode amplifier. This will become clear when the circuit is solved for the input impedance Z_{gk}.

Writing the Kirchhoff current law for the node g (Fig 13–17), we have

$$i_1 = i_2 + i_3$$

$$= e_{gk}\, j\omega C_{gk} + j\omega C_{gp}[e_{gk} - (-e_0)]$$

$$= j\omega e_{gk}\, C_{gk} + j\omega C_{gp}\, e_{gk} + j\omega C_{gp}\, e_0\,,$$

$$\frac{1}{Z_{gk}} = \frac{i_1}{e_{gk}} = j\omega(C_{gk} + C_{gp} + A C_{gp}),$$

where $A = e_0/e_{gk}$ = the amplification of the stage,

$$Z_{gk} = \frac{1}{j\omega[C_{gk} + C_{gp}(1 + A)]} = \frac{1}{j\omega C_{in}},$$

that is $C_{in} = C_{gk} + C_{gp}(1 + A).$

Therefore the actual input impedance is made up, not of C_{gk} alone, but of C_{gk} in parallel with a capacitor having a value of C_{gp} multiplied by $(1 + A)$, where A is the amplification of the stage. The importance of this result can be demonstrated by applying it to the input circuit previously described. In triodes designed more specifically for high-gain operation, A may easily be in the order of 50. For example, for a 12AX7, which is a popular high-gain triode often used for input stages, the technical data sheet shows

$$C_{gk} = 1.6 \text{ pf,} \qquad C_{gp} = 1.7 \text{ pf,} \qquad C_{pk} = 0.34 \text{ pf,}$$

$$C_{in} = C_{gk} + (1 + A)C_{gp}$$
$$= 1.6 + 51 \times 1.7$$
$$= 1.6 + 86.7 = 88.3 \text{ pf.}$$

As a result of the additional input capacitance $(1 + A)C_{gp}$, the reactance across the input of the common-cathode triode amplifier may be so low at some frequencies relative to the impedance of the circuit connected to the input that there occurs a serious reduction in signal amplitude and a distortion produced by the loss of high-frequency components.

13–15.   OUTPUT IMPEDANCE

The midfrequency linear equivalent circuit for the common-cathode connected triode is shown in Fig. 13–18. By inspection the output impedance of the tube itself is the plate resistance r_p. From the terminals C,D the circuit output impedance consists of the parallel combination of r_p and R_L. In a practical amplifier using a 12AX7 tube assume that it is operated with a load resistance of 0.3 megohm. The output impedance of the tube is r_p (62.5 K) in parallel with R_L (0.3 megohm), that is, 51.7 K.

The magnitude of the output impedance of a single stage or an entire system is important for several reasons.

1. If the objective is to transfer a voltage to a succeeding stage or device without loss due to loading, the input impedance of the system

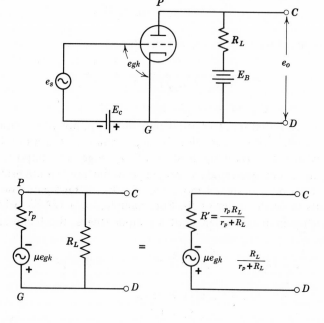

Figure 13–18.   Equivalent circuit for the output impedance of the triode amplifier.

accepting the voltage must be high compared to the output impedance of the device supplying the voltage.

2. If the objective is to transfer power from one device to another, maximum efficiency of power transfer is obtained when the input resistance of the device accepting power is equal to the output resistance of the device delivering power. If, in addition to resistance, the equivalent circuit of the source contains reactance, maximum efficiency of power transfer is obtained when the load impedance is the conjugate of the source impedance.

In both of these situations due consideration must be given to the electrical properties of any wires or cables used to connect the output of one device to the input of the other. Suppose, for example, that it is desired to connect the output of one common-cathode amplifier (which has a moderately high impedance) to the input of a similar stage by means of a shielded wire, the shield serving as a conductor to connect the common terminals of the two stages together. The capacitance per foot of such cable is considerable (eg., 5 to 20 pf), and its use is equivalent to shunting the input of the second stage with a capacitor, which may reduce the input impedance and produce the attenuation and distortion mentioned in Section 13–17. To reduce such capacitive loading, the second stage may be placed in close proximity to the first stage so that only very short connecting wires are required, or some device or circuit having a very high input impedance and very low output impedance may be connected between the output of the first stage and the input to the shielded cable. Such a device by reason of its high input impedance would not load the first stage and because of its very low output impedance would not be loaded by the capacitance of the shielded cable except at much higher frequencies for which the capacitive reactance was low in comparison to the output impedance. The cathode follower is such an impedance-transforming device.

13–16.   CATHODE FOLLOWER

The conventional triode amplifier or common-cathode circuit previously analyzed and shown in Fig. 13–8 may be rearranged, using exactly the same components, to operate as a cathode follower (Fig. 13–19). The only differences between these two circuits are that the load resistor is connected to the cathode and the battery in the grid circuit is of a different magnitude and is reversed in polarity. The plate constitutes the element common between the input and output since the two batteries E_B and E_c function only to set the operating point and offer no impedance to a-c signals.

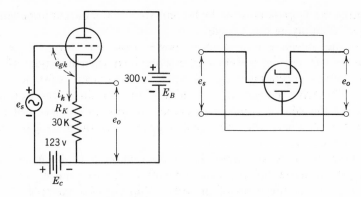

Figure 13–19.   The cathode follower.

The linear equivalent circuit may be used to calculate the gain of the cathode follower as shown in Fig. 13–20:

$$i_k = \frac{\mu e_{gk}}{r_p + R_k},$$

but

$$e_{gk} = e_s - e_0$$

$$= e_s - i_k R_k,$$

and, substituting this equation into the equation for i_k

$$i_k = \frac{\mu(e_s - i_k R_k)}{r_p + R_k},$$

and since

$$e_0 = i_k R_k,$$

$$e_0 = \frac{\mu(e_s - e_0)R_k}{r_p + R_k},$$

from which

$$G = \frac{e_0}{e_s} = \frac{\mu R_k}{r_p + (\mu + 1)R_k},$$

If the value of R_K is large with respect to r_p and μ is large compared to unity, the voltage gain of the cathode follower approaches 1.0. The useful high-input impedance characteristic of the cathode follower is obtained at the expense of voltage gain, which may be recovered in subsequent stages. The valuable function performed by the cathode follower is distortionless introduction of the signal into the amplifying system.

The gain for the cathode follower may be calculated using the values of $r_p = 11{,}000$ ohms, $\mu = 19.8$, and $R_k = 30{,}000$ ohms:

$$G = \frac{19.8 \times 30{,}000}{11{,}000 + 30{,}000(1 + 19.8)} = 0.935.$$

It is easy to see why this circuit is called a cathode follower. With an increase in input voltage which drives the grid less negative with respect to the cathode, the plate current increases. The output is the voltage drop across the cathode resistor R_K, which of course increases with the plate current. The output voltage therefore "follows" the input voltage in the same direction and has almost the same magnitude; consequently there is no phase reversal in this circuit.

13–17. INPUT IMPEDANCE OF THE CATHODE FOLLOWER

The input impedance of the cathode follower may be calculated from the linear equivalent circuit shown in Fig. 13–21. Writing the Kirchhoff current law for the node g, we obtain

$$i_1 = i_2 + i_3$$
$$= e_s j\omega C_{gp} + (e_s - e_0)j\omega C_{gk},$$

$$\frac{1}{Z_{in}} = \frac{i_1}{e_s} = j\omega[C_{gp} + C_{gk}(1 - A)]),$$

where $A = e_0/e_s =$ the voltage gain of the circuit,

$$Z_{in} = \frac{1}{j\omega[C_{gp} + C_{gk}(1 - A)]} = \frac{1}{j\omega C_{in}},$$

$$C_{in} = C_{gp} + C_{gk}(1 - A).$$

The input impedance of the cathode follower appears as C_{gp} in parallel with a capacitor having a value of $C_{gk}(1 - A)$. Because A is near unity and the value of C_{gk} is small, the contribution of $C_{gk}(1 - A)$ to the input capacitance is negligible. The input impedance is governed primarily by C_{gp}, which is on the order of a few picofarads. This is in sharp contrast to the input impedance obtained by operating the tube in the common-cathode mode. For example, it was found previously that the type 12AX7 triode, when connected as a common-cathode amplifier, exhibited an input capacitance of

$$C_{in} = C_{gk} + C_{gp}(1 + A) = 1.6 + 51 \times 1.7 = 88.3 \text{ pf.}$$

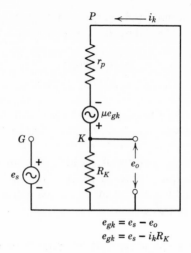

$$e_{gk} = e_s - e_o$$
$$e_{gk} = e_s - i_k R_K$$

Figure 13–20. Equivalent circuit of the cathode follower.

When this triode is connected as a cathode follower, the input capacitance is

$$C_{in} = C_{gp} + C_{gk}(1 - A) = 1.7 + 1.6(1 - 0.94) = 1.8 \text{ pf.}$$

This comparison demonstrates that one of the outstanding characteristics of the cathode follower circuit is its low input capacitance. Note, however, that this highly desirable feature was purchased at the expense of voltage gain; nevertheless, having introduced the signal into a low-capacitance circuit, amplification is easily obtained in subsequent stages.

In order to avoid degradation of the performance of a cathode follower by introducing stray capacitance across its input terminals, the wiring connecting the signal source to the cathode follower should be as short and direct as possible. This is achieved by physically locating the cathode follower as close to the source as possible, and may even

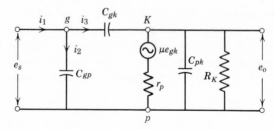

Figure 13–21. Equivalent circuit for the input impedance of the cathode follower.

involve a special layout of components which will permit attainment of this goal.

In some instances it is necessary to locate the cathode follower at a distance from the signal source and to make the interconnection with a shielded wire or cable to prevent or reduce noise pickup. As pointed out previously, considerable capacitance is inherent in shielded cable, and hence an ordinary interconnection using such cable would result in this capacitance shunting the input of the cathode follower, effectively lowering its input impedance. It is possible to use shielded cable on the input while at the same time reducing its capacitive effect to a minimum by use of the driven-shield circuit shown in Fig. 13–22. According to Donaldson (1958), the driven-shield circuit is due to Ryle although no reference is given. Attree (1949) and Bishop (1949) have also reported use of this circuit.

Figure 13–22 shows a practical cathode follower with cathode bias. The shielded cable connecting the signal source to the cathode follower input consists of an inner wire surrounded by two shields. The shield nearest the inner wire is connected to the cathode so that the potential difference between it and the central conductor is small because the cathode potential closely "follows" the grid potential. As a result of the cathode potential following the grid potential, the necessity for the source to supply a capacitive charging current is reduced, and the source works into the high impedance characteristic of the cathode follower. The potential of the inner shield does vary with respect to the outer shield, but the current required to charge this capacitance is provided by the output of the cathode follower, which is a low-impedance source easily capable of supplying this current. In this manner the driven-shield cathode follower provides shielding against outside electrical interference entering the input while at the same time preserving the high input impedance inherent in the circuit.

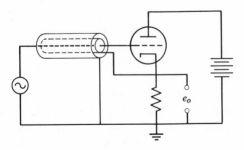

Figure 13–22.   The driven-shield cathode follower.

13–18. OUTPUT IMPEDANCE OF THE CATHODE FOLLOWER

Because the reactance of the plate-to-cathode capacitance C_{pk} is high in comparison to the plate-to-cathode impedance of the tube, the interelectrode capacitance C_{pk} can be ignored in calculating the output impedance of the cathode follower over its useful operating range. The equivalent circuit simplifies to that shown in Fig. 13–23a, which, except for rearrangement, is the same as the one in Fig. 13–20, and from which i_K is easily calculated as follows:

$$i_K = \frac{\mu e_{gk}}{r_p + R_K},$$

but $$e_{gk} = e_s - e_0 \quad \text{and} \quad e_0 = i_K R_K.$$

Therefore

$$i_K = \frac{\mu(e_s - i_K R_K)}{r_p + R_K},$$

from which $$i_K = \frac{\mu e_s/(\mu + 1)}{r_p/(\mu + 1) + R_K}.$$

This expression describes the circuit shown in Fig. 13–23b.

If the resistor R_K represents the cathode load, the cathode follower is equivalent to a generator having a voltage of $\mu/(\mu + 1)e_s$ and an internal impedance of $r_p/(\mu + 1)$ when "looking into the cathode terminal." The impedance $r_p/(\mu + 1)$ is the output impedance of the cathode follower. Observe that for tubes in which μ is large compared to unity the output impedance is very closely $r_p/\mu = 1/g_m$. For the common-cathode connection the output impedance "looking into the plate" is r_p. Therefore connecting the same tube as a cathode follower reduces its output impedance by the factor $1/(\mu + 1)$. This reduction is two orders of magnitude for a tube such as the 12AX7, in which $\mu = 100$ and $r_p = 62.5$ K. If R_k is considered an integral part of the cathode follower and an external load is connected across its terminals, the output impedance as viewed from the load terminals is even further reduced. With tubes having high μ and low r_p, very low levels of output impedance are easily obtained, thus allowing low-impedance loads such as shielded cables to be driven without loss of signal amplitude and high-frequency components.

In summary, the cathode follower is characterized by a high input impedance, low output impedance, wide bandwidth, and zero phase shift in the midfrequency range. In addition, the cathode follower theoretically provides essentially infinite power gain since with only voltage and no

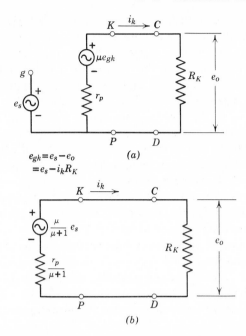

$$e_{gk} = e_s - e_o$$
$$= e_s - i_k R_K$$

(a)

(b)

Figure 13–23. Equivalent circuit for the output impedance of the cathode follower.

appreciable current at the input it is possible to control the current and voltage i.e. power supplied to a low-impedance device (such as a pen motor). The same is also true for the common-cathode amplifier although the power gain of the cathode follower is greater because of the greater difference between input and output impedance levels. These desirable characteristics more than compensate for the lack of voltage gain in the cathode follower.

13–19. MULTIELEMENT VACUUM TUBES

The large effective input capacitance and the consequent lowering of the input impedance in the triode operating in the common-cathode mode have been shown to be due to the grid-to-plate capacitance. The magnification of this capacitance at the input terminals by the factor $(1 + A)$ is a direct result of the out-of-phase relationship between the grid and plate voltages. A reduction in input capacitance can be obtained by placing an electrostatic shield between the grid and the plate, resulting in a four-element tube called a tetrode. The added screen grid is an open structure similar to the grid nearest the cathode (control grid). The screen grid is operated at a fixed positive potential and is usually bypassed to the cathode by means of a capacitor.

Locating a single screen grid between grid and plate produces undesirable curvature in the plate characteristic curves, which is eliminated by the addition of another screen-grid structure operated at cathode potential and placed between the positive screen grid and the plate. This additional structure is called the suppressor grid; the resulting five-element tube is termed a pentode. The plate characteristics of a typical pentode are shown in Fig. 13–24. It is apparent that over the useful operating range of the characteristics for any specified value of grid voltage the plate current is essentially constant regardless of the plate voltage. The plate resistance r_p is therefore very high, as is the amplification factor μ; the transconductance, however, is of the same magnitude as is encountered in triodes. A comparison of Fig. 13–24 and Fig. 13–52 shows that the current-voltage relationship for the pentode is similar to that of the transistor. These similarities are discussed in Section 13–31.

The performance of pentode amplifiers may be predicted by the graphical method in the same manner as for the triode. The equivalent circuit derived for the triode is correct for the pentode, except that r_p has such a high value it is difficult, and usually meaningless, to assign a specific value to it. Instead, it is more convenient to use a constant-current model for the

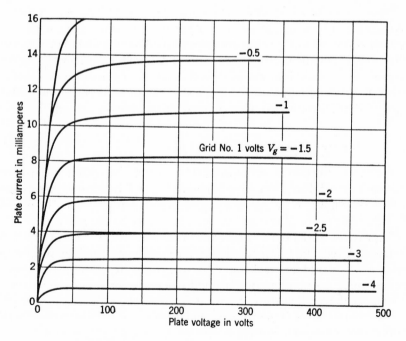

Figure 13–24. Plate characteristics of a typical pentode.

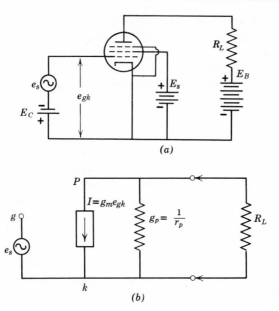

Figure 13–25. Basic pentode amplifier (*a*) and its small-signal linear equivalent circuit (*b*).

pentode equivalent. The basic pentode amplifier and its constant-current linear equivalent circuit are shown in Figs. 13–25 *a, b*. It is often possible to simplify the circuit even further, for if r_p is large compared to R_L, very little current flows through it; consequently r_p may be removed, leaving only the current source $g_m e_{gk}$ and the load resistance R_L.

Pentodes are very useful for providing a high voltage gain in a single stage. Another advantage is their low input capacitance, especially if the screen grid voltage is bypassed to the cathode. For these reasons, they have been employed in many amplifiers and other electronic circuits utilized in biomedical instrumentation. The primary disadvantage of the pentode as a voltage amplifier, in comparison to the triode, is its higher internal noise level.

The applications of the vacuum tube discussed thus far have emphasized the amplification only of voltage without requiring the tube to supply power in the output to drive current-operated devices such as galvanometers, relays, or loudspeakers. Depending upon the characteristics of particular vacuum tubes, voltage may be amplified to rather high levels with negligibly small signal power being developed. For example, a large voltage change usually appears across the load resistance in the plate circuit of a voltage amplifier in which the current change is often small. The voltage change can be effectively coupled to a succeeding stage operated with an adequate negative bias with the transfer of negligibly small power. By contrast, some devices such as galvanometers and loudspeakers, require the flow of considerable current for their operation. The substantial amounts of power that are needed can be supplied by tubes or transistors designed for this purpose.

13–20. FEEDBACK

Feedback, in the most general sense, implies the utilization of some information appearing at the output of a device to influence the information presented to the input for the purpose of exerting control over the output. As applied to amplifiers, feedback means sending back to the input a voltage derived from the output which is proportional to either (a) the output voltage or (b) the output current. The objective in first case is to cause the amplifier to maintain a constant output voltage and in the second a constant output current. The output circuit of a system possessing constant-voltage characteristics exhibits a low impedance, and a constant-current system exhibits a high impedance. These two characteristics are of considerable practical importance in many electronic devices.

Feedback can be applied in two ways: in one the voltage fed back from the output subtracts from the input, and in the other the voltage fed back adds to the input. The former is designated negative feedback; the latter, positive. Unless properly controlled, a system with positive feedback is inherently unstable; except in a few special applications, positive feedback is undesirable. On the other hand, negative feedback imparts many useful features to a system, including the following:

1. Stability of gain.
2. Increased bandwidth.
3. Reduction in noise and distortion originating within the amplifier.
4. Improved phase response (accompanying the increased bandwidth).
5. Attainment of desired impedance levels.

The classical equation, due to Black (1934), that describes the effect of feedback is easily derived from the simple system diagramed in Fig. 13–26. The triangle marked A represents an amplifier having an overall "forward" gain of A from its input terminals $B\text{-}B$ to the output terminals $C\text{-}C$. The rectangle marked β represents a system or network having a gain of β from its input terminals $D\text{-}D$ to the output terminals $E\text{-}E$. The circle marked P is a network which adds voltages coming into it to produce the voltage e_1. The voltage to be amplified (e_s) is applied to terminals $A\text{-}A$, which are the system input terminals. With switch S open, the feedback "loop"

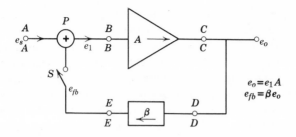

Figure 13–26. Schematic diagram of the application of feedback.

is open and $e_1 = e_s$. With switch S closed, the feedback loop is closed, and $e_1 = e_s + e_{fb}$. The "loop gain" is the gain around the system from B-B to E-E. The output voltage e_o is always $e_1 A$, that is, the product of the voltage at the *amplifier* input terminals (B-B) and the gain of the amplifier (A).

To demonstrate the changes brought about by the addition of feedback, it is necessary to compare the gain e_0/e_s for the open- and closed-loop conditions.

Open loop (S open): $\qquad\qquad e_0 = e_1 A,$

but $\qquad\qquad\qquad\qquad\qquad e_1 = e_s;$

hence $\qquad\qquad\qquad e_0 = e_s A \quad$ or $\quad \dfrac{e_0}{e_s} = A.$

Closed loop (S closed): $\quad e_0 = e_1 A,$

where $\qquad\qquad\qquad\qquad e_1 = e_s + e_{fb},$

and $\qquad\qquad e_{fb} = \beta e_0, \qquad e_0 = (e_s + e_{fb})A;$

hence $\qquad\qquad\qquad e_0 = (e_s + \beta e_0)A$

$$e_0 = \frac{A e_s}{1 - A\beta},$$

$$G = \frac{e_0}{e_s} = \frac{A}{1 - A\beta} = A\left(\frac{1}{1 - A\beta}\right), \qquad\qquad (E)$$

where G is the system gain with feedback. Equation E is the Black equation.

With the feedback loop closed, the open-loop gain A is modified by the factor $1/(1 - A\beta)$. If this factor has an absolute value greater than 1, the gain with feedback is greater than without feedback and the feedback is classified as positive. Conversely, if $1/(1 - A\beta)$ is less than 1, the feedback is negative. The magnitude of $1/(1 - A\beta)$ is determined by $|1 - A\beta|$, where $A\beta$ is the loop gain. Therefore, if $|1 - A\beta|$ is greater than 1, the feedback is negative. If $|1 - A\beta|$ is less than 1, the feedback is positive. If $|1 - A\beta|$ is zero, the system functions not as an amplifier but as an oscillator, requires no input, and generates an output at a frequency determined by the gain and phase characteristics around the loop. An application of controlled positive feedback in the "negative capacitance amplifier" for microelectrode recording is discussed in Section 13–45.

Several examples will serve to demonstrate some of the benefits resulting from negative feedback. Assume that the open-loop gain A of the amplifier in Fig. 13–26 is 1000 and that the output voltage is shifted 180 degrees with respect to the input. These facts are often expressed in the form $A = 1000\underline{|180°}$. To demonstrate the effect on gain of closing the feedback loop, assume for simplicity that the feedback network consists of a simple voltage divider made up entirely of resistors which provides 10% of the output voltage to be fed back to the input, that is, $\beta = 0.1\underline{|0°}$. The system is diagramed in Fig. 13–27. Using the Black equation, we obtain

$$G = \frac{A}{1 - A\beta}$$

$$= \frac{1000\underline{|180°}}{1 - 1000\underline{|180°}\,0.1\underline{|0°}} = \frac{1000\underline{|180°}}{1 - 100\underline{|180°}}$$

$$= \frac{1000\underline{|180°}}{1 - 100(\cos 180 + j\sin 180)} = \frac{1000\underline{|180°}}{101}$$

$$= 9.90\underline{|180°}.$$

This example shows clearly that with the addition of 10% negative feedback the magnitude of the gain has been reduced from an open-loop value of 1000 to 9.9. Although this loss of gain may appear at first to

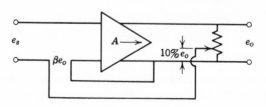

Figure 13–27. Practical application of negative (voltage) feedback.

be undesirable, certain compensating benefits are obtained, as will now be shown.

The characteristics of vacuum tubes change with time, and often a condition is reached in which the tube is still operative although the original values of the parameters μ (amplification factor), r_p (plate resistance), and g_m (transconductance) have altered considerably. The 'tube tester" is a common device used to assess the operating condition of a tube, often in broad terms such as "good," "weak," "poor," "bad," "replace." The sensitivity of the gain of a single stage of amplification to the alteration of these parameters can be evaluated from the expression $A = \mu R_L/(r_p + R_L)$, derived previously. Therefore in a single stage a change of 10% in μ will result in a 10% change in stage gain. Since the overall gain of an amplifier consisting of stages in cascade is the product of the gains of the individual stages, changes in the tube parameters of individual stages will be reflected in the overall amplifier gain.

Assume that as a result of tube aging the gain of the practical amplifier shown in Fig. 13–27 decreased 10% from $A = 1000\lfloor 180°$ to $A = 900\lfloor 180°$. With 10% feedback and applying the Black equation to determine the new gain, we obtain

$$G = \frac{A}{1 - A\beta}$$

$$= \frac{900\lfloor 180°}{1 - 900\lfloor 180° \, 0.1\lfloor 0°}$$

$$= 9.89\lfloor 180°.$$

In this example a reduction of 10% in amplifier gain resulted in a decrease of only 0.1% in system gain (from $9.90\lfloor 180°$ to $9.89\lfloor 180°$) when 10% negative feedback was employed. Even if the amplifier gain decreased by 90% (from $1000\lfloor 180°$ to $100\lfloor 180°$); the overall system gain would decrease by only 8.2% (from $9.90\lfloor 180°$ to $9.09\lfloor 180°$). The overall system gain is therefore stabilized against any factors (either long- or short-term) within the amplifier itself which affect the gain, such as changes in tube parameters or operating voltages, and the replacement of tubes or circuit components.

The effect of feedback on the phase relationship between the input and output voltages may be demonstrated by using the same system as shown in Fig. 13–26. Assume that the frequency of the input signal is such that the gain of the amplifier without feedback is $A = 707\lfloor 135°$. The amplifier itself is then operating at its high-frequency half-power point f_h, which defines the high-frequency limit of the bandwith, where the phase shift is 135 degrees.

Applying the Black equation to determine the gain and phase shift gives

$$G = \frac{A}{1 - A\beta}$$

$$= \frac{707 \underline{|135°}}{1 - 707 \underline{|135°} \; 0.1 \underline{|0°}} = 9.90 \underline{|179.5°}.$$

This shows that, even though the amplifier response is at the higher half-power point f_h, the application of 10% negative feedback results in the same system gain as is obtained with the amplifier operating in its midfrequency range, where $A = 1000 \underline{|180°}$. The application of negative feedback therefore increased the bandwidth (i. e., flat portion of the frequency response curve), which is also associated with a corresponding "correction" of the phase response toward 180 degrees. These examples serve to show that the desirable benefits of gain stabilization, increase in bandwidth, and phase response correction produced by negative feedback are obtained in proportion to the reduction of gain available in the amplifier around which the feedback is applied.

The Black equation shows even more explicitly than a numerical example why gain and phase improvement results from negative feedback. For example if the loop gain $A\beta$ is much greater than unity, the system gain G becomes

$$G = \frac{A}{1 - A\beta} \doteq \frac{A}{-A\beta} = -\frac{1}{\beta}.$$

The system gain then is a function only of the characteristics of the feedback network β. If β consists only of stable, passive, time-invariant components, such as resistors and capacitors, the overall gain of the system is likewise stable and essentially independent of the forward gain A of the amplifier so long as the loop gain $A\beta$ is very large compared to unity. This is the property which constitutes the basis for the operational amplifier.[4]

Distortion of the desired signal may be defined qualitatively as any component at the output not present at the input. "Noise" (random voltage fluctuations) is inherent in resistors, vacuum tubes, and transistors; some of these devices produce less noise than others of their kind by reason of construction and mode of operation. In a linear system noise is superimposed on the signal, and the resulting distortion is simply the linear

[4]See Section 13–24.

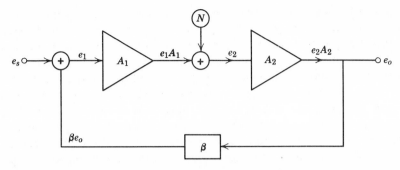

Figure 13–28. The application of feedback to reduce internal noise.

addition of noise and signal components. The degree to which the signal dominates the noise is measured by the signal-to-noise ratio (S/N). If the S/N ratio is 100, the desired signal is 100 times greater than the noise. Voltage drift, which has been mentioned as a serious problem in direct-coupled amplifiers, may also be considered as noise. In addition, signal distortions may result from nonlinearities in the characteristics of vacuum tubes, transistors, and transformers. Distortion of this type generates new frequencies related harmonically to components of the signal. Noise may also result in the production of new components of noise voltages.

The effect of feedback on the reduction of noise and distortion originating within a system can be studied with the aid of Fig. 13–28, in which the amplifier has been separated into two separate sections shown by the triangles A_1, A_2. The total amplifier gain A is A_1A_2. Assume that a source of unwanted noise signal N is introduced between A_1 and A_2 so that it adds to the output of A_1, and the sum constitutes the input e_2 to A_2. An examination of the signal paths produces the following relationships:

$$e_1 = e_s + \beta e_0,$$

$$e_2 = e_1 A_1 + N,$$

or

$$e_2 = (e_s + \beta e_0)A_1 + N.$$

The output voltage e_0 is therefore:

$$e_0 = e_2 A_2 = [(e_s + \beta e_0)A_1 + N]A_2,$$

From which

$$e_0 = \frac{e_s A_1 A_2 + N A_2}{1 - \beta A_1 A_2}$$

and finally

$$e_0 = \frac{A_1 A_2}{1 - \beta A_1 A_2}\left(e_s + \frac{N}{A_1}\right).$$

The last equation shows that the noise (distortion) in the output voltage has been reduced by the factor $1/A_1$, in which A_1 is the gain in the system before the point at which the noise or distortion enters it. If noise and distortion enter the input terminals, obviously these components will be treated as signal by the system and no amount of negative feedback will bring about improvement. If, however, some noise-free gain can be inserted ahead of the point of entry of the noise and distortion, the undesired components are attenuated in the output in inverse proportion to the amount of noise-free gain. This property is of utmost importance in reducing distortion in amplifiers, which is often produced as a result of the nonlinear vacuum tube characteristics and the large excursions of the signal in the latter stages of the amplifier.

Except for rather simple systems, it is difficult to distinguish between current and voltage feedback. Both are often used within separate loops in a single amplifier. When such distinction is possible the general characteristics produced by application of the two types of feedback are as follows.

Voltage feedback (negative)

1. Constant output voltage is maintained regardless of the magnitude of the load impedance, that is, the output impedance is reduced.

2. A voltage opposing the input signal is fed back so that the magnitude of the input signal must be increased in proportion to the amount of voltage fed back to maintain the same output. The input impedance is increased accordingly in proportion to the amount of voltage fed back and hence in proportion to the reduction in gain, noise, and distortion.

Current feedback (negative)

1. Constant output current is maintained regardless of load impedance. This is equivalent to an increase in output impedance.

2. The input impedance increases in the same manner as with voltage feedback.

The use of feedback must necessarily include recognition of the possibility of producing an unstable system. Mention has already been made of the phase shift produced in amplifiers as capacitive reactances become significant in various parts of the circuit, depending upon the frequency. It is possible for the phase shift to become such that for some frequencies the feedback will be positive rather than negative. In this condition the amplifier either (a) becomes useless as a result of continuous oscillation, (b) distorts the desired signal by increased amplification of the frequencies for which the feedback tends to be positive, or (c) shows "ringing," that is, an overshoot followed by a damped sinusoidal wave when transient phenomena such as action potentials are recorded. The third condition is characteristic of underdamped systems.

13–21. THE DIFFERENTIAL AMPLIFIER

The differential amplifier originated in the field of electrophysiology as a result of problems encountered during a decade of use of single-sided amplifiers. During this period there arose an increased desire to make simultaneous multichannel recordings of a variety of bioelectric events. Although it was possible to build more channels of amplification, complete freedom of choice in locating the electrodes on the preparation dictated that each channel have its own separate power supply, which usually consisted of large banks of batteries. Although such arrangements were used, economy frequently required operation of all channels from the same power supply. When this was done, all the channels then had one of the input terminals joined together. If multiple electrodes were placed on a preparation, all the bioelectric voltages detected were referred to the common electrode. If an event occurred at the common electrode it appeared in all channels. Thus, with such an arrangement, it was not possible to record true differences of potential between pairs of electrodes placed at will on the preparation. The meaning of this fact and its importance were called to the attention of physiologists by Adrian and Matthews (1934) and Adrian and Yamagiwa (1935).

The need for this freedom of choice was an important reason for the development of the differential amplifier. Another arose from the expanding distribution of alternating current as a source of energy. When making recordings of bioelectric events in the presence of wiring carrying alternating current, extensive shielding had to be provided. The whole preparation and the amplifier had to be placed in shielded cabinets. This requirement usually made it inconvenient to change the position of the electrodes on the preparation. In many instances it was not possible to provide adequate shielding. Because power lines are ground-referred, it became necessary to connect the shielding to a stable ground connection. When one terminal of the single-sided amplifier was grounded, it often became difficult to shield the other (the grid terminal) from power-line interference. In the differential amplifier neither input terminal is at ground potential, and because the amplifier provides an output proportional to the difference of potential between the input terminals, it matters little what the potentials of the two are; so long as they are the same, the amplifier will provide zero output.

Thus, in summary, the two main reasons for use of the differential amplifier in electrophysiology are the freedom of choice in placing the electrodes to record only the differences of potential that appear between them and the inherent rejection of voltages which appear on both input terminals, such as ground-referred interference from power lines.

The first differential amplifiers to be used in electrophysiology were, in reality, push-pull amplifiers. In the late 1920's, in the output stage of a high-quality audio amplifier it was becoming customary to use two tubes working in opposite phase (push-pull). This was achieved by coupling into such a stage with a center-tapped (input) transformer and deriving the output from the secondary of a center-tapped transformer in the plate circuit. In addition to providing low distortion, such an arrangement quadrupled the power available from the stage as compared to that obtainable with one tube operating at the same voltage. However, the push-pull mode of operation was used only in the output stage and center-tapped transformers were difficult to obtain. A method of eliminating the input transformer, which led to the development of push-pull resistance-capacity coupled amplifiers, was described by Aughtie (1929) and Davidson (1929); both had hit upon the idea of using a single-stage resistance-capacity coupled amplifier as a phase inverter. Because there were no double tubes at that time, the advantages of push-pull *RC* amplification were not used to any great extent, but the means to transfer a single-sided signal to a push-pull one had been established. Apparently unnoticed was the improvement in frequency response over that obtainable with the best transformers then or now.

One of the first push-pull *RC*-coupled amplifiers was described by Matthews (1934), who clearly called attention to the fact that the output (plate-to-plate) reflected the difference in potential between the grids. After the publication of Matthews' paper, many investigators built similar push-pull amplifiers in multichannel configurations for recording the electroencephalogram. Among them were Garceau and Forbes (1934), Adrian and Yamagiwa (1935), and Walter (1936). The amplifiers were connected to oscillographs for photographic recording. These studies were among the first to investigate the factors which influence the EEG and its clinical value.

Next to appear were two amplifiers in which only the input stage was differential; the following stages were single-sided, thereby offering the maximum economy of components in each channel. One circuit was described by Schmitt (1937); the other, by Toennies (1938). Schmitt's circuit employed two pentodes with the input signal applied to their grids. The output (single-sided) was taken from the one which functioned both as a conventional amplifier and as a mixer in which the output of the other tube modulated its screen grid. By making two simple adjustments, it was possible to balance the two sides of the amplifier to provide an output which represented the difference in potential between the grids and was relatively independent of the voltage on both grids as referred to the cathode.

Toennies' circuit employed two triodes with their cathodes joined together and returned to a negative supply through a large resistance. In the plate circuit of one tube was a resistor; in that of the other there was none. The input was applied to both grids, and the output which was presented to a single-sided amplifier derived from the tube with the resistor in its plate circuit. In essence the circuit was that of a cathode-coupled amplifier and functioned only as a differential amplifier if the cathode resistor was made large and compensation added to account for the fact that the gain of a cathode follower can never be exactly unity. With the application of such compensation, Toennies was able to balance the gain of the two sides of the amplifier to 1 part in 500, thereby creating a fairly good differential device.

At about the same time Buchtal and Nielsen (1936) and Offner (1937) called attention to some of the advantages of using push-pull construction throughout the amplifying channel: reduction of distortion, constancy of plate current for each stage (when operated in the linear part of the grid voltage-plate current characteristic), ease of obtaining bias, freedom from coupling between stages and channels through the power supply, and ability to employ a common power source for all stages. The signal is applied to both grids of the input stage, and the output is obtained from the plates of the output stage. Offner called attention to the fact that in-phase signals will be attenuated if the common-cathode resistors are made large with respect to the plate resistance of the tube. He also showed that in-phase signals will be further attenuated by feeding back the signal from the cathodes of the second stage to the grids of the first.

From that time on, many investigators described methods of attaining equal gain on each side of the push-pull amplifier to make it become truly a differential amplifier and thereby reject in-phase signals. The literature of this era describes push-pull amplifiers as balanced or symmetrical amplifiers, depending on the degree to which equality of amplification was achieved in the two sides of the device. When the gain was very nearly equal (e.g., differing by less than 1 part in 500), the push-pull amplifiers were called differential amplifiers. One of the easiest methods of obtaining this desirable characteristic was to place a large resistance in the common-cathode circuit of the first stage of the amplifier and return it to a negative supply to compensate for the large voltage drop across it, thereby providing the correct operating bias for the stage. This method, described by Matthews (1938) and Trevino and Offner (1940), works very well and is widely employed. Use of this circuit, which has been called "the long-tailed pair," requires that a large negative voltage be available. A technique for obtaining a high effective resistance in the cathode circuit without the use of a large negative voltage employs a pentode. The high plate resistance (megohms) and the low voltage drop make this method very attractive. Use of this technique was described by Goldberg (1944) and Johnston (1947).

Modern clinical electrophysiological studies such as electrocardiography, electroencephalography, and electromyography, which depend on differential amplifiers for their success, developed from the initial investigations with the amplifier circuits just described. In present-day apparatus, in addition to providing adequate gain and bandwidth, the primary goal is to achieve the highest degree of balance between the two sides of the amplifier. Achievement of this goal guarantees rejection of such in-phase signals as power line interference and signals arising from sources outside the field of the pair of recording electrodes. Although the basic techniques have been presented above, a detailed analysis of the circuits follows.

The circuit of the differential amplifier is illustrated in Fig. 13–29. In essence it consists of two symmetrical single-sided amplifiers; the electrical properties of the circuit associated with tube V_1 are exactly the same as with tube V_2. The resistors R_{g1} and R_{g2} provide a d-c path for application of grid bias to both tubes from the single battery E_c. The plate supply voltage E_B, along with the corresponding load resistors R_{L1} and R_{L2}, determine the load line for each tube. E_c determines the operating point on

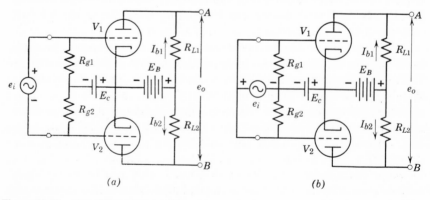

(a) (b)

Figure 13–29.   The differential amplifier: (a) out-of-phase voltage applied to input; (b) in-phase voltage applied to input.

the load line which is the same for both tubes. With no input signal ($e_i = 0$) each tube draws the same magnitude of plate current, and both tubes appear in parallel in so far as E_B is concerned. The voltage drops across R_{L_1} and R_{L_2} are equal and in the directions shown so that the potential difference between output terminals A and B is zero. Referring to Fig. 13–29a, if a voltage e_i is applied to the input terminals which causes the grid of tube V_1 to go positive while simultaneously the grid of tube V_2 is driven negatively, the plate current I_{b_1} will increase from the operating point value, thereby increasing the voltage drop across R_{L_1} and causing terminal A to become less positive than the operating point value. Conversely, making the grid of V_2 more negative decreases the current I_{b_2}, causing terminal B to become more positive than the operating point value. A potential difference then exists between the output terminals A and B with terminal B positive with respect to A. It is possible to show that the overall gain e_0/e_i is the same as would be obtained from either of the tubes operating alone.

The attractive feature of this circuit lies not in its voltage gain characteristics, but in its insensitivity to signal voltages which are simultaneoulsy in phase at both grids. For example, if the same signal voltage e_i is applied simultaneously to both grids as shown in Fig. 13–29b, the plate currents I_{b_1} and I_{b_2} will increase simultaneously by the same amount from the operating point and the voltage difference between terminals A and B will remain zero. The quantity which describes this insensitivity to in-phase grid voltages is called the common mode rejection ratio (CMRR) and is measured as the ratio of the magnitude of the in-phase voltage to the magnitude of the out-of-phase voltage required to produce the same output voltage. The CMRR is therefore the out-of-phase gain divided by the in-phase gain. In practical biological amplifiers CMRR's as high as 10,000:1 are easily obtained.

In the usual environments in which biological signals are detected it is expected that any undesirable electric and magnetic fields present will act to produce in-phase voltages at the input terminals and therefore will not produce a potential difference between the output terminals. Also, the desired bioelectric signal will present a distinct potential difference which will appear as an out-of-phase signal across the input terminals and as an amplified signal at the output terminals.

The advantage of this rejection property of the differential amplifier is illustrated in Fig. 13–30, which shows a subject connected for routine ECG recording. The 60-cycle 120-volt power wiring is the chief source of electrical interference, which is coupled into the amplifier through the capacitance existing between the "hot" side of the power line, the grid leads, and the subject or biological preparation. The interference circuit is completed through the grid resistors to ground, the "cold" side of the power line being grounded initially at the generating plant and at sub-

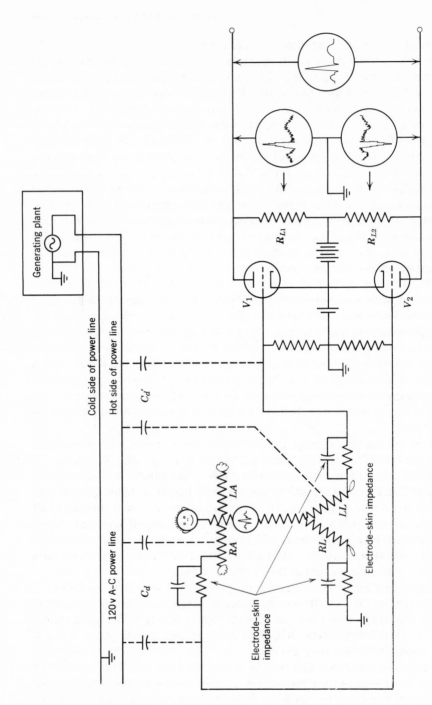

Figure 13–30. Rejection of power line interference by the differential amplifier.

sequent distribution points (Robinson, 1965). Although ground-referred domestic power-line voltages are in the vicinity of 110 and 220 volts rms, it must be remembered that the peak-to-peak values are $110 \times 2\sqrt{2}$ and $220 \times 2\sqrt{2}$, respectively. In addition, it is to be noted that when bioelectric events are to be measured the voltages presented to the electrodes are in the millivolt and microvolt range. Thus the interfering signal source, capacitively coupled through the high reactance of C_d and $C_{d'}$, is in the order of 100,000 times as large as the desired signal. If the same amount of undesired voltage is coupled to both grids through the capacitances C_d and $C_{d'}$, the undesired signal will be rejected. The best insurance for equal coupling is obtained by continuing the symmetry of the amplifier on to the external circuit by using leads of equal length and placing them in essentially the same physical location. The aim of this technique is to subject both grids to the same interference. Even when this is done it is often possible to maximize the rejection by reorienting the input leads and the subject.

A primary source of difficulty in obtaining a symmetrical input circuit is the electrode-tissue interface impedance. With the subject and the common input terminal of the amplifier connected together and grounded, undesirable voltages of different magnitudes will appear across electrodes having different electrode-tissue impedances. The actual magnitudes of these impedances are not as important as the difference in their values, because if the impedances are equal in magnitude and phase characteristics, interfering voltages equal in magnitude and phase will be presented to the amplifier input and will be rejected as determined by the CMRR of the amplifier.

The ability of a differential amplifier to reject undesired in-phase voltages can be illustrated by the following example. Let it be assumed that an amplifier has a measured CMRR of 10,000. If it is desired to record EEG signals having an average amplitude of $50\mu v$, an in-phase interference signal of $10^4 \times 50 \times 10^{-6} = 0.5$ volt would be needed to produce a noise voltage in the output equal to that produced by the desired signal, that is, under these conditions the signal-to-noise ratio would be 1:1. Reduction of the interference signal to 0.005 volt (5 millivolts) would produce an output-signal-to-noise ratio of 100, which is in most instances quite acceptable.

Because of the limited range of linearity of vacuum tubes, caution must be exercised in inferring from the value of the CMRR information concerning the maximum amplitude of the common-mode signal which may be applied and true differential action retained. For example, a CMRR of 10,000:1 does not mean that, if the desired (out-of-phase) signal is 0.1 volt, an in-phase voltage of 1000 volts could be applied to the input terminals and produce the same output as the desired signal. Certainly, for tubes of the volt-ampere ranges that have been discussed, a signal of such large magnitude would drive each tube far beyond the range of linear operation. Therefore, in order to obtain the benefits of differential amplification with common mode rejection, the undesired in-phase signal must not be of sufficient magnitude to drive either tube beyond its linear operating range. The maximum permissible value of the in-phase signal can be determined experimentally.

13–22.   COMMON MODE REJECTION RATIO

In the circuits described, a high common-mode rejection ratio was obtained by assuming that the tubes V_1 and V_2 were identical and that R_{L1} and R_{L2} were also identical. In practice it is not possible to achieve such a situation, and several circuit arrangements are made to provide a high CMRR despite small differences in tubes and components. The simplest method of achieving a high CMRR is to obtain grid bias for the first stage of the amplifier by the use of an unbypassed common cathode resistor R_k.

Having established that the desirable characteristics produced by negative feedback are obtained at the expense of system gain, it is instructive to point out that the cathode follower is an example of negative feedback because the entire output voltage is effectively fed back to modify the input. In a similar manner a certain amount of negative feedback (depending upon the relative magnitudes of R_L and R_k) occurs in a common-cathode amplifier in which the cathode resistor is left unbypassed. This feedback can be put to good use in increasing the common mode rejection in the differential amplifier. Consider the circuit shown in Fig. 13–31a. If this circuit is truly symmetrical, a given current $i_K = i_{p1} + i_{p2} = i_{K1} + i_{K2}$ will flow through R_k when $e_s = 0$ and bias the tube to the desired operating point. If a signal e_s is then applied so that terminal A is as much above ground potential as terminal B is below (i.e., v_1 and v_2 are equal in magnitude but out of phase), the current i_K will remain constant and the bias voltage will remain the same as at the operating point. If, however, an in-phase signal is applied simultaneously to both grids (i.e. v_1 and v_2 are equal and are in phase), the plate current of both tubes increases, and the voltage drop across R_K increases in the same direction as the in-phase signal (the cathodes tend to follow the grids). This constitutes negative feedback for the in-phase signal, and hence the gain of the amplifier is reduced for this signal but the desired out-of-phase signal is amplified in the usual manner.

The amount of negative feedback, and consequently of common mode rejection, is dependent directly on the magnitude of R_K. In order to make R_K large while at the same time using power supply sources of reasonable value, and to maintain the cathode and grid properly biased near ground potential,

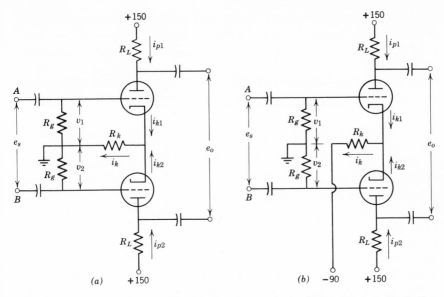

Figure 13–31.   The use of a common cathode resistor to obtain a high common mode rejection ratio.

R_K is connected not to ground but to a negative source of potential. Two tubes operated in this way constitute a "long-tailed pair." This connection is shown in Fig. 13–31b.

Because the CMRR in a truly symmetrical circuit depends upon having R_K very large (ideally, infinite), the limits of practicality are soon reached in the magnitudes of potential sources required to force the tube-operating current through such very high resistance. For some applications more practical arrangements have been sought. A relatively simple method is to replace R_K with a pentode (Goldberg, 1944; Johnston, 1947), as shown in Fig. 13–32. As was pointed out previously, the plate resistance of the pentode is very high (greater than 10^6 ohms) while the actual operating potentials on the tube elements are essentially the same as for any other vacuum tube. Therefore the pentode provides effectively a very high R_K, using a nominal plate voltage $\doteq 100$ volts, screen voltage $\doteq 75$ volts, and grid bias $\doteq -2$ volts. It should also be emphasized that, if the circuit is not truly symmetrical electrically with respect to the common terminal of the amplifier (which is usually grounded), the common mode rejection will be limited by the amount of asymmetry. Attention must be given therefore to the use of matched tubes; for example, their μ, r_p, and g_m values should be equal, and circuit components (R_L and R_g) should also be equal. Even if an extremely high CMRR is obtained for the amplifier, any asymmetry produced by variations in electrode-tissue impedances or any factor which

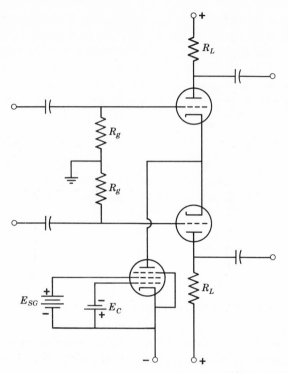

Figure 13–32. The use of a pentode in the cathode circuit to obtain a high common mode rejection ratio.

results in unequal coupling of the undesirable voltage to the two amplifier input terminals will produce an undesired voltage in the output signal.

A high CMRR in the amplifier, while obviously desirable, is, however, no panacea and cannot substitute for simple precautions such as keeping power cords away from the input circuit and using a shielded box or room. If reasonable attention is afforded to connecting living subjects and biological preparations in a symmetrical manner and if known sources of interference are physically removed or shielded against, CMRR's on the order of 10,000 are usually adequate and can easily be obtained in amplifiers without resorting to special efforts to balance tubes or to use a pentode or other constant-current device in the cathode circuit in place of a resistor.

Many penetrating analyses of the factors which underlie the attainment of a high CMRR have been presented. Obviously, if identical tubes and components are employed, the CMRR theoretically would be infinite. Even with careful matching of components and tubes, the CMRR is finite and often not high enough. For this reason serious efforts have been made to obtain a high CMRR with components of commercial tolerance. The EMI

Laboratories (1946) presented an ingenious method of obtaining a high common-cathode impedance by the use of a triode connected to make it operate as a constant-current device. Offner (1947) described a circuit with high cathode resistance and with feedback between the second and first stages of the amplifier. Although the CMRR is descriptive of the quality of a differential amplifier, it does not identify the magnitude of the in-phase signal that can be tolerated. A study of this important factor was presented by Parnum (1950).

Andrew (1958) analyzed and tested a series of interesting circuits which provide a high CMRR. All used pentodes; in one the high CMRR was achieved by battery-coupling the common-screen voltage to the common-cathode voltage obtained with a high resistance in the cathode circuit. In another circuit Andrew placed a pentode in the common cathode of the two pentodes used as the amplifying tubes; in a third version of the same circuit he battery-coupled the screens of the amplifier to the common cathodes. This circuit provided a CMRR of about 40,000 with typical tubes. A thorough analysis of the triode and pentode circuits with a high common-cathode resistor, and triodes and pentodes connected with triodes in the cathode to simulate a high common-cathode resistance, was presented by Klein (1955). An interesting study into the effect of mismatching tubes and components on the rejection ratio was presented by Dewhurst (1959), who called attention to the precautions to be taken when the CMRR is to be measured with accuracy.

Perhaps the ultimate in the achievement of a high rejection ratio was described by Salmons (1966). In his circuit a CMRR in excess of 300,000 was obtained without selected tubes or components but with the use of several compensating controls. Salmon's circuit, developed to identify the factors which limit the attainment of a high rejection ratio, consists of two triodes as input tubes with two additional cascode-connected triodes to provide a high effective cathode resistance. Two additional triodes serve as cathode followers, driving two other triodes in the plate circuits of the input tubes. Four potentiometers are employed to adjust the circuit to provide the maximum rejection ratio.

13–23. PRACTICAL AMPLIFIERS

The circuit diagram of a practical general-purpose differential amplifier for bioelectric events is shown in Fig. 13–33. Inspection of the arrangement of components reveals that it is a two-stage *RC* coupled amplifier using two pentodes as the input stage, which are capacity-coupled to two triodes that are in turn directly coupled to two triodes connected as cathode followers and constituting the output stage. The gain is provided by the first (pentode) and second (triode) stages; the cathode follower supplies an

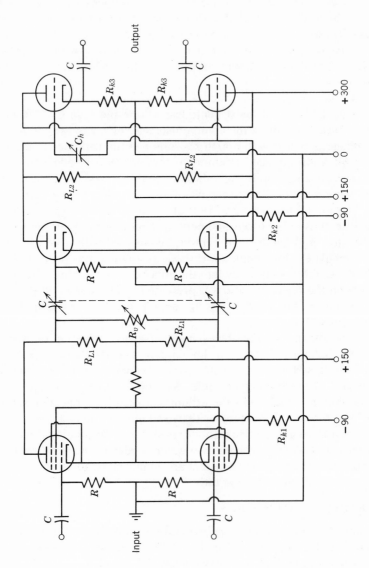

Figure 13-33. Three-stage general-purpose differential amplifier for bioelectric events.

amplification of slightly less than unity. The overall gain of the amplifier is adjustable by varying R_v connected between the plates of the input pentodes.

The low-frequency response is determined by the choice of the components used in the coupling circuits (RC). The high-frequency response is determined by the input capacitances of the tubes, the values chosen for the plate loads R_L, and the stray capacitances due to the wires interconnecting the stages. The use of pentodes for the input stage permits the attainment of a low input capacitance, and the cathode followers at the output provides a low output impedance. The low output impedance permits the use of a reasonably long, shielded cable to connect the preamplifier to the main display apparatus (oscilloscope, amplifier and pen motor, etc.) without the loss of high-frequency response. This feature is of practical significance because it permits locating the preamplifier as close as possible to the subject and minimizes the pickup of interference by allowing the use of short leads to connect the preamplifier to the preparation.

Several of the circuit design details are noteworthy. For example, the low-frequency response of the amplifier is adjustable by selection of different values of the coupling capacitor C between the first and second stages. The high frequency response is adjustable by choice of various values of C_h, which places shunt capacitances across the grids of the cathode-follower output stage. A high CMRR is obtained by the use of cathode resistors R_{K1}, R_{K2} high in value. These resistors are returned to a negative supply (-90 volts) to provide the correct operating bias for the tubes.

The operating characteristics of the amplifier are dependent on the tubes and the components employed. With matched pentodes and components in the input stage and the use of 2-μf coupling capacitors C and 2-megohm resistors R, the overall time constant is 2 seconds and the low-frequency response extends to 0.08 cps. The high-frequency response extends to 10,000 cps. The CMRR is in the vicinity of 10,000.

Differential amplifier circuits are by no means restricted to applications with vacuum tubes. Many differential amplifiers have been built using transistors. Because of their small size, low current consumption, and existence in complementary forms, the possible circuit arrangements are numerous and techniques to obtain a high rejection ratio, such as those used by Salmons, become practical. A good review and analysis of many of the circuits was presented by Middlebrook (1963).

13–24.   OPERATIONAL AMPLIFIERS

An operational amplifier consists basically of a very-high-gain direct-coupled amplifier which is modified by the connection of specific passive circuit elements to the input and to an external feedback loop. Because of the high gain in the amplifier, the output of the system so formed is a function of the electrical behavior of the input and feedback elements, appropriate selection of which permits carrying out many mathematical operations such as addition, subtraction, differentiation, and integration, as well as the generation of many special functions. Because the addition of simple passive circuit components makes possible a great variety of functions, operational amplifiers are becoming widely used in the creation of many electronic measuring and control devices.

A block diagram of an operational amplifier is shown in Fig. 13–34. The high-gain amplifier is represented by the triangle A, and the input and feedback elements are designated Z_i and Z_o, respectively. Although an ideal high-gain direct-coupled amplifier would possess, among other attributes, infinite gain, infinite input impedance, and zero output impedance, practical amplifiers obviously do not meet these criteria. Amplifiers suitable for operational use are, however, characterized by high gain (greater than 20,000 for direct current), high input impedance (0.1 to 10 megohms), and low output impedance (a few hundred ohms). These fundamental ("open-loop") characteristics of the operational amplifier may appear to fall rather short of the ideal; nevertheless, when it is connected with input and feedback elements ("closed loop") to perform a special function, the input impedance can be made much greater or can be set to a value determined by the input element; also, the output impedance may be reduced from the open-loop value to the order of 0.01 ohm. These changes in impedance characteristics are obtained at the expense of overall gain.

A few of the possibilities offered by the operational amplifier are described by analysis of the circuit of Fig. 13–34, in which the input impedance element is Z_i and the feedback impedance element is Z_o, e_i and e_o are the input and output voltages, respectively. The amplifier A is usually constructed with two input terminals in addition to a terminal common to both input and output. The common terminal is seldom shown explicitly in schematic representations of the operational amplifier. Connection to it is indicated by the standard symbol for ground or earth, and it is customary to refer

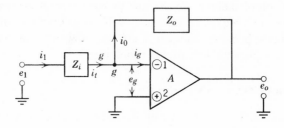

Figure 13–34. The operational amplifier.

to input and output voltages relative to ground even though the common terminal may or may not be connected physically or electrically to ground. For voltages measured relative to ground, terminal 1 is "inverting," that is, the phase from input to output is reversed 180 degrees, while a voltage applied between terminal 2 and ground appears at the output without being shifted in phase. For many applications terminal 2 is grounded as shown. Point g is called the "summing" point, and because of the very high gain of the amplifier, g is at "virtual" ground, that is, $e_g \doteq 0$. Because of the very low value of e_g, i_g flowing into terminal 1 is likewise very low and can be neglected. Writing the Kirchhoff current equation for node g, we have

$$i_0 + i_g = i_t,$$

but $$i_g = 0 \quad \text{and} \quad i_t = i_1.$$

hence $$i_0 = i_t \tag{F}$$

and $$\frac{e_g - e_0}{Z_0} = \frac{e_i - e_g}{Z_i},$$

but $$e_g = 0.$$

therefore $$-\frac{e_0}{Z_0} = \frac{e_i}{Z_i},$$

and $$e_0 = -\frac{Z_0}{Z_i} e_i.$$

The output voltage is seen to be determined by the impedance elements Z_o and Z_i. Accordingly, if Z_o and Z_i consist of resistors, the gain of the system is set by the ratio of the resistance values.

A practical circuit for summing several input voltages is shown in Fig. 13–35a. In this circuit Z_o consists of the single resistor R_0, while the input impedance Z_i is composed of the three resistors R_1, R_2, and R_3, which are connected to individual sources of voltage e_1, e_2, and e_3. The output voltage e_o of this circuit may be calculated by applying equation F as follows.

Recalling that $$i_0 = i_t,$$

but $$i_t = i_1 + i_2 + i_3$$

so that

$$i_t = \frac{e_1}{R_1} + \frac{e_2}{R_2} + \frac{e_3}{R_3}$$

and

$$i_0 = -\frac{e_0}{R_0},$$

we have

$$-\frac{e_0}{R_0} = \frac{e_1}{R_1} + \frac{e_2}{R_2} + \frac{e_3}{R_3},$$

$$-e_0 = e_1 \frac{R_0}{R_1} + e_2 \frac{R_0}{R_2} + e_3 \frac{R_0}{R_3}$$

or

$$e_0 = -R_0 \left(\frac{e_1}{R_1} + \frac{e_2}{R_2} + \frac{e_3}{R_3} \right).$$

By setting various resistance ratios: R_0/R_1, R_0/R_2, and R_0/R_3, the desired gain (either greater or less than unity) can be given to each input voltage. For example, direct summation of the input voltages (i.e., $e_0 = e_1 + e_2 + e_3$) requires only that all resistances be equal. If it is desired that the output

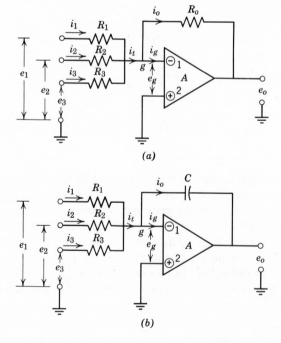

(a)

(b)

Figure 13–35. Use of the operational amplifier for summation (a) and integration and summation (b).

voltage e_0 be given by the expression

$$e_0 = \tfrac{1}{2}e_1 + e_2 + 2e_3,$$

the resistance values of R_0, R_1, R_2, and R_3 could be 1, 2, 1, and 0.5 megohms, respectively.

Figure 13–34 can be converted to an integrating circuit by making the input element Z_i a resistor having a value of R ohms and the feedback element Z_o a capacitor C with a value of C farads. Again the output voltage may be calculated by using equation F:

$$i_0 = i_t,$$

$$C\frac{d(e_g - e_0)}{dt} = \frac{e_1 - e_g}{R}$$

$$e_g = 0,$$

$$-C\frac{de_0}{dt} = \frac{e_1}{R},$$

$$de_0 = -\frac{e_1}{RC}\,dt,$$

$$e_0 = -\frac{1}{RC}\int e_1\,dt.$$

This choice of circuit elements produces a system in which the output voltage is the time integral of the input voltage, and the system gain is $-(1/RC)$. The values for R and C may be chosen to produce desired signal levels, for example, if $C = 1.0$ mf and $R = 1$ megohm, $RC = 1.0$ and the system provides unity gain with a phase shift of 180 degrees.

Several inputs may be integrated and summed simultaneously. A circuit for accomplishing this is shown in Fig. 13–35b. The output voltage is given by

$$e_0 = -\left(\frac{1}{CR_1}\int e_1\,dt + \frac{1}{CR_2}\int e_2\,dt + \frac{1}{CR_3}\int e_3\,dt\right).$$

In a similar manner it is easy to show that, if the impedance elements are interchanged (i.e., $Z_i = C$ and $Z_o = R$), a differentiating circuit results and the output voltage is $e_o = RC\,(de_1/dt)$. Because of the high values required of e_o for representation of the derivatives of rapidly changing input voltages, the practical range of e_o may be exceeded when differentiation is attempted with this simple circuit. Practical circuits for alleviating this difficulty are shown in the applications manuals listed in the references at the end of the chapter.

A group of operational amplifiers, suitably arranged so that the desired input and feedback elements may be connected easily for each amplifier and the amplifiers themselves interconnected, constitutes an analog computer. Such a device is extremely useful for the rapid solution of linear differential equations. In addition it permits "on-line" manipulation of parameters to study their relative effectiveness in determining a solution (output). For example, a very simple arrangement of operational amplifiers may be used to "solve" the second-order differential equation describing rectilinear and rotary motion in the damped spring-mass system discussed in Chapter 12. The literature contains many examples of the use of analog computers for the solution of biological problems and for the construction of models simulating physiological systems. The discussions presented by Randall (1962), Grodins (1963), and Milhorn (1966) will be found to be of considerable interest to the life scientist.

Another application of operational amplifiers in the life sciences involves the generation of derived functions. For example, Rushmer (1961) employed a group of operational amplifiers to generate other functions which were processed to produce desired information. The arrangement he used is diagramed in Fig. 13–36. Starting with three physiological variables—direct ventricular blood pressure, aortic flow velocity, and ventricular diameter—he utilized the operations of differentiation, integration, and multiplication to produce other signals representing aortic flow, flow per stroke, myocardial "power," and "work per stroke."

At least one manufacturer[5] makes available a simple experimental unit useful in carrying out many operations. It contains several high-gain operational amplifiers with power supply and convenient terminal boards for plugging in desired input and feedback elements and for interconnecting the amplifiers. A picture of such a combination of operational amplifiers, called a manifold, is shown in Fig. 13–37. A small manifold of this type permits the investigator to connect many useful special-purpose circuits, some of which are shown in Fig. 13–38.

13–25. SOLID-STATE ELECTRONICS

In recent years solid-state devices such as the diode, the transistor, and integrated circuitry have revolutionized the concepts of nearly all electronic

[5] Philbrick Researches, Inc., Dedham, Mass.

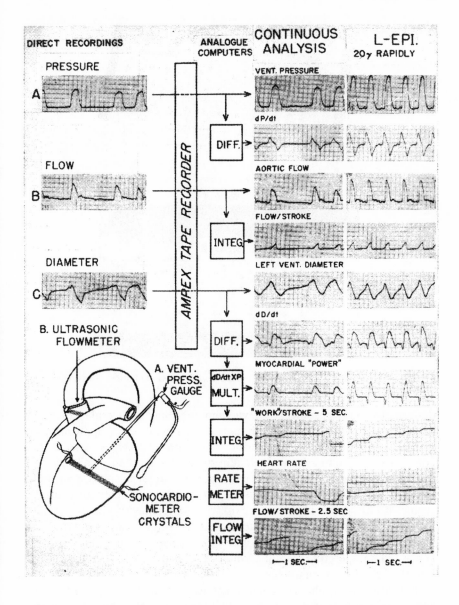

Figure 13–36. Use of operational amplifiers for computation and production of derived functions. (From R. F. Rushmer, Cardiovascular Dynamics, 2nd Ed., W. B. Saunders Co., Philadelphia Pa., 1961. By permission.)

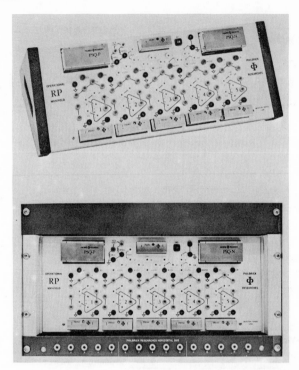

Figure 13–37. Operational amplifier manifold. (Courtesy Philbrick Researches, Inc., Dedham, Mass.)

designs. In many instances the vacuum tube has been replaced in new equipment by these devices, although there remain some applications in which the vacuum tube is superior. The main advantages of solid-state components in comparison to vacuum tubes include their small size, light weight, greater efficiency, extreme resistance to physical shock, and ability to operate with low voltage and current. In addition, no cathode heating is required. Two series of transistors exist with complementary characteristics, one operating from a positive supply and the other from a negative. The vacuum tube still retains advantages with respect to the amount of noise generated, temperature stability, voltage excursion, power-handling capabilities, variation in characteristics caused by manufacturing processes, amplification at ultrahigh frequency, and less sensitivity to radiation such as gamma rays and neutrons. Both vacuum tube and solid-state technologies are undergoing rapid changes, each seeking to overcome its defects and to improve its inherent advantages. For this reason it is wise to avoid categorical statements regarding the advantages and disadvantages of the two types.

13–26. SEMICONDUCTORS

Certain solid materials, called semiconductors, exhibit unique electrical characteristics which permit their use in the construction of devices, such as diodes and transistors, in which current can be controlled. The most important semiconductor materials are germanium and silicon. The designation semiconductor is descriptive because these materials have resistivity values in the range between those of conductors and of non-conductors (insulators). For example, silver, one of the best conductors, has a resistivity of 1.59×10^{-6} ohm cm, and fused quartz, one of the best insulators, 5×10^{18} ohm cm. Pure germanium and silicon have resistivity values of the order of 60 and 60,000 ohm cm, respectively. It is not the fact that these materials are poor conductors which renders them useful; rather it is their behavior with regard to the electron energy levels associated with their crystal structure. Figure 13–39 shows the normal crystal structure of germanium, in which each atom assumes its place by sharing its four valence electrons. The actual structure is, of course, three dimensional rather than two as shown. If an electric field is produced within such a crystal, as by the application of electrodes connected to a source of voltage, no conduction (movement of electric charge) would be expected because there are no charge carriers free to move. This situation is in contrast to the one found in a good conductor such as silver, in which the charge carriers (electrons) are not associated with any particular atom but are free to move under the influence of an electric field.

The differences between good conductors, semiconductors, and insulators are explained by quantum theory in terms of the energy levels of the electrons in these three types of material. The energy levels of interest, designated the valence band, the forbidden band, and the conduction band, are illustrated in Fig. 13–40. For an electron to participate in the conduction process it must acquire sufficient energy (photic or thermal) to become free of the valence band and to move into the conduction band. The conduction band and valence band overlap in good conductors; hence electrons are always available for conduction. In semiconductors and insulators, the two bands are separated by a "forbidden" band which defines a range of energy levels wherein the electrons are denied on the basis of quantum characteristics of the particular material. Accordingly, semiconductors differ from insulators by the width of the forbidden energy band. The forbidden band in semiconductors is sufficiently narrow so that thermal energies acquired at room temperature are adequate to permit some electrons to enter the conduction band. In an insulator the forbidden band is sufficiently wide to prevent the availability of conduction electrons.

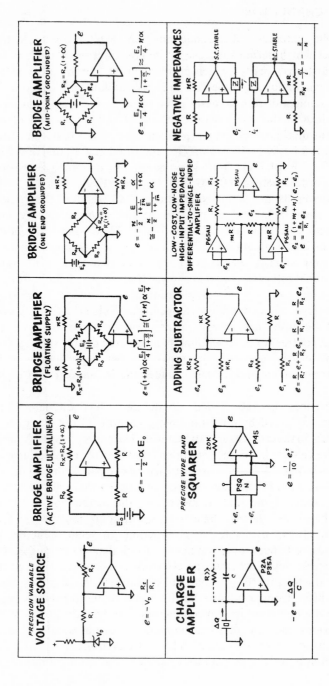

Figure 13-38. Miscellaneous circuit arrangements for use with operational amplifiers. (Courtesy Philbrick Researches, Inc., Dedham, Mass.)

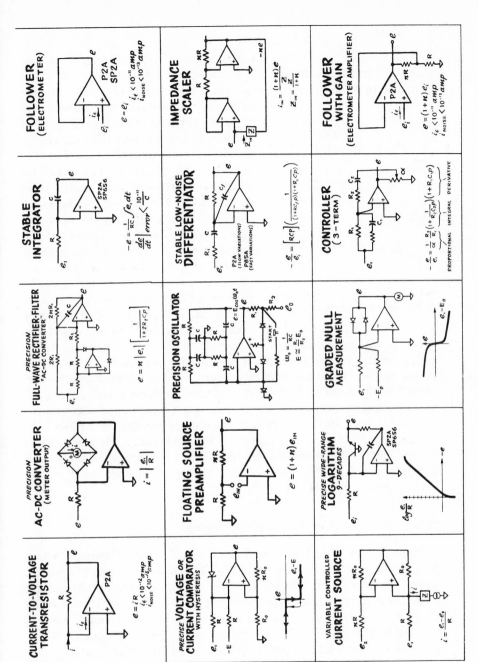

FOLLOWER (ELECTROMETER)

P2A
SP2A

$e = e_i$; $i_\epsilon < 10^{-11}$ amp
$i_{NOISE} < 10^{-13}$ amp

IMPEDANCE SCALER

$i_{IN} = \frac{(1+n)e}{Z}$
$Z_{IN} = \frac{Z}{1+n}$

FOLLOWER WITH GAIN (ELECTROMETER AMPLIFIER)

P2A

$e = (1+n)e_i$;
$i_\epsilon < 10^{-11}$ amp
$i_{NOISE} < 10^{-13}$ amp

STABLE INTEGRATOR

SP2A
SP656

$-e = \frac{1}{RC}\int e_i\, dt$
$\frac{de}{dt}\Big|error < \frac{10^{-11}}{C}$

STABLE LOW-NOISE DIFFERENTIATOR

P2A (SLOW VARIATIONS)
P85A (FAST VARIATIONS)

$-\frac{e}{e_i} = [RCp]\left(\frac{1}{(1+R_iC_ip)(1+R_iC_ip)}\right)$

CONTROLLER (3-TERM)

$-\frac{e}{e_i} = \frac{1}{\alpha}\frac{R_2}{R_1}\left(1+\frac{1}{R_2C_2p}\right)(1+R_1C_1p)$
PROPORTIONAL   INTEGRAL   DERIVATIVE

PRECISION
FULL-WAVE RECTIFIER-FILTER "AC-DC CONVERTER"

$e = n|e_i|\left|\frac{1}{1+2R_fC_fp}\right|$

PRECISION OSCILLATOR

$G = E\cos\omega_o t$
START = $\frac{1}{TP}$
$\omega_o = \frac{1}{RC}$
$E \simeq \frac{R_1}{R_2}E_o$

GRADED NULL MEASUREMENT

$e_i - E_0$

PRECISION
AC-DC CONVERTER (METER OUTPUT)

$i = \left|\frac{e_i}{R}\right|$

FLOATING SOURCE PREAMPLIFIER

$e = (1+n)e_{IN}$

PRECISE WIDE-RANGE
LOGARITHM 9-DECADES

SP2A
SP656

$\log\frac{e_i}{R}$
$-e$

CURRENT-TO-VOLTAGE TRANSRESISTOR

P2A

$e = iR$; $i_\epsilon < 10^{-12}$ amp
$i_{NOISE} < 10^{-13}$ amp

PRECISE **VOLTAGE** or **CURRENT COMPARATOR** WITH HYSTERESIS

$e_i - E$

VARIABLE CONTROLLED CURRENT SOURCE

$i = \frac{e_2 - e_1}{R}$

Figure 13-38. (continued)

387

If, by the absorption of energy, a covalent bond is disrupted, the release of an electron for conduction leaves a positive charge "uncovered" in the outer shell of the germanium atom, as illustrated in Fig. 13–41. The absence of an electron creates a "hole," which may be considered equivalent to a positive particle having the same electrical charge as the electron. Conduction can then take place by the application of an electric field which will cause a movement of either holes or electrons. Conduction produced by charge carriers created by absorption of photic or thermal energy in pure germanium and silicon is called intrinsic conduction, because it is a characteristic of these materials and determines the measured resistivity. The generation of charge carriers by absorption of photic or thermal energy can be put to use for measuring these forms of energy with solid-state devices especially designed for this purpose; however, in transistors for other applications, such as in amplifiers, charge carriers created in this manner are undesirable because they constitute components of current which are not related to the desired signal and hence contribute "noise." Pure germanium and silicon are not used in the construction of diodes and transistors; very small but known amounts of specific "impurities" are added. The addition of an "impurity" material, called "doping," lowers the resistivities of the germanium and silicon and produces either an N (negative) or a P (positive) type of material, depending upon the characteristics of the impurity added.

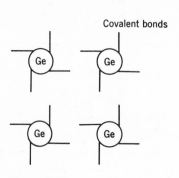

Figure 13–39. Structure of germanium showing covalent electrons.

13–27. N-AND P-TYPE SEMICONDUCTORS

Figure 13–42a shows the result of "doping" pure germanium with a pentavalent element such as antimony. The antimony atom is found to assume a place in the crystal structure by sharing four of its valence electrons with the germanium atoms. An excess electron remains and is available for conduction. The antimony is said to be a "donor" material because it donates electrons to the material, thereby producing N-type germanium in which the negative electron is the "majority" carrier.

The converse situation occurs if a trivalent element such as indium is added (Fig. 13–42b). The indium atom, having only three valence electrons to share, has a deficit of one electron, and hence a "hole" is created which may be filled by accepting an electron from a neighboring germanium atom.

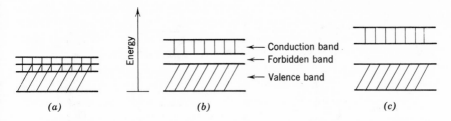

Figure 13–40.   Energy levels of a good conductor (*a*), semiconductor (*b*), and insulator (*c*).

In so doing, the hole is transferred to the vicinity of the germanium atom contributing the electron, so that, although the charged particle actually moving in the material is the electron, the effect is the same as if an equivalent positive charge (the hole) were moving in the opposite direction. Indium is called an "acceptor" material because it must accept an electron to fill completely a position in the crystal structure. Doping germanium with indium produces a *p*-type material in which the positive hole is the majority carrier.

Doping silicon or germanium with selected impurities, in quantities of a few parts per million, lowers the resistivity of the pure material considerably. For example, doped germanium and silicon suitable for diodes and transistors have resistivities of about 2 ohm cm; the undoped values are approximately 60 and 60,000 ohm cm, respectively.

13–28.   THE *P-N* JUNCTION

The joining of *P*- and *N*-type materials to form a continuous crystal structure produces a junction with the charge distribution shown in Fig. 13–43. After an initial combination of holes and electrons an equilibrium is reached and a potential barrier to further charge transfer is created by

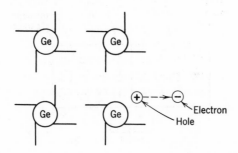

Figure 13–41.   The creation of a hole-electron pair in germanium.

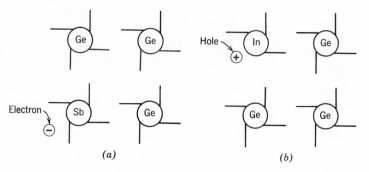

Figure 13–42. The creation of N- and P-type germanium by (a) pentavalent and (b) trivalent doping.

the ionic layers consisting of atoms bound (not free to move) in the crystal structure which have either lost electrons (antimony) or gained electrons (indium). The region between the ionic layers is void of charge carriers and is called the depletion region. The electrical potential across the depletion region has the polarity depicted by the battery shown in Fig. 13–43 and presents a potential barrier which the majority carriers in either material must overcome in order to move across the junction.

13–29. DIODE ACTION

The manner in which the P-N junction functions to conduct current in one direction (diode action) is illustrated in Fig. 13–44. Figure 13–44a shows the effect upon majority carriers resulting from the establishment

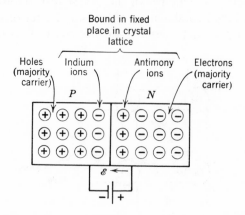

Figure 13–43. The electric field across a P-N junction.

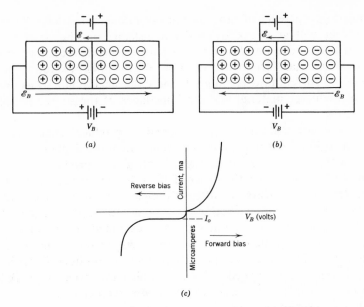

Figure 13–44. The *P–N* junction: (*a*) forward bias; (*b*) reverse bias; (*c*) current-voltage characteristics.

of an electric field $\mathscr{E}_B$ within the material (and across the junction) by connecting the *P*-type material to the positive terminal of a battery and the *N*-type material to the negative terminal. The junction is then said to be forward biased. $\mathscr{E}_B$ is in opposition to the field $\mathscr{E}$ across the junction, and if it exceeds $\mathscr{E}$ the holes and electrons will move towards and across the junction and a continuous current will flow around the loop. Conversely, if the polarity of the battery is reversed (Fig. 13–44*b*) and the junction is reverse biased, the electric field established is in the same direction as $\mathscr{E}$ and has the effect of widening the depletion region. As a consequence no current flows by the movement of majority carriers, but it must be remembered that any hole-electron pairs produced by absorption of photic or thermal energy will create minority carriers (holes in *N*-type material, electrons in *P*-type) which will find the field direction favorable for movement through the material and across the junction.

Figure 13–44c shows the form of a typical *P-N* junction (diode) current-voltage characteristic. Observe that the current with forward bias is measured in milliamperes, while the reverse current is in microamperes. The reverse current displays a steady value I_0 over a large portion of its range. This is the saturation current and is produced by the collection of free charge carriers created by the absorption of photic or thermal energy. As the reverse voltage is increased, a sharp increase in current is obtained, denoting the occurrence of either avalanche or Zener breakdown. These are two distinct voltage breakdowns distinguishable on the basis of their change with temperature. Which type occurs is dependent upon the doping of the two materials forming the junction. When either breakdown occurs, the resulting current flow is limited by only the small ohmic resistance of the semiconductor material and the impedance of the source of voltage applied to it.

Semiconductor materials may be doped to produce narrow or wide depletion regions. Zener breakdown occurs when the depletion region is so narrow that a relatively small applied voltage can produce a very high electric field intensity (on the order of 10^6 volts/cm) across the depletion region. The field intensity is sufficiently high to cause valence electrons to break away from atoms fixed in the crystal lattice and produce current flow. The absorption of thermal energy, exhibited by an increase in temperature of the semiconductor, imparts energy to the valence electrons and thereby reduces the field intensity required to produce Zener break-down; therefore the applied voltage at which this type of breakdown occurs (Zener voltage) decreases with increased temperature.

Avalanche breakdown occurs at junctions having depletion regions so wide that, before the electric field intensity reaches the level necessary to produce Zener breakdown, valence electrons are removed by bombardment from accelerated minority carriers. The electrons released by bombardment are in turn accelerated to cause an avalanche of change carriers. The applied voltage required to produce avalanche breakdown increases with

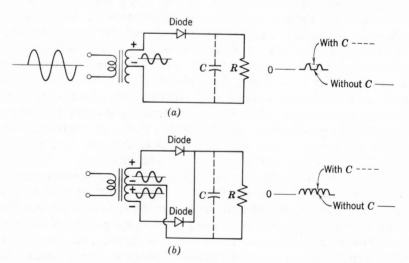

(a)

(b)

Figure 13-45. The use of a diode to obtain half-wave (a) and full-wave (b) rectification.

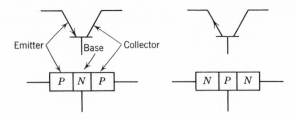

Figure 13–46. The *PNP* and *NPN* transistors.

temperature because the electron mean free path in the semiconductor is decreased as a result of frequent collisions, preventing acquisition by the electrons of sufficient kinetic energy to liberate a valence electron.

P-N junctions, suitably doped to produce Zener breakdown, are often called Zener diodes and are widely used as voltage reference devices because of the essentially constant voltage maintained independently of current after initiation of breakdown. Figures 13–45*a,b* show the use of the forward bias characteristic of the *P-N* junction to create half- and full-wave circuits to rectify a sinusoidal voltage waveform. These circuits are used extensively to rectify a-c voltage from power mains, which, after filtering with capacitors and other components, may be used to replace batteries to supply d-c power for the operation of electronic devices. A similar arrangement is used to "detect" a waveform which has been superimposed upon a sinusoidal carrier wave form by some scheme of modulation. (See Section 13–38.)

13–30.   TRANSISTORS

The basic transistor consists of two *P-N* junctions arranged in either the *PNP* or the *NPN* configuration as shown in Fig. 13–46. The three elements of the transistor are designated emitter, base, and collector. The corresponding triode analogs are cathode, grid, and plate. Observe that the *PNP* and *NPN* schematic designations differ only by the direction of the emitter arrow. The arbitrarily assigned directions for positive conventional current and voltage are shown in Fig. 13–47. Actual currents and voltages opposite to these are arbitrarily designated as negative.

The functioning of a transistor can be understood from the *NPN* connection illustrated in Fig. 13–48. With the battery connections shown, the emitter-base junction is forward biased and the collector-base junction is reverse biased. Considering each junction as an independent diode, it might at first be expected that the current would be large around the emitter-base loop and negligible around the collector-base loop. The

PNP or *NPN*

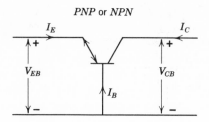

Figure 13-47. Convention for designating positive current and voltage.

current flow is established as follows. The electric field across the emitter-base junction is in such a direction as to move the electrons from the emitter and the holes from the base toward the junction and across it. If the junction has been purposely constructed so that the density of electrons in the emitter greatly exceeds the density of holes in the base and the physical distance of the base region is short, many emitter electrons appear in the base and, being minority carriers in this region, encounter a strong field that sweeps them on into the collector, which is connected to the positive terminal of the battery V_{CB}. If the base is constructed thin in dimension and low in hole density, the electrons from the emitter will have minimal time and opportunity to recombine with holes. In a properly designed transistor, the base current (which results from the recombination of holes and electrons across the emitter-base junction) is very small.

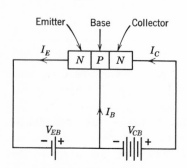

Figure 13-48. The common-base circuit.

It is possible to write the relationship between the currents as $I_E = I_B + I_C$, where I_E, I_B and I_C are the emitter, base, and collector currents, respectively. Therefore, if I_B is small compared to I_E and I_C, $I_E \doteq I_C$. It is important to note that in a typical transistor the emitter voltage V_{EB} required to produce a given emitter current I_E is usually very low (on the order of a few hundred millivolts), whereas the collector voltage V_{CB} may be several volts. If then $I_E = I_C$, the power level in passing from emitter loop to collector loop is greatly increased so that the transistor is an active device providing power gain. If power gain is present it is possible to have either voltage gain or current gain, or both.

Like the triode vacuum tube, the transistor possesses three elements and hence three terminals with which to form two input and two output terminals. One element must be common to both input and output. The connection in Fig. 13–48 shows the base common. The common-base circuit has as its vacuum tube analog the common-grid circuit. These two circuits are quite useful for certain applications but are not generally selected for amplification because the input impedance is very low. The common-base circuit has been discussed here because it provides the easiest route to an understanding of transistor function. The most useful basic transistor circuits are the common-emitter and common-collector, which have as their vacuum tube analogs the common-cathode and common-plate (cathode follower) circuits, respectively.

13–31. TRANSISTOR CHARACTERISTICS

Figures 13–49a and 13–49b show *NPN* and *PNP* transistors connected to batteries to apply forward bias to the base-emitter junction and reverse bias to the collector-base junction. Meters in the base and collector

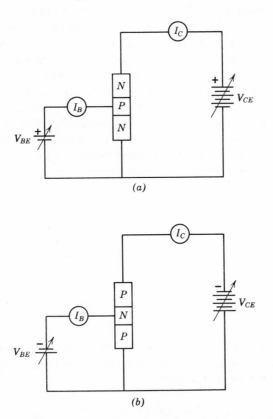

Figure 13–49.   Circuit for measurement of transistor characteristics.

circuits are shown to indicate that the base and collector currents are to be measured. Note that the emitter is common to both base and collector circuits. If the base current I_B is set to specific values by adjustment of the base-emitter voltage V_{BE}, and the collector current I_C is measured as the collector-emitter voltage V_{CE} is varied, data are obtained for plotting two characteristic curves of the transistor. The collector characteristics are obtained by plotting I_C versus V_{CE} with I_B as the parameter. The base characteristic is obtained by plotting I_B versus V_{BE} with V_{CE} as the parameter. This relationship I_B versus V_{BE} shows very little change for various values of V_{CE}, and therefore a single curve representing the average is sufficient and has value in indicating the appropriate voltage required to bias the base to a desired current.

These static characteristics for a typical *PNP* transistor are shown in Figs. 13–50*a* and 13–50*b*. Observe the similarity between the quantities used to describe the vacuum tube plate characteristics, that is, collector current corresponds to plate current, collector-emitter voltage to plate-cathode voltage, and base current to grid-cathode voltage. Note also the similarity of the transistor collector characteristics to the plate characteristics of the pentode. Use of the average base characteristic permits the base current to be translated into base-emitter voltage so that a complete correspondence of voltage to voltage and current to current can be made between the two devices. It is, however, standard practice to show the base current as the parameter on the collector characteristics as in Fig. 13–50*a*. This practice emphasizes the fact that the transistor is fundamentally a device which is operated by a current presented to the input, while the vacuum tube is operated by an input voltage.

13–32.   CURRENT GAIN

From the transistor static collector characteristics (Fig. 13–50*a*) it is possible to define the transistor parameter β just as μ was found for the vacuum tube:

$$\beta = \frac{\Delta I_C}{\Delta I_B}\bigg|_{V_{CE}}$$

Drawing a vertical line on the characteristic Fig. 13–50*a* (along which V_{CE} is constant), we can find corresponding values of ΔI_C and ΔI_B and evaluate them at a given point. In the figure

$$\beta = \frac{\Delta I_C}{\Delta I_B} = \frac{(46 - 18) \times 10^{-3}}{(0.6 - 0.2) \times 10^{-3}} = 70.$$

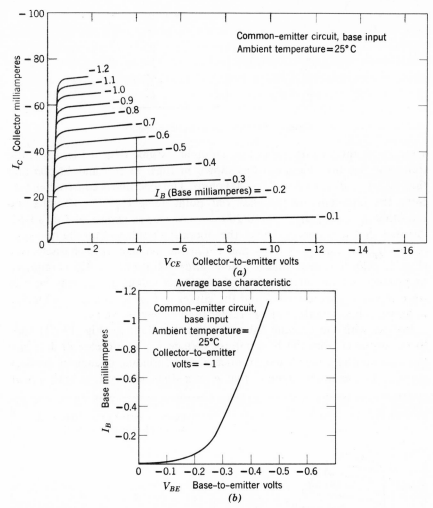

Figure 13–50. Typical collector (*a*) and base (*b*) characteristics (common-emitter circuit). (Courtesy Radio Corporation of America.)

The quantity β is the forward current gain for the transistor operated as a common-emitter circuit. Just as in the case of the vacuum tube, in which the useful voltage gain was always less than the amplification factor of the tube, the useful current gain with the transistor is less than β.

13–33. COMMON-EMITTER AMPLIFIER

Figure 13–51 shows the basic circuit for the common-emitter amplifier. The procedure for graphical analysis of the operation of the circuit is the

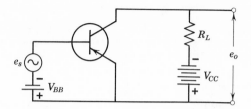

Figure 13–51.   Common emitter amplifier.

same as for the vacuum tube. For example, assume that in Fig. 13–51 the transistor has the characteristics shown in Figs. 13–50a and 13–50b and that $V_{CC} = -10$ volts and $R_L = 200$ ohms. The load line is constructed between the intercepts on the axes, one point being $V_{CC} = -10$ volts and the other $I_C = V_{CC}/R_L = -10/200 = -50$ ma, as shown in Fig. 13–52. Assume that it is desired to set the operating point so that the no-signal ($e_s = 0$) base current is -0.4 ma. From the average base characteristic (Fig. 13–50b) it is seen that a base-emitter voltage of -0.325 is required to produce a base current of -0.4 ma. Other values of V_{BB} may be read from the base characteristic, and the curves in Fig. 13–50a can be labeled in terms of base-emitter voltage rather than current as shown.

Just as with the vacuum tube, the signal voltage e_s (Fig. 13–51) adds to or subtracts from the bias battery voltage V_{BB} to increase or decrease the base-emitter current and produce a corresponding change in the base current. For example, assume that e_s is a sinusoidal voltage with a peak

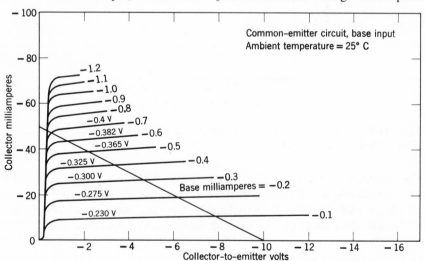

Figure 13–52. Graphical analysis of the common-emitter amplifier, showing average collector characteristics.

value of 0.025 volt. The base-emitter voltage will therefore vary about the operating point value of 0.325 volt to a maximum of 0.350 and a minimum of 0.300 volt. The corresponding changes in collector-emitter voltage, which constitutes the output signal voltage, are -2.1 to -4.7 volts. The magnitude of the voltage gain in this case is

$$G = \frac{4.7 - 2.1}{0.050} = 52.$$

Two characteristics of the common-emitter amplifier are apparent from this analysis: (a) the circuit provides voltage gain, and (b) the phase of the output voltage is 180 degrees out of phase with respect to the input voltage. This circuit configuration presents many of the same input and output impedance problems as exist with the common-cathode vacuum tube circuit which are reduced or eliminated by the transistor counterpart to the cathode follower, the emitter follower, or the common-collector circuit.

13–34.   THE EMITTER FOLLOWER

The basic emitter follower circuit is shown in Fig. 13–53. The input signal e_s is applied between the base and the collector, and the output is obtained across the resistor in the emitter circuit. Just as with the cathode follower, the voltage gain of this circuit is less than unity. The emitter follower has a high input impedance, a very low output impedance, and no phase shift from input to output. The primary application of the emitter follower is impedance transformation.

13–35.   TRANSISTOR-BIASING CIRCUITS

The use of a battery to bias the transistor to the operating point is inconvenient, and some other biasing arrangement is desirable. Proper

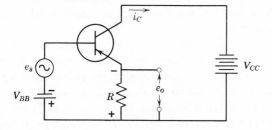

Figure 13–53.   The emitter follower circuit.

transistor biasing presents problems which are not encountered in vacuum tubes. These problems arise as a result of two factors: (1) the sensitivity of transistor characteristics (and hence parameters) to temperature, and (2) the variation between characteristics in transistors of the same type. The effect of temperature on transistor collector characteristics is to shift all curves upward; therefore for a given load resistance (and hence a fixed load line) the static value of collector current is increased with temperature. In some circuits a rise in temperature produces an increase in current, which in turn results in greater heating at the collector-base junction. Regenerative heating of this kind can produce "thermal runaway" and possible destruction of the transistor. Stable operation of a transistor circuit is dependent primarily upon temperature stability, and the most important requirement of any biasing arrangement is to provide operating stability. It is possible to design circuits utilizing some form of negative feedback which will ensure that the transistor cannot "run away." An analysis of these systems is beyond the scope of this introductory presentation and can be found in many electronic texts or handbooks.

Several conventional biasing arrangements are shown in Fig. 13–54. The circuit in Fig. 13–54a is perhaps the simplest to understand and will serve to illustrate the general principle of biasing the transistor from a single source of power. The resistance network consisting of R_1 and R_2 forms a voltage-dividing network across the voltage supply V_{cc} with the base connected to the midpoint A. The load line is determined by $(R_L + R_3)$. The operating point is set by selection of the ratio of R_1 to R_2. In using this method of bias, it is important that the current through R_1 and R_2 be at least five times larger than the base current I_B so that changes in the base current do not alter the bias appreciably. The input impedance of this circuit consists of R_1 and R_2 in parallel with the impedance from the base to the common terminal. The latter impedance consists of the base-to-emitter resistance in series with the emitter resistance R_3, and if R_3 is bypassed with a capacitor this impedance is only that from base to emitter, which is at most several hundred ohms. If R_3 is left unbypassed negative feedback results and the input impedance, as seen at the base terminal of the transistor itself without any additional circuitry such as bias networks, is $(\beta + 1)R_3$.

Figures 13–54b–e illustrate other popular biasing methods. In Fig. 13–54b the bias is derived from the collector voltage. Although bias is obtained by the use of a single resistor, negative feedback is inherent with this connection. A similar method, which includes the base-emitter resistance and the resistance in the emitter circuit R_3, is shown in Fig. 13–54c. In Fig. 13–54d the bias current is derived from a voltage divider connected

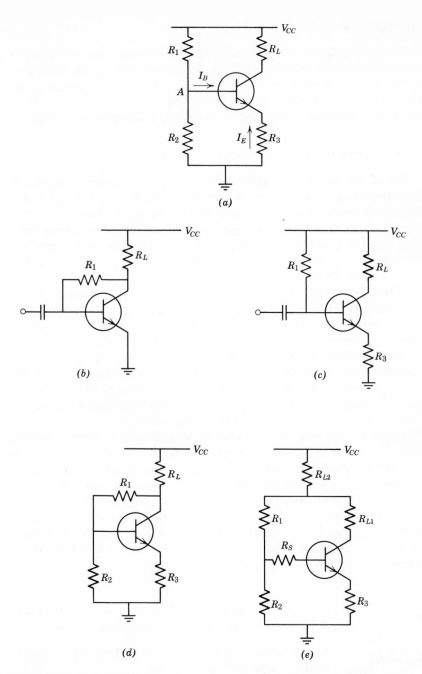

Figure 13–54. Transistor biasing circuits. (From G. E. Transistor Manual, 7th Ed., General Electric Co., Syracuse, N.Y.)

between the collector and the lower end of the emitter resistor. Collector-to-base feedback is present with this connection, as it is with that shown in Fig. 13–54e, in which the voltage divider is connected to a point on the collector load resistor ($R_{L1} + R_{L2}$). Note, however, that in d and e feedback is also present because of the use of an unbypassed emitter resistor (R_3).

13–36. TRANSISTOR EQUIVALENT CIRCUITS

The small-signal linear equivalent circuit for the vacuum tube consists of a simple single-loop circuit in which the plate current may be calculated for any specified value of grid-to-cathode voltage. The simplicity of the circuit results from the assumption that insignificant grid current flows with negative grid bias. In contrast to the vacuum tube, input current in the transistor cannot be neglected and the equivalent circuit requires two current loops instead of one.

A practical equivalent circuit is derived on the basis of standard four-terminal network theory which describes the behavior of a four-terminal "black box" in terms of open- and short-circuit measurements of the input and output voltages and currents. The most convenient equivalent circuit is obtained by using a combination of both open- and short-circuit parameters which are designated "hybrid" or h-parameters. One possible linear a-c equivalent circuit for a transistor is shown in Fig. 13–55. It is seen to consist of two current loops, one of which contains an equivalent voltage source $h_1 v_2$ and the other on equivalent current source $h_{21} i_1$. Observe that the magnitude of each of these sources is determined by a quantity present in the other circuit; that is, the voltage source $h_{12} v_2$ in the first loop is dependent upon the voltage in second loop, while the current source $h_{21} i_1$ is dependent upon the current i_1 in the first loop. This demonstrates the bidirectional nature of the transistor as a circuit element in contrast to the essentially unidirectional behavior of the vacuum tube.

The h-parameters are listed in many transistor technical data sheets or may be measured directly. In conjunction with Fig. 13–55, the h-parameters are defined as follows:

$$h_{11} = \frac{v_1}{i_1}\bigg|_{v_2=0} = \text{the impedance appearing across the input terminals with the output terminals shorted to signal frequencies.}$$

$$h_{22} = \frac{i_2}{v_2}\bigg|_{i_1=0} = \text{the admittance looking into the output terminals with the input terminals open circuited.}$$

$$h_{12} = \frac{v_1}{v_2}\bigg|_{i_1=0} = \text{the feedback voltage ratio, where } v_1 \text{ is produced by an applied } v_2 \text{ with the input terminals open circuited.}$$

$$h_{21} = \frac{i_2}{i_1}\bigg|_{v_2=0} =$$ the ratio i_2/i_1, where i_2 is produced by a given i_1 with the output terminals shorted to signal frequencies.

It should be borne in mind that different sets of h-parameters will be defined, depending upon whether the transistor is connected common emitter, common collector, or common base. Once the appropriate set of parameters is known, the linear equivalent circuit of Fig. 13–55 may be used to study the results of driving complex loads with the transistor in the same manner as with the vacuum tube. It is apparent that transistor circuit analysis is much more complex than its vacuum tube counterpart.

Since transistors are current-operated devices, the impedance values associated with them are generally lower than those of vacuum tubes but may be made to compare favorably with vacuum tube values through ingenuity in circuit design. A qualitative comparison of the three basic transistor circuits is shown in Fig. 13–56.

13–37. PRACTICAL TRANSISTOR AMPLIFIER CIRCUITS

A practical common-emitter, RC-coupled transistor amplifier consisting of two similar stages is shown in Fig. 13–57. Each transistor is biased by the voltage-dividing network consisting of 100-K and 10-K resistors connected in series across the 12-volt battery. The gain for the circuit shown is approximately 170, and the input impedance is about 1300 ohms. The input impedance is determined by the parallel combination of the 100-K, 10-K, and the base-emitter resistances. The maximum possible value of input impedance for this circuit, which would be obtained with zero base current, is the parallel equivalent of 10 K ohms in parallel with 100 K ohms or 9.1 K ohms. By leaving the 1-K emitter resistor unbypassed, the impedance "looking" into the base can be increased by the factor $(1 + \beta) R_K$. The β for the type 2N1414 transistor is approximately 34, so that $(1 + \beta) R_K$ is $(1 + 34)10^3 = 35,000$ ohms. This value in parallel with 9.1 K

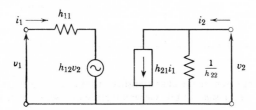

Figure 13–55. Transistor linear equivalent circuit.

	Common base (CB)
Transistor as a Device (Arrows indicate electron current flow. Loads not shown.)	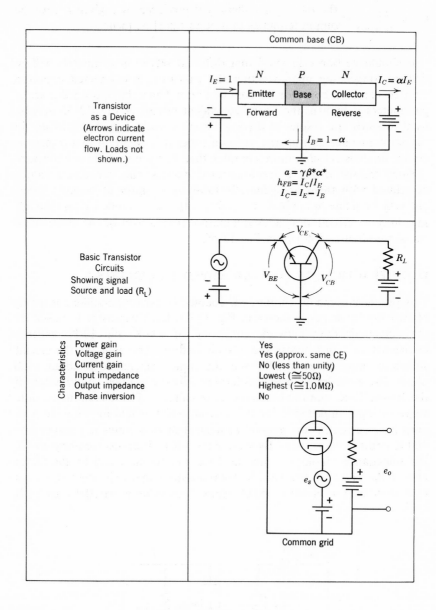
Basic Transistor Circuits Showing signal Source and load (R_L)	
Characteristics Power gain Voltage gain Current gain Input impedance Output impedance Phase inversion	Yes Yes (approx. same CE) No (less than unity) Lowest ($\cong 50\,\Omega$) Highest ($\cong 1.0\,M\Omega$) No

Figure 13–56. Comparison of the characteristics of transistor and vacuum-tube circuits. (From *G. E. Transistor Manual*, 7th Ed., General Electric Co., Syracuse, N.Y.)

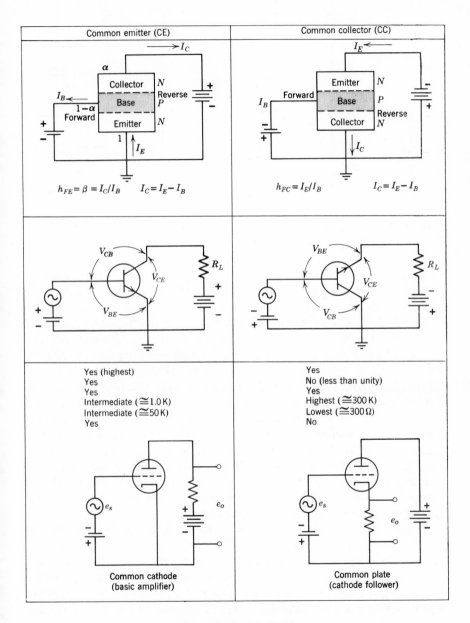

Common emitter (CE)	Common collector (CC)
$h_{FE} = \beta = I_C/I_B \quad I_C = I_E - I_B$	$h_{FC} = I_E/I_B \quad I_C = I_E - I_B$

Yes (highest)
Yes
Yes
Intermediate ($\cong 1.0\,K$)
Intermediate ($\cong 50\,K$)
Yes

Yes
No (less than unity)
Yes
Highest ($\cong 300\,K$)
Lowest ($\cong 300\,\Omega$)
No

Common cathode
(basic amplifier)

Common plate
(cathode follower)

Figure 13–56. (*continued*)

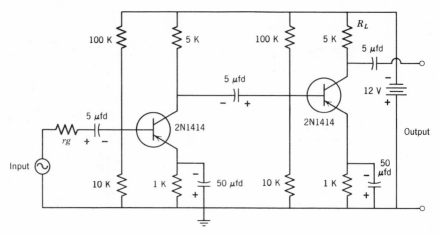

Figure 13–57. Two-stage *RC*-coupled transistor amplifier. (From *G. E. Transistor Manual*, 7th Ed., General Electric Co., Syracuse, N.Y.)

produces an input impedance of 7.2 K. Leaving the emitter resistor unbypassed reduces the gain of the amplifier, which must be considered in relation to any benefit derived from the increase in input impedance.

Figure 13–58 shows a transistorized preamplifier developed by Kado and Adey (1961) for field study of the electroencephalogram. This amplifier uses two indentical emitter followers to obtain a high input impedance (300,000 ohms). This is followed by three similar common-emitter stages of differential amplification. The last stage is a single transistor operated as a common-emitter amplifier to provide "single ended" rather than balanced output for driving a single-sided or unbalanced amplifier after the signal level has been amplified several hundred-fold. The frequency response reported is 3.5 to 78 cps between 3-db points, and the CMRR is 560 : 1. The gain is variable from 10,000 to 36,000. This amplifier was designed and constructed to operate under severe physical stresses. After assembly and testing it was encapsulated in a high-impact epoxy resin, using vacuum techniques to form a solid, shock-resistant unit.

Another example of a low-noise, biological preamplifier, reported by Schuler et al. (1966), is shown in Fig. 13–59. In addition to the usual two terminals (*A*, *B*) connected to the subject, this input stage makes use of an additional "interference reference" electrode *R*, which is applied to the subject near the signal electrodes *A* and *B* to acquire the interference signal common to electrodes connected to terminals *A* and *B*. The purpose of electrode *R* is to eliminate the need for discriminating against ground-referred interference signals in the first stage, in which the desired signal level may be in the microvolt range. Common-mode rejection is then

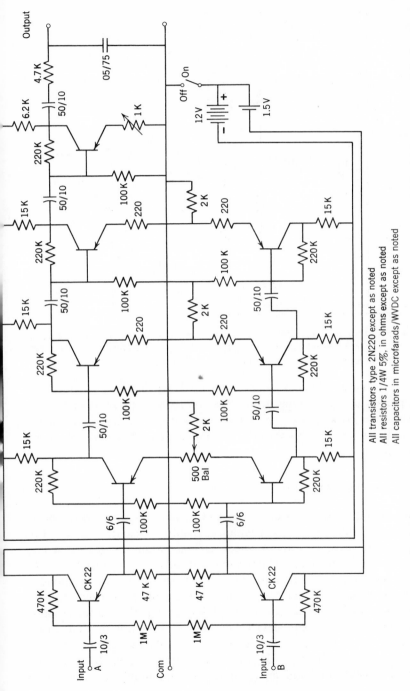

Figure 13–58. Differential amplifier for EEG, using transistors. (From R. T. Kado and W. R. Adey, *Digest of the International Conference on Medical Electronics*, 1961, Institute of Electrical and Electronic Engineers.)

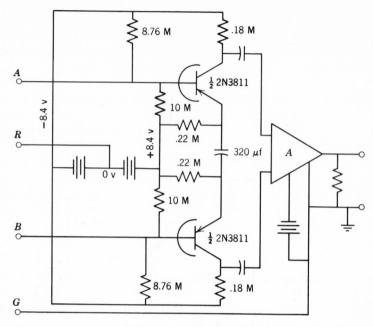

Figure 13–59. Low-noise preamplifier designed to minimize effect of unequal electrode impedances. [From G. Schuler et al., *Science* **154** (3953): 1191–1192 (1966). Copyright, 1966, by the American Association for the Advancement of Science.]

obtained in the amplifier *A* at the millivolt level. Because the undesired signal picked up through electrode *R* is common to the other electrodes, the first stage provides extremely high common mode input impedance, which reduces considerably the effect of impedance unbalance at the signal electrodes.

13–38. CARRIER AMPLIFIERS

Many of the transducers discussed in Chapter 4, such as those based on changes in inductance or capacitance, require sinusoidal a-c excitation for operation. Also, resistive devices such as strain gauges often may be utilized more effectively if operated with alternating current. In bio-medical research it is often desirable or necessary to use transducers excited by alternating current to measure steady or slowly changing events. Devices known as carrier amplifiers permit the amplification of slowly changing (low-frequency) events and those containing static (d-c) components by means of stable, high-gain a-c amplifiers. Carrier amplifiers possess the advantage of operating over a very narrow band of frequencies so that it is possible to build an amplifier for optimum operation over a particular narrow frequency range. By so limiting the bandwidth requirements of the amplifier, noise, either internal or external to the device, which falls outside the passband of the amplifier does not appear in the output. The ratio of signal to noise is increased accordingly.

The principle underlying the carrier amplifier consists of causing the lower-frequency event to modulate a high-frequency (carrier) signal used to energize the transducer. After amplification the modulated carrier is subjected to an appropriate detection process for recovery of the desired low-frequency modulating signal.

The principle of the carrier amplifier, as employed with strain gauge transducers arranged in a Wheatstone bridge configuration, is shown in Fig. 13–60. The bridge may be made up, for example, of one or more strain gauge elements suitably arranged to sense strain and connected to provide temperature compensation. For illustration purposes, assume that the strain gauge bridge is excited from a 1000-cps sinusoidal source and is not balanced to null but rather is slightly offset to provide a 1000-cps voltage of 10 mv peak when the strain gauge Rs is in the arbitrarily designated no-strain or "zero" position. Assume also that the relationship between strain gauge movement and the corresponding change in resistance is known and is linear. If then the strain gauge is displaced mechanically in a sinusoidal manner at a low frequency rate (e.g., 1 cps), the change in resistance will be sinusoidal, and, if the input impedance of

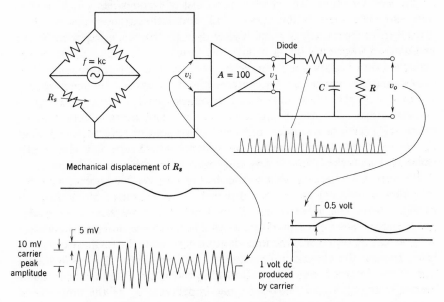

Figure 13–60.   Principle employed in the carrier amplifier.

the amplifier is very high with respect to the resistance of the bridge, the amplifier will not load the bridge (draw current). The amplitude of the 1000-cps output voltage from the bridge will be modulated sinusoidally by the resistance change. Assume that the modulation changes the bridge output from 10 mv for zero displacement to 15 mv for maximum displacement in one direction and to 5 mv for maximum displacement in the opposite direction, as shown in Fig. 13–60. If the gain of the amplifier is 100, the variations in the voltage v_1 appearing at the amplifier output terminals are similar in form but 100 times larger in amplitude. A diode is utilized at the output of the amplifier to convert the voltage v_1 into undirectional pulsations having a fundamental frequency of 1000 cps. The pulsations are smoothed by the RC circuit, which, if it possesses a suitable time constant, effectively short-circuits the carrier and higher-frequency components and leaves only the steady (d-c) component and the slowly alternating (1-cps) components. In order to ensure faithful reproduction of the input signal, the carrier frequency should be at least 10 times that of the highest significant frequency component contained in the signal, that is, many carrier cycles must occur in regions where the input signal changes rapidly.

Thus, by use of the carrier principle, the characteristics of d-c amplification may be obtained with a-c amplifiers. Another outstanding advantage of the carrier system lies in the use of narrow-band filters which may be sharply tuned to pass only the carrier frequency and the sidebands generated by the desired signal. The sidebands consist of frequencies which are the sum and difference of the carrier and modulation frequencies, so that, if the carrier frequency is much higher than the highest component in the modulation frequency (as is usually the case), the carrier and sidebands occupy a very narrow spectrum centered about the carrier frequency. The use of a narrow bandpass filter centered about the carrier frequency greatly attenuates all other frequencies and increases correspondingly the signal-to-noise ratio. The use of carrier amplifiers with narrow-band filtering operating at different carrier frequencies also permits several such devices to be operated simultaneously in systems which are not electrically isolated. This technique is widely employed in long-distance telephony.

The impedance pneumograph described in Chapter 9 is another example of a device utilizing the carrier principle. It is shown in block diagram in Fig. 13–61. The input terminals to which the transthoracic electrodes are connected are represented by a and b. The total transthoracic impedance is $Z_0 + \Delta Z$; Z_0 represents the impedance measured at the resting expiratory level, and ΔZ the change in impedance with inspiration. It is easily shown that, if the internal impedance R_k of the driving oscillator is made much greater than $Z_0 + \Delta Z$, and the input impedance Z_a of the amplifier is large in comparison to $Z_0 + \Delta Z$, the current through the subject is essentially

Impedance pneumograph

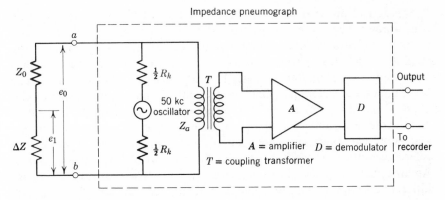

Figure 13-61. The impedance pneumograph. Z_0 = transthoracic impedance at resting expiratory level, ΔZ = change in transthoracic impedance with respiration, R_k = added resistance to make oscillator approximate a constant current source = 200 K, Z_a = input impedance of amplifier = 50 K. [From L. E. Baker et al., *Am. J. Med. Electron.* 4(2): 73-77 (1965).]

constant over a wide range of Z_0; therefore the voltage across the subject e_0 is a function only of Z_0 and ΔZ. If Z_0 is constant, the change in e_0 is dependent solely upon ΔZ. The baseline (d-c component) is determined by Z_0. After demodulation the nonrespiratory direct voltage produced by the current through Z_0 may be "bucked out," leaving in the output only the voltage variations derived from the transthoracic impedance change accompanying the respiratory act.

13-39. PHASE-SENSITIVE DETECTOR

The use of a linear variable differential transformer (LVDT) for transducing displacement is shown in Fig. 4-2 and described in Chapter 4. It is recognized that the arrangement illustrated constitutes a carrier system. As previously pointed out, use of a diode detector to recover the signal from the carrier will not provide information as to the direction of displacement if the system is initially adjusted for zero-signal output at the balance or zero-displacement position of the LVDT core. Just as with the bridge circuit, it is possible to initially set the core to an arbitrary point on either side of the zero position and obtain directional information so long as displacement is restricted to the chosen side of the zero point. Although this manner of operation is adequate in many instances, it does not utilize the full range of core displacement available with the LVDT. The use of a phase-sensitive detector permits setting the LVDT core to its center position and determining directional changes regardless of which side of center the core is displaced.

A practical phase detector is shown in Fig. 13–62. Its basic operation is as follows. The same voltage from the oscillator that excites the LVDT is also applied to a phase-compensating device; this does not alter the magnitude but does permit control of the phase of the voltage, which is then applied as a reference signal to the primary of transformer T_2. The function of the reference signal is to control conduction of the diodes $D_1, D_2, D_3,$ and D_4. For example, when point C is positive, point D is negative and the diodes D_3 and D_4 conduct, while diodes D_1 and D_2 are nonconducting and represent essentially open circuits. On the next half cycle of the reference voltage, D_1 and D_2 conduct while D_3 and D_4 are nonconducting. Assume that the phase-shift compensation has been set so that the phase difference between the signal voltage to be detected and the reference voltage is zero. The amplitudes of the two voltages will, therefore, rise and fall together. Assume also that point C is positive and point D is negative so that D_3 and D_4 are conducting. If point B is then positive, signal current will flow from point B to point R and divide equally between the paths $RSCN$ and $RQDN$. The two equal parts of the signal current flowing in opposite directions in the secondary of transformer T_2 will produce no net effect in the magnetic circuit of T_2. The currents are brought together at point N to produce the total load current I_L which flows from point N to point M through load resistor R_L. On the next half cycle, conditions are altered so that point D is positive and point C negative; diodes D_1 and D_2 conduct

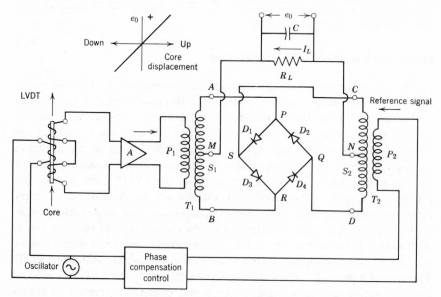

Figure 13–62.   Phase-sensitive detector circuit.

while D_3 and D_4 are nonconducting. On the signal side, point A is then positive and point B negative. The two signal current paths are $APSCN$ and $APQDN$. Again the currents are collected at N and flow in the same direction as before through R_L.

The system functions therefore as a full wave rectifier. The capacitor C bypasses the carrier frequency and provides a d-c voltage (e_0) that is a function of the magnitude of the signal voltage, which in turn depends upon the position of the LVDT core. Therefore, as the core is moved away from zero position in one directon (i.e., upward), the magnitude of the voltage presented to amplifier A increases and a corresponding increase in output voltage e_0 is obtained. If the core is moved away from zero position in the other direction (i.e., downward), the magnitude of the voltage presented to amplifier A will vary with core position just as before; however, the phase of the voltage will be exactly opposite to what existed on the other side of the zero position. This will cause the signal currents in the diodes to flow in the opposite direction so that the direction of I_L is likewise reversed. Therefore, the exact position of the LVDT core can be determined by the magnitude and polarity of the output voltage e_0.

13–40.   THE CHOPPER AMPLIFIER

The chopper amplifier is a narrow-band a-c amplifier providing stable d-c gain with a high signal-to-noise ratio. It is especially useful for providing essential drift-free amplification of d-c and slowly changing voltages. This device is a carrier amplifier that generates its own carrier, which is modulated by the signal.

The basic operation of the chopper amplifier may be understood from Fig. 13–63a. The chopper S_1 alternately connects the input terminal C of the a-c amplifier to the reference terminal B, which is usually connected to ground. When connected to B, the amplifier input terminals are short circuited and the input voltage is zero. The input to the amplifier consists therefore of an a-c voltage varying from zero to the value of the input voltage existing when the signal is connected (S_1 open). By this process a steady d-c or slowly varying signal is "chopped" into a train of pulses having a frequency equal to the rate of the chopper. After amplification the chopped signal is rectified with a diode. The rectified signal is then filtered, and the d-c and slowly varying signal components are recovered (Fig. 13–63a).

Instead of rectifying the output of the amplifier with a diode, as shown in Fig. 13–63a, a second chopper contact operating synchronously with the first may be used, as shown in Fig. 13–63b.

Mechanical choppers are electromagnetically operated switches which

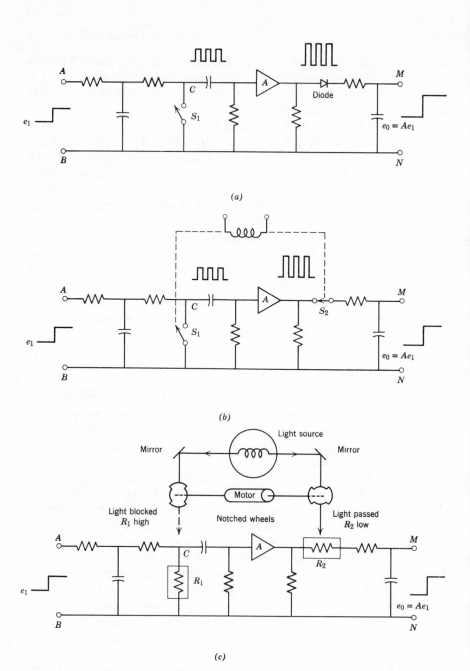

Figure 13-63. Chopper amplifiers using (a) diode rectifier, (b) synchronous mechanical choppers, (c) alternately illuminated photoconductors.

are limited in their rapidity of movement by inertial considerations. They are available in 60- and 400-cycle units. These devices have a finite life.

Chopping with semiconductor switches is now used with subsequent increase in possible chopping rate. Such devices are not subject to mechanical wear and have an extremely long life. Semiconductor choppers may be in the form of a conventional transistor which is switched from the conducting to nonconducting state (i.e., operated in the switching mode) or a photoconductor which displays a large increase in conductance when exposed to radiant energy. Such a device may be switched very rapidly between essentially an open circuit and a relatively low value of resistance by alternately exposing it to and shielding it from a source of radiant energy; this is easily accomplished by use of a shutter arrangement, as illustrated in Fig. 13–63c.

It is apparent that the response time of the chopper amplifier is governed by the chopping or sampling rate. For faithful reproduction of a signal by this means (or in any carrier system) it is important that the signal being chopped not change appreciably between samples. For example, if the signal is changing slowly, and there occurs a sharp notch, it is necessary to use a high chopping rate, that is, many cycles of the chopper are required to sample the notch. A rule of thumb commonly applied is that the sampling rate should be at least ten times greater than the highest sinusoidal frequency component of the signal. Therefore, for a 60-cycle chopper (chopping at the rate of 60 per second), an upper sinusoidal frequency limit of 6 cps is dictated.

13-41. CHOPPER STABILIZATION OF D-C AMPLIFIERS

The problem of drift in d-c amplifiers has been mentioned previously. With careful design, correct selection of components, and proper operation, the drift can be held to a few millivolts per hour, which is quite adequate for many applications. Computing circuits and long operating time requirements usually necessitate greater stability. One of the methods used for this purpose employs a chopper amplifier in conjunction with a wide-band d-c amplifier. With such a system, d-c drift can be reduced to less than 1 μv/day.

It will be recalled from Section 13–24 that the d-c amplifier used for operational purposes normally has two input terminals and a common terminal. One terminal is called the inverting terminal (designated by a minus sign) because a signal applied between it and the common lead will appear at the output inverted (i.e., shifted by 180 degrees). The other input terminal is noninverting (designated by a plus sign); a signal applied between it and the common terminal appears at the output in phase with the input. The manner in which a chopper amplifier is utilized to provide stable d-c amplification is shown in Fig. 13–64. The main amplifier A is a wide-band d-c amplifier which has its inverting input capacitively coupled to the system input so that this portion of the main amplifier responds only to the a-c components, which are passed by the RC-coupling network. On the other hand, the output of chopper amplifier B, which responds to d-c and low-frequency signal components, is connected directly to the noninverting input of the main amplifier. The a-c signals are amplified by the main amplifier only, whereas the d-c and low-frequency components are amplified by both amplifiers in cascade. The chopper amplifier provides drift-free d-c amplification. With drift considered as "noise" (i.e., an undesired change in grid voltage), the placing of the drift-free gain of the chopper amplifier ahead of the source of d-c drift in the main amplifier attenuates the drift in the main amplifier output in proportion to the amount of drift-free gain provided. The principle underlying this technique is discussed in Section 13–20.

13–42. THE LOADING PROBLEM

The amplification of a voltage for purposes of measurement and recording has been discussed in the foregoing sections of this chapter. If amplification is to be faithful, it is necessary, among other things, that the input impedance of the amplifier be large compared to the impedance of the voltage source to ensure that no significant amount of current is drawn from the source. The degree of loading can be specified in terms of the amount of current drawn, that is, zero current corresponds to zero loading. If the entire circuit (including the source) is purely resistive, and loading occurs, the voltage appearing across the input terminals of the amplifier is of the same waveform as is produced by the source, but is merely reduced in amplitude.

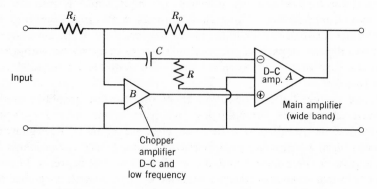

Figure 13–64. Chopper stabilization of a d-c amplifier.

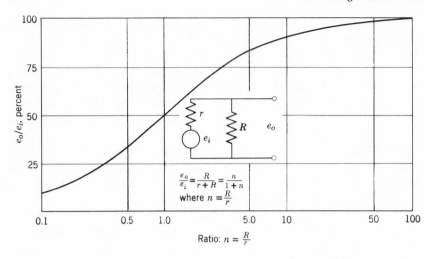

Figure 13–65. The effect of input impedance on the voltage measured from a source e_i.

Figure 13–65 shows the manner in which the source voltage e_i would be divided between the input resistance R of the amplifier and the internal resistance r of the source for various ratios (n) of these two resistances. From this figure it is seen that, when the input impedance of the amplifier R is made high with respect to that of the source r, the ratio e_o/e_i approaches 1.0, that is, virtually all of the voltage of the source is presented to the amplifier input terminals. Under such a condition the amplifier input circuit does not "load" the source of voltage. If the circuit is not purely resistive but contains a reactive component also, the impedances of both the source and the amplifier are frequency dependent. The degree of loading must then be assessed from the ratio of the magnitudes of the impedances evaluated over the desired operating frequency range. For example, if the impedance of a source Z_s is purely resistive but the amplifier input impedance Z_i consists of a resistance shunted by a capacitance, the magnitude of Z_i will decrease inversely with increasing frequency while Z_s remains constant. Loading may then occur at higher frequencies as the ratio Z_i/Z_s decreases. The capacitive reactance also introduces phase shift, which likewise is frequency dependent. Therefore, for frequencies at which loading occurs, the voltage presented to the amplifier input will be not only attenuated but also shifted in phase. Both of these factors contribute to distortion of the voltage to be amplified. Just as in a purely resistive circuit, the complications produced by loading are avoided by making the amplifier input impedance at least 100 times larger than the impedance of the voltage source.

The loading problem as it applies specifically to the recording of bio-electric events is discussed in Chapter 10, and records are presented which display the type of distortion of a bioelectric event brought about by loading. It is also pointed out in Chapter 10 that the loading is not purely resistive because the electrode-tissue interface adds capacitive reactance to the circuit. This reactive component produces attenuation of signal components as a function of frequency and imposes a phase shift of signal components.

As electrodes are made smaller, there is a corresponding necessity to make amplifier input impedances larger. The need for amplifier input stages having input impedances on the order of several thousand megohms is encountered in all electrophysiological studies employing micro-electrodes. In striving for such high values of input impedance, in addition to the inevitable shunting effect of interelectrode capacitances in vacuum tubes and junction capacitances in transistors, the important role of leakage current must be considered. In microelectrode studies, not only is it important that no current flow in the input circuit because of the signal distortion that might result, but also current must be prevented from flowing through the electrode and into the living cell to ensure that no alteration in cell behavior occurs. It has been reported by MacNichol and Wagner (1954) that currents in the range of 10^{-10} ampere alter the excitability of most cells. These investigators placed the maximum permissible value of current at 10^{-12} ampere. In practice, it is desirable to limit the current to considerably less than this value. This range of current sets rigid requirements for the vacuum tube or transistor and the associated input circuitry.

In examining the vacuum tube it was assumed that no current would flow in the grid circuit if the grid were biased negatively with respect to the cathode. Careful measurement reveals that a very small current does flow even in the absence of an alternating signal which can produce current flow through interelectrode and stray capacitances. Some of the possible sources of grid current are the following:

1. Electrons from the cathode striking the grid despite its being negative in relation to the cathode.
2. Current leakage from grid to cathode and grid to plate (or grid to other elements in a multielement tube).
3. Collection of positive ions by the grid. Positive ions may be emitted from the cathode or produced by electron collision with residual gas molecules within the tube.
4. Emission of electrons from the grid because of absorbed thermal energy from the cathode or from absorption of photic energy from light emission from the cathode and x-rays produced by electrons striking the plate.

Although the grid current in most negatively biased vacuum tubes is small (10^{-8} to 10^{-10} ampere), it can be measured by an ingenious method due to Nottingham (1929), using the simple instrumentation shown in Fig. 13–66a. With switch S in position 1 and the plate voltage E_b held constant, the plate current I_b is measured for various values of grid voltage E_c, and the grid characteristic I_b versus E_c is plotted. With the switch in position 1, $v_{gk} = E_c$. If no grid current I_g flows, placing the switch in position 2 (which includes a high resistance R), will result in exactly the same curve because, with $I_g = 0$ no voltage drop would occur across R. With values of R in the range of 10 to 1000 megohms (such as would be encountered at a microelectrode-tissue interface), it is found that the two E_c versus I_b curves do not coincide, but resemble those shown in Fig. 13–66b. It is apparent from these two curves that grid current flowing through R changes the grid-to-cathode voltage. Only at point A is the grid current zero. Upon examining the curve with R inserted, it is seen that, to the right of point A, v_{gk} is actually more

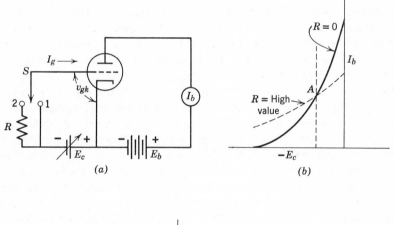

(a)

(b)

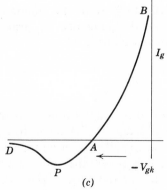

(c)

Figure 13–66.   Determination of grid current in the vacuum tube.

negative than the applied grid voltage E_c because the plate current is less than is obtained when $v_{gk} = E_c$. This occurs for conventional current flowing into the grid and is defined as positive grid current. Conversely, to the left of point A, the direction of current flow is reversed and v_{gk} is less negative than the applied voltage. Conventional current in this direction (out of the grid) is called negative grid current.

By measuring the difference between the two curves in volts and knowing the magnitude of R, the grid current I_g and the true grid-to-cathode voltage V_{gk} may be calculated, and a grid current I_g versus grid voltage V_{gk} curve may be plotted as shown in Fig. 13–66c. The reciprocal of the slope of this curve at any point is a measure of the input resistance of the tube at that point.

It is of interest to observe that, while there is no grid current at point A, the value of grid resistance $R_g = \Delta V_{gk}/\Delta I_g$ is positive. If the bias is chosen for operation in the region of point P, where the curve is flat, a small change in grid voltage produces no change in grid current; therefore, the input resistance is theoretically infinite. However, there still remains the leakage resistance of the tube, and at this point there is a flow of grid current. Between points P and D the grid resistance is negative. Under such a circumstance the grid circuit might operate as a source of energy and conceivably create some sort of instability.

In practice with conventional tubes, choice of the operating point is a compromise between the maximum permissible grid current and the minimum allowable input impedance. Low grid current is obtained by operating the filament and plate at reduced voltages and shielding the tube from environmental light. Discussions of the methods to lower grid current have been presented by Gabus (1937), Crawford (1948), and Bishop (1949). There are vacuum tubes called electrometer tubes which are specially constructed and operated to minimize grid current and provide maximum grid resistance. Nottingham (1929), Metcalf and Thompson (1930), and Nielsen (1947) have presented excellent analyses of the components of grid current and showed analytically the influence of grid circuit resistance upon the effective input impedance of the tube.

13–43. THE ELECTROMETER TUBE

An electrometer tube is constructed and operated in such a manner as to reduce current leakage between the grid and other elements by isolating the grid terminal and providing long leakage paths. To ensure the integrity of this insulation, the external surface between the tube terminals is kept free of moisture, oils, and foreign material which could provide a conductive path. The tube is also placed in a sealed enclosure containing a desiccant to absorb any moisture which might enter. The tube is operated with low voltages between elements to minimize the production of positive ions from residual gas and to reduce the production of x-rays by the plate. The heater voltage is also held to a minimum to reduce the thermal energy which might reach the grid and produce electron emission. In operation the tube is fully shielded from external light and external magnetic and electric fields.

The grid current for a typical electrometer tube is on the order of 10^{-14} ampere but with special attention to all operating precautions can be kept as low as 10^{-17} ampere. The resulting calculated grid (input) resistance is approximately 10^{14} ohms. When the tube is connected in an amplifier circuit the actual input impedance may be reduced a few orders of magnitude because of circuit parameters and the interelectrode capacitance. The effect of interelectrode capacitance can be minimized by use of the negative input capacitance circuit, which will be discussed subsequently.

Electrometer tubes are available as triodes, tetrodes, and pentodes. The tetrode electrometer is not operated in the same manner as the conventional tetrode described in Section 13–19, in which the first grid (nearest the cathode) is the signal or control grid and is maintained at a negative potential relative to the cathode, while the second grid structure (the screen) is operated at a relatively high positive potential. In the electrometer tetrode the first grid is operated at a low positive voltage which attracts electrons from the cathode to form a virtual cathode or electron source for the tube, while at the same time it repels positive ions emitted from the heated cathode. The second grid functions as the control grid. Electrometer tetrodes, which are sometimes called space-charge electrometers, permit achievement of the lowest possible grid currents. An application of a four-element electrometer to measure the potential produced by charge collected in an ionization chamber is shown in Fig. 13–67.

Some of the specifications for a typical electrometer triode (VX55) are as follows:

Operating	Plate voltage	$E_b = 7.5$ volts
Point	Grid bias	$E_c = -2.2$ volts
	Plate current	$I_b = 95\ \mu$a
	Transconductance	$g_m = 110$ micromhos
	Grid current	$I_g = 5 \times 10^{-14}$ ampere
	Amplification factor	$\mu = 2.1$
Direct interelectrode capacities		
	Grid to plate	$C_{gp} = 2.0$ pf
	Grid to filament	$C_{gf} = 2.0$ pf
	Plate to filament	$C_{pf} = 1.5$ pf

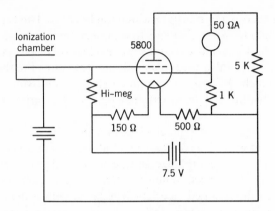

Figure 13–67. Modified DuBridge-Brown circuit showing application of tetrode electrometer tube. [From D. L. Collins, *Instruments* **26**:11 (1953). By permission.]

The dimensions and electrical data for a miniature pentode electrometer are shown in Fig. 13–68. Note that this tube may be operated as a triode for some applications and that data for this connection are also given.

Electrometer tubes find application in any situation requiring extremely high input impedance for the measurement of electrostatic potentials or very small currents (less than 10^{-13} ampere). Typical uses are in the measurement of potentials produced in ionization chambers, pH meters, and photoemissive devices. Good accounts of the characteristics of electrometer tubes and the operating characteristics of amplifiers constructed with these tubes have been presented by Keithley (1952, 1962), Victoreen (1949), and Collins (1953).

13–44. FIELD EFFECT TRANSISTOR

The field effect transistor (FET) solves some of the problems in providing a very high input impedance in transistor circuitry. In contrast to the transistors having two junctions (base-emitter) and (collector-emitter), this device has only a single junction and is often called a unipolar field effect transistor. The principle of the FET is illustrated in Fig. 13–69, which shows a single slab of N material embedded in a block of P material. One end of the N slab is designated the source, and the other end the drain. The N material between source and drain is constructed to provide a narrow channel. The current to be controlled is supplied from voltage source V_1. The charge carriers (electrons in the N-type material) enter at the source terminal and leave by the drain terminal. Variation of voltage V_2, applied between the gate terminal and the source, causes the width of the depletion regions at the P-N junctions to change, effectively

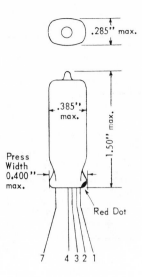

.285" max.

.385" max.

1.50" max.

Press Width 0.400" max.

Red Dot

7   4 3 2 1

ELECTRICAL DATA

DIRECT INTERELECTRODE CAPACITANCES: ($\mu\mu$fd.) **Unshielded**

Control Grid to All	2.2
Control Grid to Screen Grid and Plate	2.0

RATINGS - ABSOLUTE MAXIMUM VALUES:

Filament Voltage (dc) ●	1.25 ± 20% volts
Plate Voltage	22.5 volts
Screen Grid Voltage	22.5 volts
Total Cathode Current	300 μAdc

CHARACTERISTICS AND TYPICAL OPERATION:

	Triode ■	Pentode	
Filament Voltage	1.25	1.25	volts
Filament Current	10	10	ma.
Plate Voltage	10.5	8.5	volts
Screen Grid Voltage	----	4.5	volts
Control Grid Voltage	-3	-2	volts
Plate Current	200	6.0	μa.
Screen Grid Current	----	3.6	μa.
Amplification Factor	1.8	----	
Transconductance	175	14	μmhos
Plate Resistance (approx.)	----	8	meg.
Maximum Control Grid Current	2.5×10^{-13}	----	amp.
Nominal Control Grid Current		3×10^{-15}	amp.

● *For use with batteries having an initial voltage of 1.55 volts max.*

■ *Screen Grid connected to plate*

Figure 13–68. Dimensions and electrical data for type CK5886 subminiature electrometer pentode. (Courtesy Raytheon Co.)

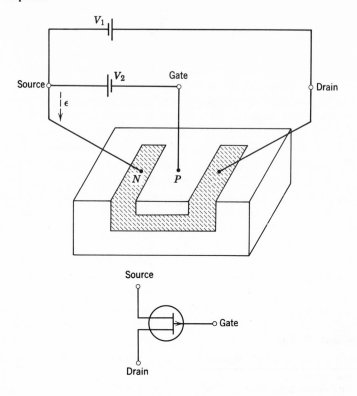

Figure 13–69. The field effect transistor.

modifying the width of the active conduction channel. V_2 may be made large enough to completely "pinch off" the channel.

The operation of the device is as follows. Assume that the voltage V_2, between the gate and the source, is zero, that is, the gate and the source are connected together directly. If the drain-to-source voltage V_1 is then increased, current will flow in the channel and produce a potential drop along the N material from drain to source with the regions nearest the drain terminal being more positive than those closer to the source. Reverse bias of the P-N junction is greater therefore in the vicinity of the drain, and the extent of the depletion regions will be greater at this location. At the drain end of the channel, the depletion regions from the top and bottom may actually touch and produce the condition known as "pinch-off." The drain-source voltage at which this occurs (with $V_2 = 0$) is termed the pinch-off voltage and is given the symbol V_p. Once pinch-off has been reached, the source-drain voltage may be increased with no corresponding increase in current until, at higher values, avalanche breakdown occurs. Current continues to flow after pinch-off is reached because the pinch-off potential still exists from the source to the point of pinch-off in the channel; hence electrons flow from the source to the pinch-off point and on into the depletion region, to be collected at the drain.

If the gate-to-source voltage V_2 is applied to further reverse-bias the junction, the voltage drop along the channel necessary to cause pinch-off will not be as great and will be produced by a lower drain current. Accordingly the gate-source voltage may be used to control the drain current. A typical set of drain characteristics for a P-channel FET is shown in Fig. 13–70a. These characteristics indicate that the drain current is essentially constant over a wide range of drain voltage, and hence the source-drain circuit has a high internal impedance.

The input or control voltage V_2 operates into a circuit of very high impedance, on the order of 10^{10} ohms. The input impedance is high because the only current which flows in the gate-source circuit is the saturation current of the reverse-biased gate-source junction. Typical input characteristics, also for a P-channel FET, are shown in Fig. 13–70b.

The metal oxide silicon field effect transistor (MOS-FET) operates on essentially the same principle as just described but possesses even greater input resistance because the gate is insulated from the source-drain path by a thin layer of silicon dioxide, which is an excellent insulator. Input leakage current is usually less than 10^{-15} ampere. As would be expected, much attention has been given to the various types of FET's for use in all circuits in which a very high input impedance is required. Because the input impedance of these devices can be made to approach or even exceed that of electrometer tubes, it is often assumed that the tube can be replaced in all such circuit applications. There is evidence[6] to show, however, that the vacuum tube (electrometer) is still superior for input stages facing high-impedance signal sources such as those encountered in microelectrode recording in biological systems.

An application of an insulated-gate FET to measure the potential difference between a glass electrode and a reference electrode in the determination of pH as described in Chapter 10 is shown in Fig. 13–71. The input impedance of the circuit is approximately 10^{14} ohms, which is far in excess of that needed for use with glass electrodes.

Table 13–1 is a summary of the basic characteristics of vacuum tubes, conventional transistors, and field effect transistors. The values shown are typical; actual values depend upon the particular type of tube or transistor and the circuit in which it is used.

[6] *Insight*, Fall, 1966, Argonaut Associates, Inc., Beaverton, Ore.

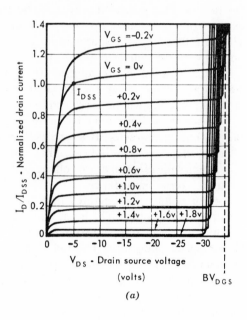

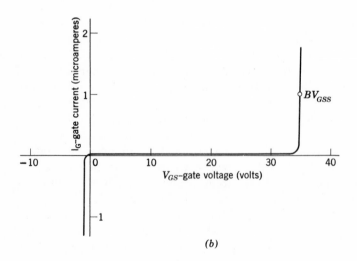

Figure 13–70. Typical drain (*a*) and input (*b*) curves of a field effect transistor. (Courtesy Siliconix Inc., Sunnyvale, Calif.)

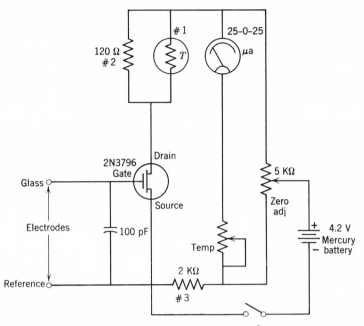

Figure 13–71.   pH meter employing a field effect transistor. [From J. K. Jacobsen, *Anal. Chem.* **38**:1975 (1966). By permission.]

13–45.   INPUT STAGES FOR MICROELECTRODES

The characteristics of microelectrodes for recording membrane and action potentials from single cells are discussed in Chapter 11, and the lumped parameter electrical equivalent circuits derived. It was pointed out in Chapter 11 that the equivalent circuits for both metal and pipette microelectrodes consist of resistance and capacitance and are therefore frequency dependent and capable of distorting the potential produced by the bioelectric generator even before this potential is presented to an amplifier. Obviously, if the electrode itself is capable of introducing distortion, it is important that the amplifier not make additional contributions but instead, provide some compensation to overcome the limitations imposed by the electrode. From the discussion of the loading problem presented in Section 13–42, it is apparent that faithful recording of bioelectric activity with microelectrodes is directed toward two ideal goals: (1) making the input impedance of the amplifier extremely high so that minimal loading is produced, and (2) rendering the complete circuit, consisting of specimen, electrode, and amplifier, as nearly resistive as possible to prevent the occurrence of frequency-dependent distortion. The steps taken toward realizing these goals will now be examined.

Table 13-1 Summary of Basic Characteristics of Vacuum Tubes, Conventional Transistors, and Field Effect Transistors

	Input Impedance	Control	Output Impedance
Vacuum Tube	Basically high since the grid is operated negatively and grid current is in many applications negligible.	Voltage controlled	Moderate to low (Triode) 10 to 60K High – essentially a current source $\simeq 1$ megohm (Pentode)
Conventional Transistor	Fundamentally low input impedance because the input loop is a forward biased diode. $\simeq 1.0K$	Current controlled	Moderate to high $\simeq 50K$
Field Effect Transistor (FET)	Very high, since input loop is a reverse biased junction. $\simeq 10^{10}$ to 10^{15} ohms	Voltage controlled	High but can be made moderate by manufacturing techniques $\simeq 1$ megohm

428

The electrical equivalent circuit of a micropipette connected to a vacuum tube is shown in Fig. 13–72, where R_e is the resistance of the electrode, C_e is the electrode capacitance, C_w the shunt capacitance produced by circuit wiring, and C_{in} the input capacitance of the vacuum tube produced by the interelectrode capacitances and dependent upon the mode of operation of the tube. In Section 13–14 the input capacitance of a triode operating in the common-cathode mode was shown to be $C_{in} = C_{gk} + C_{gp} (1 + A)$, where C_{gk} is the grid-to-cathode capacitance, C_{gp} the grid-to-plate capacitance, and A the voltage gain of the stage. For most tubes C_{gk} and C_{gp} are nearly equal. This expression shows that, even if the stage produced a gain of zero (which would render it useless), C_{in} would still be given by the sum of C_{gk} and C_{gp}. For most triodes operated as low-gain amplifiers, the effect of C_{gk} and C_{gp} is too great to seriously consider the common-cathode connection as providing a truly high impedance input. It was also shown in Section 13–17 that for the triode connected as a cathode follower (common-plate connection) the effective input capacitance was given by $C_{in} = C_{gp} + C_{gk} (1 - A)$. In most practical cathode followers the gain A can easily be made greater than 0.9; therefore the contribution of C_{gk} is reduced accordingly. If A can be made equal to unity, the contribution of C_{gk} can be reduced to zero. Truly then, the triode connected as a cathode follower is far superior to the common-cathode connection when the goal is to provide an input circuit with low input capacitance.

The use of a tetrode or pentode connected as a conventional amplifier (common cathode) provides good voltage gain and reduces the input capacitance to a value comparable to that which would be obtained in the triode amplifier if the gain A could be reduced to zero. Certainly the use of a tetrode or pentode represents a step in the right direction toward providing an input stage with high impedance and gain. Harris and Bishop (1949) and Solms et al. (1953) described interesting low-capacitance input circuits in which the screen grid was connected to the cathode through a

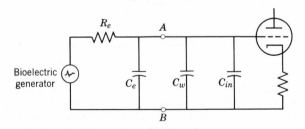

Figure 13–72. Electrical equivalent circuit of micropipette connected to the input of a vacuum tube: R_e = resistance of electrode; C_e = capacitance of electrode, C_w = wiring capacitance; C_{in} = vacuum-tube input capacitance.

battery rather than connected to a fixed potential relative to the common point of the circuit. This technique allows the screen voltage to follow the cathode voltage and thereby reduces the effect of the grid-to-screen capacitance.

Bak (1958) combined the attractive features of the pentode tube and the cathode follower circuit. By amplifying the cathode voltage (output signal) and applying it to the screen grid, he was able to obtain a simple input stage with unity gain, an input impedance of 10^{12} ohms (at direct current), uniform frequency response from direct current to 700 kc, and an input capacitance of 0.3 pf. Bak's circuit is shown in Fig. 13–73.

A useful low-input capacitance circuit described by Krakauer (1953) is a variant of the cathode follower circuit. It employs an electrometer triode (5803) as an input tube followed by an ordinary triode, the grid of which is connected to the cathode of the input tube. The plate supply voltage of the electrometer tube is derived from the cathode of the second stage.

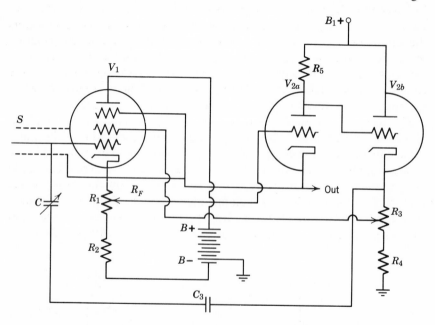

Figure 13–73. The unity gain cathode follower. V_1 = Z729 British A. F. pentode, $V_{2a} = 12AU7$ ($\frac{1}{2}$), $V_{2b} = 12AU7$ ($\frac{1}{2}$), C = 1.5 to 7.5 $\mu\mu f$, $C_3 = 250$ $\mu\mu f$, $R_1 = 10$ K pot., R_F = Part of R_1 between tap and cathode, $R_2 = 75$ K, comp. 1 watt, $R_3 = 5$ K pot., $R_4 = 33$ K, comp. 1 watt, $R_5 = 390$ K, comp. $\frac{1}{4}$ watt, S = driven shield, $B_1+ = 110$ volts, B– = 45 volts, B+ = 45 volts. All filaments 6 volts, battery operated. *Note.* Capacitor C_3 is not a critical value and may be increased or decreased, depending upon the maximal grid to ground capacity to be neutralized in any practical application. [From A. F. Bak, *EEG Clin. Neurophysiol.* **10**:745–748 (1958). By permission.]

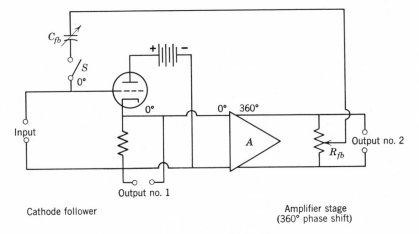

Figure 13–74. Principle employed in the negative-capacity (positive-feedback) amplifier.

This circuit achieved an input capacitance of 0.1 pf. A circuit using the same principle, which provided an input resistance of 50 megohms with a rise time of 14 μs, was reported by Haapanen and Ottison (1954).

As is evident from the foregoing descriptions of ingenious circuitry, considerable success has been achieved in reducing the input capacitance and raising the input impedance of the amplifier input stage; however, none of these procedures provides the capability of compensating for capacitance introduced by the wires necessary to connect the amplifier input to the microelectrode or the capacitance of the electrode itself. Compensation for the total circuit capacitance can be achieved by the adoption of the neutralized input capacity amplifier developed for microsecond pulse measurements (Bell, 1949). In the literature pertaining to microelectrode recording, amplifiers utilizing this technique are often called negative-capacity amplifiers. The principle of operation is illustrated in Fig. 13–74, which shows a cathode follower input stage operating into an amplifier A providing 360 degrees of phase shift. Controlled positive feedback is applied to raise the impedance by using in-phase voltage from the output to raise the voltage at the amplifier input in response to an increase in signal voltage. When the input voltage is raised in this manner, the signal voltage is not required to drive current into the input circuit; a feedback voltage is used to supply current to the input capacitance rather than having it provided by the signal source (see Fig. 13-72). The input capacitance is therefore canceled and effectively removed as a factor tending to lower the input impedance.

Solms et al. (1953) reported a comprehensive analysis of the problems encountered in microelectrode recording and presented a practical

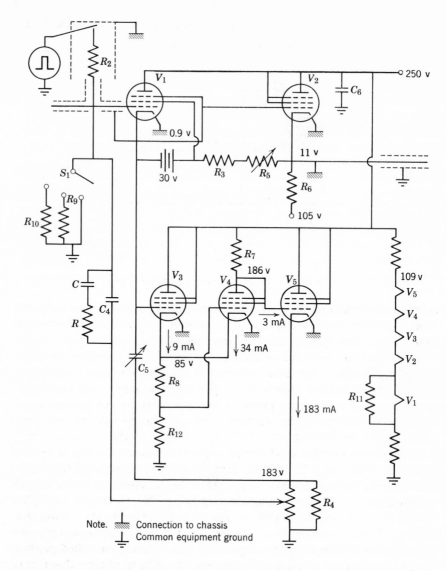

Figure 13–75. Negative-capacity amplifier employing a pentode cathode follower. All five tubes are type 12SJ7. There is no grid leak on V_1 under recording conditions. R_{10} is connected when measuring electrode resistance. R_9 is connected during grid current measurement. The maximum gain of the feedback amplifier is 2.5. Approximate operating currents and voltages are shown in the diagram. All voltages are indicated with respect to the common equipment ground. The resistances shown in series with the heaters are, in part, heaters of the associated amplifiers. The heaters should be properly arranged to avoid exceeding the heater-cathode potential rating for V_5.

Parts list: $R_1 = 10$ megohms, $\frac{1}{2}$ watt; $R_2 = 25$ megohms, $\frac{1}{2}$ watt; $R_3 = 33,000$ ohms, 2 watts; $R_4 = 20,000$-ohm wire-wound potentiometer, 2 watts, paralleled by two 10,000-ohm, 2-watt compensated amplifier constructed entirely of pentodes and utilizing the "negative-capacitance" principle. Their circuit is shown in Fig. 13–75. Woodbury (1953) reported another version of the negative-capacity amplifier, in which an electrometer tube input stage employing positive feedback (negative capacity) reduced the total effective input capacitance to less than 1.0 pf. He also stated that with this amplifier the use of a 30-megohm electrode with a 30 μs time constant would reproduce accurately all but the fastest potential changes encountered in the action potential spike of nerve. MacNichol and Wagner (1954) devised a circuit using remotely controlled positive feedback, which permitted mounting the preamplifier close to the biological preparation.

With the development of the transistor, it was only natural that the device be utilized in bioelectric amplifiers, and many such applications have been reported; however, the relatively low input impedance of conventional transistors prevents their use in input stages required to have a very high impedance value. By various circuit arrangements it is possible to construct an input stage with selected conventional transistors that will attain an impedance of perhaps 5 megohms. This value is not sufficiently high to compete with an ordinary vacuum tube, particularly in view of the elaborate circuitry required to obtain this characteristic with the conventional transistor. The first high-input-impedance amplifiers utilizing transistors employed vacuum tubes as the input element to obtain the necessary high impedance. Subsequent transistor stages were then used to amplify the output of the tube to the desired level.

The circuit of Johnstone and Pugsley (1960), shown in Fig. 13–76, is an excellent example of this technique and incorporates several principles previously described. For example, the signal to be amplified is applied directly to the grid of the ME 1400 pentode electrometer. No grid resistor is used. The tube operates as a cathode follower with a transistor in the cathode to act as a constant-current device which causes the gain of the cathode follower to approach unity and thereby reduces the effect of the capacitance between grid and cathode. Any other capacitance in the input circuit is reduced by the application of positive feedback. The feedback arrangement in this circuit is somewhat unique because the feedback voltage

resistors in series: total resistance 10,000 ohms; R_5 = 20,000-ohm wire-wound potentiometer, 2 watts; R_6 = Two 47,000 ohm, 2-watt resistors in parallel; R_7 = 10,000 ohms, 1 watt; R_8 = 470 ohms, 1 watt; R_9 = 100 megohms; R_{10} = 5-megohm precision resistor, 1% tolerance; R_{11} = 470-ohm and 1000-ohm, $\frac{1}{2}$-watt resistors in parallel: total resistance 320 ohms; R_{12} = 220 ohms, 1 watt; C = 1 $\mu\mu$f; C_4 = 4 $\mu\mu$f; C_5 = 75-$\mu\mu$f variable air capacitor, rotor connected to cathode of V_5; C_6 = 40-μf, 450-volt electrolytic; S_1 = 1 circuit, 4-position ceramic rotary switch. [From S. J. Solms et al., *Rev. Sci. Instr.* **24**:960–967 (1953). By permission.]

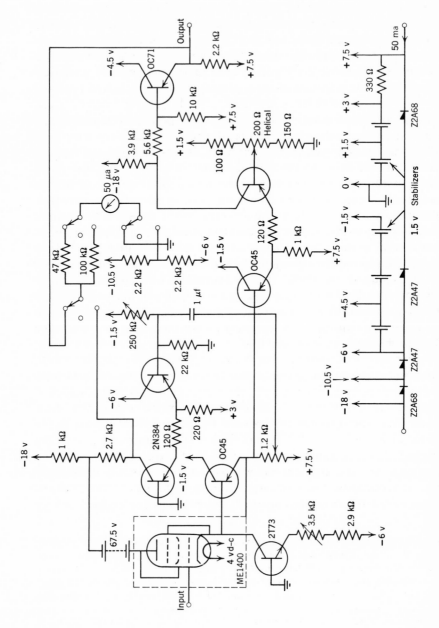

Figure 13-76. Electrometer-tube negative-capacitance amplifier using transistors. [From B. M. Johnston and I. D. Pugsley. *Electron. Eng.* **32**:422–424 (1960). By permission.]

is applied to the plate rather than the input grid. The grid, cathode, and plate potentials therefore all change together in the same direction so that the effect of the capacitance between them is minimized. The specifications and performance data shown in Table 13–2 were reported for this amplifier.

Pugsley (1963) has described another circuit employing a triode electrometer in conjunction with transistors, which employs controlled positive feedback to produce a unity-gain cathode follower. The feature of negative capacitance is not provided as a part of the device, but terminals are supplied to allow an external amplifier to be used for this purpose.

The field effect transistor, the solid-state counterpart of the vacuum tube electrometer, has been used to replace the vacuum tube as the input device in high-impedance circuits which were otherwise solid state. At this writing it is difficult to assess the degree to which the FET is able to compete with the vacuum tube electrometer. Webb (1965) reported an amplifier allegedly designed for microelectrode recording, although no records or data of actual intracellular recording were given. Using FET's, Richards (1965) developed a differential amplifier which he stated was unsuitable for refined biophysical measurements because of a high noise level at low frequencies and a lower input impedance compared with vacuum tubes. Fein (1964) reported an amplifier in which insulated-gate FET's were employed in a unity-gain follower circuit with input capacity neutralization. Fein stated that this device was in routine service in his laboratory, presumably for the measurement of nerve and muscle cell potentials, which he cited as being the principal purpose of amplifiers of this type. The performance reported, in the form of photographs of square-wave tests using a 22-megohm resistor to simulate the electrode resistance,

Table 13–2   Specifications and Performance Data for the
Johnstone—Pugsley Amplifier

Input impedance	10^{11} ohms
Gain	10
Noise	100 μv (peak-to-peak)
Drift	100 mv/hour

Source Impedance (ohms)	Rise Time (μs)	Bandwidth (kc)	Overshoot (%)	Feedback
0	2	150	5	Without
50×10^6 (typical microelectrode)	400	0.9	0	Without
50×10^6	80	4.5	0	With

indicated that this amplifier would perform well with microelectrodes having a similar resistance value.

Amplifiers employing vacuum tube electrometers and designed specifically for microelectrode recording are available commercially from at least two manufacturers.[7] At this time there can be purchased an all-solid-state amplifier utilizing FET's.[8] The input impedance of the commercial instruments which use electrometer vacuum tubes is approximately 10^{10} ohms. With one instrument, electrode impedances as high as 500 megohms can be accommodated, and shunt capacitances as great as 500 pf can be compensated. The grid current is less than 10^{-13} ampere, and the nominal bandwidth is 50 kc, depending upon the electrode impedance and shunt capacity. Specifications for the all-solid-state amplifier show an input impedance of 10^{13} ohms with a leakage current of 2×10^{-13} ampere. It is also stated that any high-impedance probe (microelectrode) may be compensated to obtain a rise time in the range of 1.5 to 15 μs.

It has been pointed out that, despite all efforts to reduce the input capacitance of the amplifier, some capacitance, such as that produced by the wiring to the preparation and the electrode itself, is inevitable. The need to compensate for this external capacitance requires use of positive feedback, as employed in the negative-capacity amplifier. Unless carefully controlled, positive feedback can lead to unstable circuit operation, and just as a distorted record of bioelectric activity can result from insufficient compensation for the residual capacitance; so also can a false record be produced by overcompensation. The effect of compensation on waveform restoration is shown in Fig. 13–77a by a sequence of waveforms corresponding to increasing amounts of positive feedback.

The equivalent electrical system is shown in Fig. 13–77b, in which R_s represents the total resistance associated with the electrode and C_s is the total shunt capacitance to be compensated. This illustration is due to Amatniek (1958), whose report is recommended for a detailed description and analysis of the problems encountered in microelectrode recording with such amplifiers. These waveforms were produced by incrementally increasing the compensation by raising the positive feedback, and observing the resulting modifications to a 500-μs square pulse. Trace 1 in Fig. 13–77a shows the output waveform with minimum positive feedback. Increasing amounts of feedback produced a shorter rise time, and traces 2 and 3 show the limits of optimum adjustment because further increases in feedback produce first overshoot, then ringing, and finally continuous

---

[7] Argonaut Associates, Inc., Beaverton, Ore., and Grass Instruments, Quincy, Mass.

[8] Instrumentation Laboratory, Inc., Watertown, Mass.

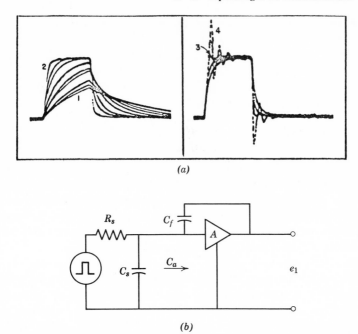

(a)

(b)

Figure 13-77. The effect of negative-capacity compensation (positive feedback on rise time. [From E. Amatniek, *IRE Trans. Med. Electron.* **10**:3–14 (1958). By permission.]

oscillation (not shown). Amatniek also pointed out that, with optimum compensation, the distortion he attributed to the generation of a negative impedance that is not purely capacitive may in fact approximate a negative capacitance only over a limited bandwidth.

Having demonstrated the degree to which waveform restoration is possible in a system simulating the resistance and capacitance of the microelectrode, it is appropriate to inquire about the means of carrying out such a procedure with electrodes inserted in the cell under examination. As discussed by Amatniek (1958), the usual method is to insert a square-wave calibrating signal either in series with the preparation or in parallel via a very high resistance. Feedback is then adjusted to produce the best restored square wave in the amplifier output.

Amatniek's concept of the electrical circuit existing when a microelectrode impales a cell suspended in a liquid medium is shown in Fig. 13–78. The bioelectric generators e_b containing internal resistance R_b are assumed to exist within the membrane. The membrane capacitance C_b is between the electrolytes inside and outside the cell with the membrane acting as a dielectric. These components—e_b, R_b, and C_b—are assumed

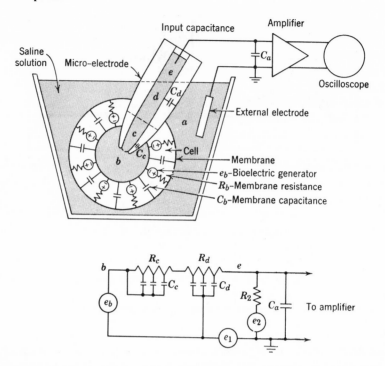

Figure 13–78. Equivalent circuit for a single cell impaled by a micropipette. [From E. Amatniek, *IRE Trans. Med. Electron.* **10**:3–14 (1958). By permission.]

to be uniformly distributed. The intracellular fluid b contacts the inner surface of the membrane and the tip of the microelectrode. For purposes of analysis the microelectrode has been divided into three regions: (1) the portion c within the cell which contains most of the resistance R_c and some capacitance C_c distributed along R_c; (2) the portion d which contains some resistance R_d but is characterized primarily by the capacitance C_d between the electrolyte filling the microelectrode and the liquid in contact with the extracellular fluid a; and (3) the region e contributing no significant resistance or capacitance. The equivalent circuit is completed by adding capacitor C_a, which represents the capacitance produced by wiring and amplifier input capacitance. To adjust the input stage for compensation, a square-wave test signal may be introduced either in series with the preparation, as depicted by the voltage source e_1, or in parallel through a very high resistance R_2 as indicated by e_2. Amatniek (1958) pointed out that, even if identical square waves could be applied at the three locations: e_1, e_2, or the cell itself e_b, different waveforms would be presented to the amplifier because of the different circuits viewed from these locations. It is of course not possible to know accurately the waveform of the bioelectric generator e_b, so the question as to what degree of compensation for reproduction of test square waves e_1 or e_2 approaches optimum for e_b remains largely unresolved.

Yang et al. (1958) have analyzed the effect of "negative-capacitance" compensation on the intrinsic response time of the amplifier and have investigated a method of inserting a test signal into the amplifier grid in order to adjust the compensation while the electrode is in place in a cell. Lettvin et al. (1958) have reported a direct-coupled input stage for use with microelectrodes which incorporates the compensating arrangement described by Yang. A circuit which provides a method of testing for optimum positive feedback and for measuring electrode resistance has been described by Frank and Becker (1964).

The application of proper compensation is obviously a complex subject. A standard for its specification has been proposed by Amatniek (1961); however, this standard has not been in existence long enough to be evaluated. Therefore, at this time manufacturers are reluctant to specify procedures for adjustment of negative capacity amplifiers. One manufacturer[9] provides a source of compensating voltage from a terminal on the amplifier but does not supply a control. The reason for doing so is stated as follows:

"We do not incorporate a capacitive neutralizing control on the P6 and P7 because we feel the experimenter should understand these principles well enough to improvise neutralizing controls specific to the experiment. If not properly handled, the use of such a circuit can easily give misleading results. So can its omission with electrodes above a few megohms. No satisfactory test, practical from the standpoint of production manufacture, has been devised to determine the proper amount of neutralizing voltage for a particular experiment. So we feel that omission as opposed to overcompensation is the lesser of the two evils."

Other manufacturers provide an adjustment control for applying compensation and leave the proper use of it to the investigator.

13-46.   THE VIBRATING REED ELECTROMETER

A vibrating reed electrometer (VRE) is a carrier amplifier having extremely high input impedance (on the order of 10^{16} ohms). It is useful for measurements in radioactivity, mass spectrometry. pH, and cation determination. It is also employed in determining the electrical insulating properties of materials and can serve for the measurement of stable cell membrane potentials. Although the extremely high input impedance would

[9] Grass Instruments, Quincy, Mass.

appear to make the VRE ideal for microelectrode recording with increasingly smaller microelectrodes, its slow response time (on the order of 0.5 second or more) limits its application for recording rapid voltage changes such as single-cell action potentials.

The extremely high input impedance of the VRE is obtained by the absence of any direct conducting path between the input terminals. This is in contrast to the direct-coupled vacuum tube electrometer, in which it was found paradoxically that either some leakage grid current flowed in the input circuit, even though the actual grid-to-cathode resistance could be adjusted to appear infinite, or if the leakage current were adjusted to zero, the grid-to-cathode resistance was not infinite. The only d-c conducting path in the VRE is that afforded by leakage across the terminals and components, which may be insulated to the degree permitted by the state-of-the-art and consistent with a feasible physical arrangement of parts and electrical components.

The basic operation of the circuit is illustrated in Fig. 13–79. The voltage to be measured (e_{in}) is applied across the input terminals and causes charge to be transferred through the resistance R to the vibrating reed capacitor C. The product RC is the time constant of the input system and controls the rate at which charge may be transferred. This, of course, governs the response time of the instrument. The capacitance of C is changed periodically (450 cps) by means of electromechanical vibrating action which varies the spacing between the metallic plates constituting C. With a fixed charge Q on the plates, the voltage across the capacitor follows the variations in capacitance in accordance with the basic relationship for the capacitor: $V = Q/C$. The voltage developed across C is coupled into the preamplifier by the small capacitor C_1. After amplification by the preamplifier and main amplifier it is then rectified by a phase-sensitive detector,[10] filtered, and presented to the output terminals for appropriate recording. In addition to voltage measurement, a feedback circuit is provided in commercial electrometers for measuring very small currents. Some applications and specifications for a VRE as given by one manufacturer[11] are as follows:

1. Through the measurement of ion currents, carbon 14 activity may be measured to 5×10^{-15} curie per milligram of $BaCO_3$ and tritium activity to as low as 10^{-11} curie per milligram of hydrogen.

2. In mass spectrometry, ion currents as small as 10^{-17} ampere may be detected.

---

[10] See Section 13–39.
[11] Cary Instruments, Applied Physics Corporation, Monrovia, Calif.

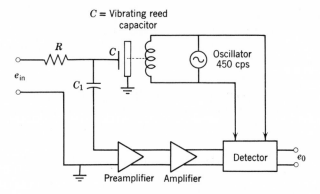

Figure 13–79.   Principle of the vibrating reed electrometer.

3. When used with a suitable glass electrode, pH changes to 0.0005 pH may be detected.

4. In the measurement of electrical properties such as dielectric characteristics of insulating materials and semiconductors, currents as small as 10^{-17} ampere, charges to 5×10^{-16} coulomb, and voltages as low as 20 μv may be detected.

13–47.   THE TREND IN AMPLIFIER TECHNOLOGY

The present trend in all electronic circuitry (including amplifiers) is toward ever-smaller, integrated, solid-state circuits. Integrated circuits make use of techniques which permit the formation of transistors, diodes, capacitors, and resistors on a single, solid, monolithic silicon chip by deposition and etching of layers of appropriate materials. The finished product appears physically as a single piece of solid material with the internal connections between the "deposited" components completed by pathways etched as the material layers are laid down. The only connecting wires are those required to provide terminals external to the integrated circuit.

The compactness of integrated circuits presently obtainable appears fantastic to investigators who began their work some years ago with large vacuum tubes, transistors, and individual components which required wired interconnections. For example, an entire operational amplifier consisting of 14 transistors, 3 diodes, and 15 resistors is available in a cylindrical container 0.335 inch in diameter and 0.180 inch high. The need for most of the space inside the container is dictated, not by the size of the integrated circuit itself, but by the necessity of connecting wires to the appropriate points within the circuit and stabilizing them mechanically for external connection. The cost of these devices is very low, in many cases far less than that of a single transistor only a few years ago. It is impossible to forecast the extent which such "packaging density" will reach in the near future. That it will increase is inevitable. It would appear therefore that in the future the knowledge required to apply these devices will shift from details of single-component function to emphasis on the terminal behavior of systems. This trend has been recognized by the authors, and the preceeding material has been selected on the basis of providing a balanced presentation of individual device characteristics and system function to cover present-day needs, as well as an appreciation of the integral operation and terminal behavior of the compact systems which are already appearing in the field of biomedical instrumentation.

REFERENCES

Adrian, E. D. 1926. The impulses produced by sensory nerve endings. Part 1. *J. Physiol.* **61**:49–72.

Adrian, E. D. 1931. Potential changes in the isolated nervous system of *Dytiscus marginalis*. *J. Physiol.* **72**:132–151.

Adrian, E. D., and B. H. C. Matthews. 1934. The investigation of potential waves in the cortex. *J. Physiol.* **81**:440–471.

Adrian, E. D., and K. Yamagiwa. 1935. The origin of the Berger rhythm. *Brain* **55**:323–351.

Alley, C. L., and K. W. Atwood. 1966. *Electronic Engineering*. New York: John Wiley & Sons.

Amatniek, E. 1958. Measurement of bioelectric potentials with microelectrodes and neutralized capacity amplifiers. *IRE Trans. Med. Electron.* **10**:3–14.

Amatniek, E. 1961. Input capacity neutralization characteristics, a proposed standard. *Digest of the 1961 International Conference on Medical Electronics*. McGregor and Werner. Washington, D.C.:

Andrew, A. M. 1958. Differential amplifier design. *Wireless Eng.* **32**:73–79.

Attree, V. H. 1949. Reducing the effect of capacitance in screened cable. *Electron. Eng.* **21**:100.

Aughtie, F. 1929. Push-pull amplification: the use of resistance-capacity coupling. *Wireless Eng.* **6**:307–309.

Bak, A. F. 1958. A unity gain cathode follower. *EEG Clin. Neurophysiol.* **10**:745–748.

Bell, P. R. 1949. *Negative-Capacity Amplifier*, M.I.T. Radiation Laboratory Series, Vol. 19, App. A. New York: McGraw-Hill Book Co.

Bishop, P. O. 1949. A high impedance input stage for a valve amplifier. *Electron. Eng.* **21**:469–470.

Black, H. S. 1934. Stabilized feedback amplifiers. *Bell System Tech. J.* **13**:1–18.

Boas, E. P. 1928. The cardiotachometer. *Arch. Intern. Med.* **41**:403–414.

Buchtal, F., and J. O. Nielsen. 1936. Ein neuer Gegentakt-Gleichstromverstarker zum Kathodenstrahloszillographen zur Verwendung in der Elektrophysiologie. *Skand. Arch. Physiol.* **74**:202–322.

Collins, D. L. 1953. Electrometer tubes. *Instruments* **26**:11–13.

Crawford, K. D. E. 1948. H. F. Pentodes in electrometer circuits. *Electron. Eng.* **20**:227–231.

Daly, I. de B., and K. E. Shellshear. 1920–21. The use of thermionic valves with the string galvanometer. *J. Physiol.* **54**:287–291.

Davidson, F. G. 1929. Push-pull amplification. *Wireless Eng.* **6**:437–438.

Dewhurst, D. J. 1959. The design of balanced amplifiers using components of commercial tolerance. *Electron. Eng.* **30**:355–357.

Donaldson, P. E. K. 1958. *Electronic Apparatus for Biological Research.* London: Butterworth's Scientific Publications.

E.M.I. Laboratories. 1946. Balanced output amplifiers of highly stable and accurate balance. *Electron. Eng.* **18**:189.

Fein, H. 1964. Solid-state electrometers with input-capacitance neutralization. *IEEE Trans. Bio-Med. Eng.* **BME-11**:13–18.

Forbes, A., and C. Thacher. 1920. Amplification of action currents with the electron tube in recording with the string galvanometer. *Am. J. Physiol.* **52**:409–471.

Forbes, A., H. Davis, and J. H. Emerson. 1931. An amplifier, string galvanometer and photographic camera designed for the study of action currents in nerve. *Rev. Sci. Instrs.* **2**:1–15.

Frank, K., and M. C. Becker. 1964. Microelectrodes for recording and stimulation. Chap. 2 in *Physical Techniques in Biological Research* (W. L. Nastuk, Ed.), Vol. 5, part A. New York: Academic Press.

Gabus, G. H., and M. L. Pool. 1937. A portable unit using an RCA 954 tube. *Rev. Sci. Instrs.* **8**:196–198.

Garceau, E. L., and A. Forbes, 1934. A direct coupled amplifier for action currents. *Rev. Sci. Instrs.* **5**:10–13.

Gasser, H. S., and J. Erlanger. 1922. A study of the action currents of nerve with the cathode ray oscillograph. *Am. J. Physiol.* **62**:496–524.

Gasser, H. S., and H. S. Newcomer. 1921. Physiological action currents in the phrenic nerve. An application of the thermionic vacuum tube to nerve physiology. *Am. J. Physiol.* **57**:1–26.

Goldberg, H. 1944. Bioelectric-research apparatus. *Proc. IRE* **32**:330–336.

Grodins, F. S. 1963. *Control Theory and Biological Systems.* New York: Columbia University Press.

Haapanen, L., and D. Ottison. 1954. A frequency compensated input circuit for recording with microelectrodes. *Acta Physiol. Scand.*, 32, Suppl. **115**:271–280.

Harris, E. J., and P. O. Bishop. 1949. Design and limitations of D.C. amplifiers. *Elect. Eng.* **21**:355–359.

Huxley, A. F., and R. Stampfli. 1949. Evidence for saltatory conduction in peripheral myelinated nerve fibers. *J. Physiol.* **108**:315–339.

Johnston, D. L. 1947. Electro-encephalograph amplifier. *Wireless Eng.* **24**:237–242.

Johnstone, B. M., and I. D. Pugsley. 1960. A negative capacitance preamplifier for electrophysiological use. *Electron. Eng.* **32**:422–424.

Kado, R. T., and W. R. Adey. 1961. A transistorized preamplifier for field study of EEG. *Digest of the International Conference on Medical Electronics.* Washington, D.C.: McGregor and Werner.

Keithley, J. F. 1952. Vacuum-tube electrometer applications. *Instruments* **25**:458.

Keithley, J. F. 1962. Electrometer measurements. *Instrs. Control Systems* **35**:74–81.

Klein, G. 1955. Rejection factor of difference amplifiers. *Philips Res. Rept.* **10**:241–259.

Krakauer, W. 1953. Electrometer triode follower. *Rev. Sci. Instrs.* **24**:496–530.

Lettvin, J. Y., B. Howland, and R. C. Gesteland. 1958. Footnotes on a headstage. *IRE Trans. Med. Electron.* **PGME-10**:26–28.

Levine, I. 1960. High input impedance transistor circuits. *Electronics* **33**:50–52.

MacNichol, E. F., Jr., and T. Bickart. 1958. The use of transistors in physiological amplifiers. *IRE Trans. Med. Electron.* **10**:15–24.

MacNichol, E. F., Jr., and H. G. Wagner. 1954. A high impedance circuit suitable for electrophysiological recording from micropipette electrodes. *Naval Med. Res. Inst.* **12**:97–118.

Marvin, H. B. 1953. Personal communication of July 23.

Matthews, B. H. C. 1928. A new electrical recording system for physiological work. *J. Physiol.* **65**:225–242.

Matthews, B. H. C. 1934. A special purpose amplifier. *J. Physiol.* **81**:28P–29P.

Matthews, B. H. C. 1938. A simple universal amplifier. *J. Physiol.* **93**:23P–27P.

Metcalf, G. F. and B. J. Thompson. 1930. A low grid current vacuum tube. *Phys. Rev.* **36**:1489–1494.

Middlebrook, R. D. 1963. *Differential Amplifiers*. New York: John Wiley & Sons.

Milhorn, H. T. 1966. *The Application of Control Theory to Physiological Systems*. Philadelphia: W. B. Saunders Co.

Nastuk, W. L., and A. L. Hodgkin. 1950. The electrical activity of single muscle fibers. *J. Cellular Comp. Physiol.* **35**:39–72.

Nielsen, C. E. 1947. Measurement of small currents. *Rev. Sci. Instrs.* **18**: 18–31.

Nottingham, W. B. 1929. A note on the high grid resistor amplifier. *J. Franklin Inst.* **208**:469–474.

Offner, F. F. 1937. Push-pull resistance coupled amplifiers. *Rev. Sci. Instr.* **8**:20–21.

Offner, F. F. 1947. Balanced amplifiers. *Proc. IRE* **35**:306–310.

Parnum, D. H. 1950. Transmission factors of differential amplifiers. *Wireless Eng.* **27**:125–129.

Pugsley, I. D. 1963. A pre-amplifier for use with microelectrodes. *Electron. Eng.* **35**:788–791.

Randall, J. E. 1962. *Elements of Biophysics*, 2nd Ed. Chicago: Year Book Medical Publishers.

Richards, J. C. S. 1965. A D.C. differential amplifier using field effect transistors. *Electron. Eng.* **37**:598–601.

Robinson, T. A. 1965. The role of grounding in eliminating electronic interference. *IEEE Spectrum.* **2**:85–89.

Rosenberg, H. 1927. Neue Untersuchungen uber den Aktionsstrome des Nerven. *Arch. ges. Physiol.* **216**:300–307.

Rushmer, R. F. 1961. *Cardiovascular Dynamics*, 2nd Ed. Philadelphia: W. B. Saunders, Co.

Salmons, S. 1966. The achievement of high overall rejection in difference amplifiers. *Electronic Eng.* **38**:218–221.

Schmitt, O. H. 1937. A simple differential amplifier. *Rev. Sci. Instr.* **8**:126–127.

Schuler, G., G. Park, and J. P. Ertl. 1966. Low-noise, interference-resistant amplifier suitable for biological signals. *Science* **154**:1191–1192.

Solms, S. J., W. L. Nastuk, and J. T. Alexander. 1953. Development of a high fidelity preamplifier for use in the recording of bioelectric potentials with intracellular electrodes. *Rev. Sci. Instr.* **24**:960–967.

Toennies, J. F. 1938. Differential amplifier. *Rev. Sci. Instr.* **9**:95–97.

Trevino, S. N., and F. F. Offner. 1940. An AC operated DC amplifier with large current output. *Rev. Sci. Instr.* **11**:412–415.

Upton, M. *Electronics for Everyone*. 1957. New York: New American Library.

Victoreen, J. A. 1949. Electrometer tubes for the measurement of small currents. *Proc. IRE* **37**:432–441.

Walter, W. G. 1936. The location of cerebral tumors by electroencephalography. *Lancet* **2**:305–308.

Webb, R. E. 1965. Field effect transistors for biological amplifiers. *Electron. Eng.* 37: 803–805.

Williams, H. B. 1924. The Einthoven string galvanometer, a theoretical and experimental study. Part 1. *J. Opt. Soc. Am.* and *Rev. Sci. Instrs.* 9:129–172. Part 2. 1926, 13:313–382.

Woodbury, J. W. 1953. Recording central nervous activity with intracellular ultramicro-electrodes: use of negative-capacity amplifier to improve transient response. *Fed. Proc.* 12:159.

Yang, C. C. 1958. J. P. Hervey, and P. F. Smith. On amplifiers used for microelectrode work. *IRE Trans. Med. Electron.* PGME-10:25.

14

Criteria for the Faithful Reproduction of an Event

For the familiar three-part system (transducer, processor, and reproducer) used to measure the time course of a physiological event, it is possible to set forth general conditions which, if satisfied, will guarantee faithful reproduction of the event. It is necessary either to appropriately impose these same conditions on the three parts of the channel or to incorporate any necessary compensation so that the overall system will meet the criteria if the individual parts do not. In such a system three criteria must be fulfilled. Because of the extreme importance of these criteria, their meaning must be clearly understood. Despite the fact that many of the underlying factors are of necessity technical and complex, simple examples can be chosen to illustrate their importance.

Any system designed for faithful reproduction of an event must possess these characteristics:

1. Amplitude linearity.
2. Adequate bandwidth.
3. Phase linearity.

The first requisite, amplitude linearity, calls for the input-output characteristic to be linear in the working range. If, for example, the input is doubled, say in the positive direction, the output indication also must be doubled. If the operating range extends into the reverse direction, negative inputs must be reproduced by a linear output indication in the reverse direction.

14-1. FOURIER SERIES

Before the second and third criteria can be discussed it is necessary to establish the relationship between sine waves and waves of nonsinusoidal

446

form. All periodic waves of nonsinusoidal form are designated complex waves. By the use of the Fourier series it is possible to show that any periodic complex wave can be dissected into a series of sine and cosine waves which, when added, will reproduce the original complex wave. The sine and cosine waves which have the same frequency as the complex wave constitute the components of the fundamental or first harmonic. Those having twice and thrice the frequency constitute the second and third harmonics, etc.

These facts may be stated by saying that a periodic complex wave can be represented by an infinite series consisting of a constant, plus harmonically related sine and cosine waves. Expressed mathematically, the series for the function $F(t)$ may be written as follows:

$$F(t) = \frac{a_0}{2} + a_1 \cos wt + a_2 \cos 2wt + a_3 \cos 3wt + \ldots + a_n \cos nwt$$

$$+ b_1 \sin wt + b_2 \sin 2wt + b_3 \sin 3wt + \ldots + b_n \sin nwt,$$

in which
$$a_n = (1/\pi) \int_0^{2\pi} F(t) \cos nwt \, dt,$$

$$b_n = (1/\pi) \int_0^{2\pi} F(t) \sin nwt \, dt,$$

and $w = 2\pi f$ (where f is the fundamental frequency of the complex wave in cycles per second).

In order to use the series to describe a waveform it is necessary to calculate the coefficients $a_0 \ldots a_n$ and $b_0 \ldots b_n$, some of which may be zero. However, for purposes of this study it is neither necessary nor profitable to perform the calculations to demonstrate the validity of the series. Many waves have been analyzed and the coefficients published. Selection of two examples, the square wave and the blood pressure curve, will suffice to show the value of the concept.

One of the most difficult waveforms to reproduce is the square wave, shown in Fig. 14–1a, which instantaneously changes its value from zero to a fixed value, maintains this value for a time before reversing itself below zero by the same amount and for the same time, and then returns abruptly to zero again. When this wave is analyzed for its harmonic content, some of the coefficients are zero and the series reduces to the fundamental and an infinite series of odd harmonics in which the amplitudes of the higher-frequency components decrease, that is, these components contribute less to the resynthesis of the original wave. Table 14–1 lists a few of the harmonic amplitudes for the square wave.

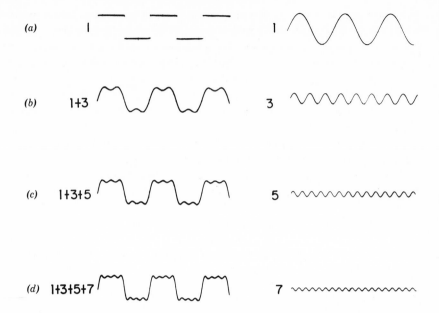

Figure 14–1. Synthesis of a square wave.

In Fig. 14–1*b* the first and the third harmonic components have been summated to yield the curve labeled 1 + 3. In this case, even with only two components, the beginnings of the square wave are apparent. When the first, third, and fifth components are summated (Fig. 14–1*c*), a better representation of the original wave is obtained (1 + 3 + 5). By adding the first, third, fifth, and seventh components, an even better likeness of the original wave is obtained, as shown by Fig. 14–1*d* (1 + 3 + 5 + 7). Adding more and more harmonics would further improve the reproduction; the addition of an infinite number of the ever-diminishing-amplitude high-frequency components would reconstitute the original wave.

Table 14–1   Harmonic Amplitudes of Square Wave

Harmonic	Amplitude (%)
Fundamental	100
3rd	33
5th	20
7th	14

The arterial pressure pulse is a good example of the utilitarian value of harmonic analysis. Hansen (1949), using a high-fidelity system, recorded the arterial pulse wave and applied harmonic analysis to it. His data (redrawn) are plotted in Fig. 14–2a and show the degree of fidelity obtainable by summating the first six harmonics. The arterial pressure waveform is designated (a), and the waveform resulting from summing the first six harmonics is labeled (b). It is also to be noted that the amplitudes of the higher-frequency components are progressively smaller with increasing harmonic numbers, the sixth being present with an amplitude of slightly more than 10%. Figure 14–2b illustrates this point.

To obtain a more faithful reproduction, addition of many more of the smaller-and-smaller-amplitude high-frequency components would be necessary. Thus, the amount of frequency response required is closely related to the degree of fidelity desired.

From these relatively simple examples two very important conclusions can be drawn. The first is that the frequency of the periodic complex wave determines the frequency of the fundamental component. The second is that the fidelity of reproduction of the quickly changing parts of the wave is determined by the number of high-frequency components added. Thus the bandwidth required for reproduction of the two waves analyzed would extend from below the fundamental frequency of the complex wave to the highest harmonic deemed important for adequate reproduction of the sharp portions of the complex wave.

Note that, in the two examples cited, the waves chosen were symmetrical about the time axis. If they were not, the analysis would have shown the same components with one notable exception: the constant a_0 would have a value other than zero, for a_0 is the average amplitude over a complete period. It is easily proved mathematically, and indeed is obvious, that a train of unidirectional pulses must have an average value other than zero. In the case of the arterial pressure wave, a_0 would be the mean pressure. Therefore, to reproduce a train of unidirectional pulses, it is necessary to provide a uniform frequency response extending from zero cycles per second to a value high enough for full reproduction of the highest harmonic deemed important. In practice, the high-frequency response is made to include the tenth harmonic and sometimes higher harmonics.

14–2.   AMPLITUDE AND PHASE DISTORTION

Perhaps of more importance than the cases in which the criteria are satisfied are those in which some criteria are not met. The following examples illustrate some of the possible types of distortion. Because

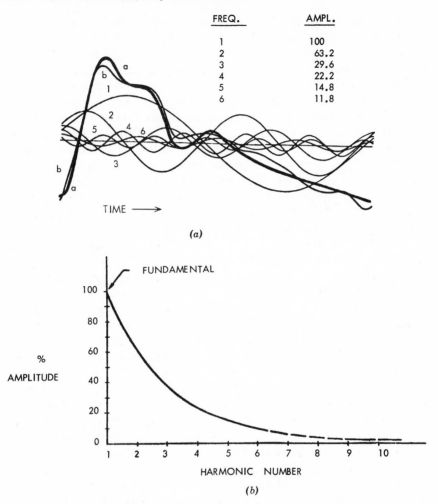

FREQ.	AMPL.
1	100
2	63.2
3	29.6
4	22.2
5	14.8
6	11.8

(a)

(b)

Figure 14–2. (a) Fourier analysis of a blood pressure curve; (b) harmonic amplitudes of components of a blood pressure pulse. (From data obtained by A. T. Hansen, Pressure Measurement in the Human Organism, Technisk Forlag, Copenhagen, 1949. By permission.)

the square wave is one of the most difficult to reproduce, it is useful to examine the effects of alteration of the amplitudes of the harmonics on the reproduction of this waveform. Terman (1943) showed that, if only the low-frequency components are attenuated, the square wave will have a concave top as sketched in Fig. 14–3a. On the other hand, if the low-frequency components are enhanced, the top of the square wave will be convex as in Fig. 14–3b.

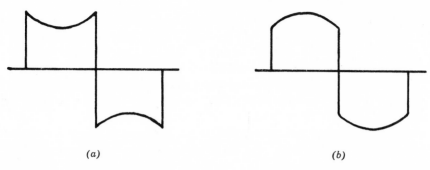

(a)   (b)

Figure 14-3. Amplitude distortion: (a) loss of low-frequency response (no phase distortion); (b) increased amplification of low frequencies (no phase distortion). (From F. E. Terman, Radio Engineers Handbook, 1st Ed., McGraw-Hill Book Co., New York, By permission.)

If the harmonics are present in their proper amplitudes but are merely displaced in time, a characteristic type of distortion occurs. Time displacement is not customarily expressed in seconds; it is usually stated in angular measure (radians or degrees) as a phase lag or lead. For example, if the time displacement for a given frequency f is t, and since the period T corresponds to 360 degrees, the phase lag or lead $\emptyset$ in degrees is $t/T \times 360$ degrees. The fact that $T = 1/f$ permits expressing the phase lag or lead in terms of frequency, that is, $\emptyset = tf \times 360$ degrees. Thus, with equal time displacements for all frequency components $(t = k)$, $\emptyset = kf$, that is, the phase lag or lead must be linear with frequency. It is also possible to state this requirement by specifying that, in relation to some reference (such as the fundamental), the components must be transmitted through the system in such a manner that they bear exactly the same phase relationship one to another, at the output as existed at the input.

Figure 14-4 illustrates the effect of phase distortion on the reproduction of the square wave. In this illustration the harmonic components are

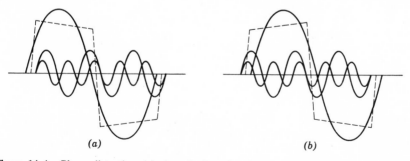

(a)   (b)

Figure 14-4. Phase distortion: (a) phase leads at low frequency (no amplitude distortion); (b) phase lags at low frequency (no amplitude distortion).

present in their correct amplitudes, but time displacements have been caused to occur. In Fig. 14–4a, the fundamental leads the higher harmonics, and in Fig. 14–4b the reverse condition exists. In each case the resulting reproduction is shown by the dotted lines.

Phase distortion can be present when only minimal loss of amplitude response occurs. Terman (1943) called attention to the fact that in many networks, such as those used to couple amplifier stages, when the low-frequency sine-wave response is 99.94% a 2-degree phase-shift error is encountered which results in a 10% tilt to the top of the square wave of the same frequency.

Because phase shift and loss of amplitude response are usually inseparable, it is often difficult to appreciate the effect of each of these types of distortion. To demonstrate the practical importance of this fact Geddes (1951) constructed a variable-frequency oscillator which produced a sine wave having a notch at its peak positive amplitude. The location of the notch (square pulse) was fixed, but the frequency of the complex wave was variable. This wave was used to test electroencephalographs to estimate their ability to reproduce faithfully the familiar spike-and-wave complex found in recordings from patients with petit-mal epilepsy.

The wave was applied to one of several EEG machines meeting existing standards; the frequency was varied and the output recorded. Figure 14–5a is a sketch of the input wave form. The reproduction at various frequencies

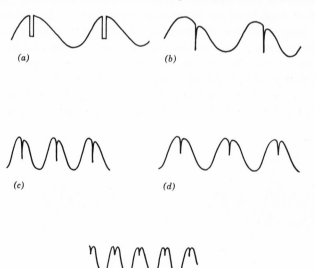

(a)   (b)

(c)   (d)

(e)

Figure 14–5. Amplitude phase distortion.

is shown in Figs. 14–5*b–e*. In Fig. 14–5*b*, recorded at 1 cps, it is obvious that there is a 45-degree phase shift. Increasing the frequency to 2 and 3 cps, as shown in Figs. 14–5*c* and 14–5*d*, places the spike more nearly in its correct position, where it appears when the frequency is 6 cps. However, it is to be noted that, although the phase distortion is minimal (Fig. 14–5*e*), at 6 cps, the amplitude of the spike has decreased because the system had inadequate high-frequency response to pass the high frequency components contained in the spike.

The practical significance of phase distortion was demonstrated by Saunders and Jell (1959), who recorded the effect in a unique way by using two identical channels of an EEG machine. The output of the first channel was attenuated and fed into the second; the output of both channels appeared on the same record. They first tested the system for phase distortion, using a 3-cps sine wave. On a typical EEG machine in which a 3-cps sine wave was attenuated insignificantly, they recorded a time delay between channels amounting to 51.3 ms or 55.4 degrees. It is to be noted that this testing technique demonstrated the phase shift in the second channel only. Next, in a practical study, stimulus-response waves, eye-blink artifacts, and spike-and-wave patterns were observed to exhibit time distortions when the recordings from the two channels were compared. A time separation of 75 ms between the spike and wave recorded on the first channel was reduced to 63 ms after passing through the second channel.

From the examples given it is apparent that the three criteria—amplitude linearity, frequency response, and phase linearity—must be satisfied to guarantee the faithful reproduction of an event. Amplitude linearity occurs when output and input are proportional. Frequency response is usually described in terms of bandwidth, which is designated as the frequency range between the lowest and highest sine-wave frequencies at which a satisfactory amplitude response is obtained. It is also frequently designated as the spectrum between the two frequencies at which the output amplitude has fallen to 70% of the mid-frequency response. In some instances the 50, 90, or 95% points are specified.

14-3.   THE STEP FUNCTION

For practical testing of a system, the step function is of considerable value. It is a waveform which changes abruptly from one level to another and is frequently employed as a calibration signal in many bioelectric recording instruments. Since the sine-wave frequency response curves of most devices are given by equipment manufacturers, it is illuminating to apply the step function to systems with known frequency response curves in order to determine the relationship between sinusoidal and step-function response.

If the step function shown in Fig. 14–6a is applied to a simple system that does not possess a sine-wave frequency response extending to zero cycles per second (Fig. 14–6b) but has an infinite high-frequency response, the reproduced wave is of exponential form and is as diagramed in Fig. 14–6c. The decay time is described as the time taken for the amplitude to fall from 100% to 37% amplitude. This time, measured in seconds, is called the time constant. The time constant is related to the sine-wave frequency response by the following relationship:

$$T = \frac{1}{2\pi f_L},$$

where T is time constant in seconds, and f_L is frequency on the sine-wave curve at which the response is 70%.

Often in the recording of physiological and bioelectric events, as a result of the intermittent activity of a variety of cells and organs, short-duration asymmetrical (with respect to the time axis) or completely monophasic pulses are presented to the reproducing apparatus. A harmonic analysis of such waveforms reveals the presence of a first term (a_0) in the Fourier series. Therefore, faithful reproduction of such events requires the use of a system with a frequency response extending to zero

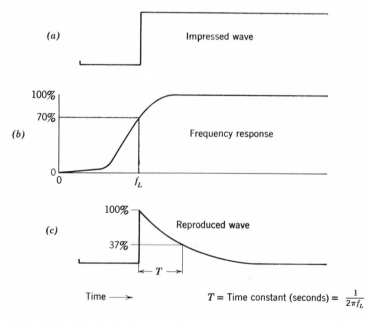

Figure 14–6.   Relationship between time constant and low-frequency response.

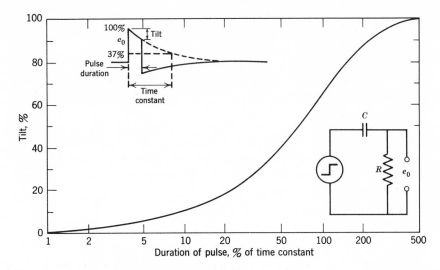

Figure 14-7.   Square pulse response.

cycles per second, that is, a d-c response. Frequently it is not practical to meet this requirement. Under many circumstances a reasonable reproduction of the event can be obtained with a processing system having a time constant which is very long with respect to the duration of the event. This technique is employed in the instruments which record many of the bioelectric events, such as the ECG, EEG, and EMG.

The effect of time constant on the reproduction of a single monophasic flat-topped pulse is illustrated in Fig. 14-7. In this diagram the percentage drop (tilt) on the top of the reproduced wave is compared with the ratio of the duration of the pulse to the time constant of the circuit passing it. For simplicity of illustration, the calculations were based on a single-section R-C circuit.

It is readily apparent that a 10% tilt is encountered if the duration of the pulse is approximately one tenth of the time constant of the circuit. Increasing the time constant of the circuit or decreasing the pulse duration would reduce the percentage tilt.

It is to be noted that there is also an undershoot following the pulse. The amount is equal to the amount of the tilt. If the pulse duration is many times longer than the time constant, the familiar biphasic condenser charge and discharge current wave is seen.

To further improve the reproduction of short-duration square pulses when using amplifiers without d-c response, phase- and amplitude-compensating networks are often added which are designed to flatten the top of the pulse. This technique is employed in most ECG amplifiers. A good treatment of this subject is given by Valley and Wallman (1948) in the chapter of their book dealing with pulse amplifiers.

If the step function (Fig. 14–8a) is impressed on a simple system having a low-frequency response extending to zero cycles per second and a high-frequency response not extending to an infinitely high frequency (Fig. 14–8b), the type of response shown in Fig. 14–8c is encountered. It can be seen that the reproduced wave does not attain its final value instantly but takes a finite time to reach it. This rise or response time is frequently described as the time in seconds for the amplitude to rise from 10% to 90% of its final value. The rise time is related to the high-frequency sine-wave response by the following expression:

$$t = \frac{1}{kf_h},$$

where t is rise time (10 to 90%) in seconds; f_h is frequency on the sine-wave response curve where the response has fallen to 70%; and k depends on

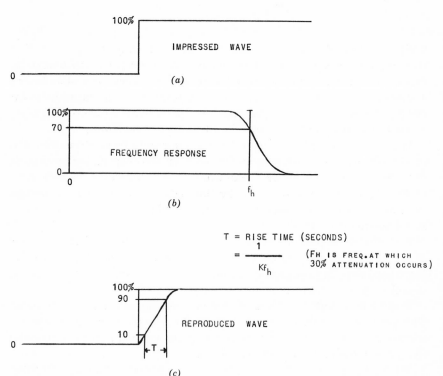

Figure 14–8.   The effect of high-frequency response on the reproduction of a step function.

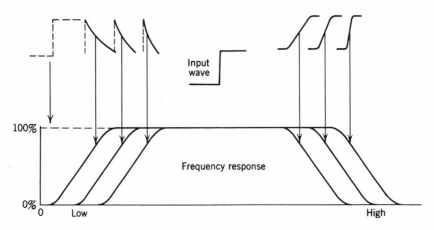

Figure 14-9. The effect of low- and high-frequency response on the reproduction of a step function.

the circuit configuration and hence the rate at which the high-frequency response decreases with increasing frequency (high-frequency roll-off); in many circuits, k varies between 2 and 3.

From the above it is obvious that increasing f_h, that is, improving the high-frequency response, shortens the rise time. Figure 14-9 summarizes how low-frequency and high-frequency responses affect the reproduction of a step function.

From this discussion it is readily apparent that the sharp portions of a complex wave dictate the high-frequency response required for its faithful reproduction. The required low-frequency response is determined by the fundamental frequency of the complex wave and by the presence or absence of an average value. If the complex waveform possesses an average value, the required low-frequency response must extend to zero cycles per second (i.e., the system must provide d-c response) if baseline information is to be retained.

14-4. DAMPED RESONANT SYSTEMS

Frequently, in the course of measuring physiological events, the phenomenon of resonance is encountered. Basic to this phenomenon is the presence of at least two real or apparent energy-storage elements between which energy is continuously transferred. In the case of electrical components, capacitance and inductance are the real storage elements. It is also possible for the resonance phenomenon to exist in amplifier circuits which contain no inductive elements. Systems of this type show "ringing" or a tendency toward oscillation at a frequency for which there is a component of positive feedback around all or part of the circuit. (See Chap. 13, Sec. 20).

Resonance may also be purely mechanical, as in the case of devices possessing elasticity and mass. Two examples of such mechanical devices are blood pressure manometers, in which an elastic diaphragm or Bourdon tube is distorted by pressure, and moving-coil recorders, in which a torsion rod or spring returns the movement to its baseline when the signal is removed. The actual motion of the moving element (and hence its capabilities as a transducer or reproducer) depends on three factors—inertia, elasticity or stiffness, and damping—and is described in mathematical terms by the interrelationship between them. *Inertia* is a measure of the force required to set the mass in motion or to alter its direction once it is in motion. Stiffness describes the rigidity of the system. It is defined in terms of the force required to deflect the moving member unit distance from its position of equilibrium. *Damping* is a measure of the frictional force acting on the mass. The frictional force is directed opposite to the direction of displacement of the mass. It is usually assumed that the magnitude of the frictional force varies directly with velocity, that is, the damping is viscous. Damping may be present as fluid resistance, or it may exist as an electrically induced force.

Simple mechanical systems can be described in terms of one-to-one electrical analogs because the behavior of both systems is expressed by the same mathematical equations. Inertia, damping, and stiffness determine the behavior of mechanical systems. In a series electrical circuit these quantities correspond to inductance, resistance, and capacitance, respectively.

Because the dynamic behavior of mechanical systems is so important in physiological measurements, the interrelationship between inertia, damping, and stiffness must be appreciated to understand how the characteristics of a given system can be altered under various conditions of measurement. Many devices can be well represented by a simple system involving only one degree of freedom (i.e., a system which can be completely characterized in terms of a single variable). Two simple mechanical models can be used to illustrate the behavior of most of these devices under the influence of a unit-step of force and a constant-amplitude variable-frequency sinusoidal force.

Consider a mass M free to move on a frictionless horizontal surface coupled to a fixed support by a spring. Connected to the mass is a rod terminated by a vane dipping into a reservoir of fluid, providing viscous damping. Figure 14–10a is a sketch of such a system in which the mass M is free to move in a left- or right-hand direction only. If a force is applied to move the weight from its position of equilibrium and then is removed, the mass will return to its original position slowly or rapidly and may overshoot and oscillate about the position of equilibrium several times before coming to rest, as shown in the figure. The type of motion executed depends upon the relationship between the mass, stiffness, and damping.

Another simple example of the same phenomenon is shown in Fig. 14–10b, which illustrates the essential components of a recording pen or galvanometer having a mass with a given moment of inertia coupled to an elastic torsion rod. If a deflecting torque is applied to cause rotation and is then removed, the system will return to its position of equilibrium slowly or rapidly, as in the previous case, depending upon the relationship between

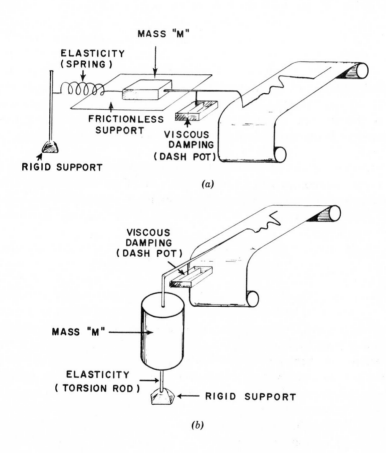

Figure 14–10. Transient response of lightly damped systems.

the same three quantities. The example of Fig. 14–10*a* deals with translation and describes the operation of blood pressure transducers and similar devices; that of Fig. 14–10*b* illustrates devices such as recording galvanometers in which rotary motion exists. Nonetheless if the mass, stiffness, and coefficient of damping are time invariant, the displacement in both cases is described by a linear differential equation of the second order and first degree. The following expressions describe the resultant motion:

Translation $\qquad M\dfrac{d^2x}{dt^2} + K_1\dfrac{dx}{dt} + K_2\,x = $ sum of applied forces.

Rotation $\qquad I\dfrac{d^2\phi}{dt^2} + K_1\dfrac{d\phi}{dt} + K_2\,\phi = $ sum of applied torques.

In these equations M and I are the mass-inertial components; M is the mass and I is the moment of inertia. K_1 is the viscous damping force, K_2 is the stiffness or restoring force usually represented by a spring constant, x is the linear displacement, ϕ is the angular displacement, and t is time.

Note the similarity between the two expressions just given and the following equation, which represents the sum of the voltage drops across an inductance L, resistance R, and capacitance C in a series circuit:

$$L\frac{d^2q}{dt^2} + R\frac{dq}{dt} + \frac{q}{C} = \text{applied voltage,}$$

where q is the charge, dq/dt is the rate of change of charge which is current i, and $d^2q/dt^2 = di/dt$.

Because the behavior of the mechanical systems is described by the same form of mathematical expression as that representing the electrical circuit, the electric circuit is called an analog of either mechanical system. Thus the behavior of these simple mechanical systems, and of others more complicated, can be investigated by the use of simple electrical components. The inertial components (M and I) are represented by the inductance L, the damping force K_1 by resistance R, and the stiffness of the mechanical systems K_2 by the reciprocal of capacitance. The displacement (x or) has as its analog the charge q. Hence, in the electrical simulation, the voltage across the capacitance describes x or ϕ.

Because these equations are of similar form the solutions are the same except for the letter designation of terms. A mathematical solution to the above equations may be difficult to carry out, depending upon the time function required to describe the applied force. A graphic solution, however, is easily obtained from the electrical analog if the desired forcing function can be generated. The electrical analog also provides a convenient means of changing parameters, thus permitting the behavior of such systems under a variety of conditions to be demonstrated easily. Hence, the mathematical ability necessary to solve the equations directly is not essential for an appreciation of the importance of the individual circuit elements in determining the response of the system to many different inputs. A description of the response to two different applied forces—(1) a step function and (2) a variable-frequency sine wave—will enable the reader to understand the behavior of a simple system under a variety of operating conditions.

The first, and probably the most important condition, is the particular interrelationship between the quantities which provides just enough damping so that the motion is nonoscillatory when a step force is applied or removed, that is, the moving element deflects or returns to its position of equilibrium as rapidly as possible without overshoot. Such a condition is called critical damping. Less damping results in a more rapid motion with overshoot. If the damping is reduced to zero, an oscillatory condition is produced. Although in actual practice it is never possible to achieve zero damping, a lightly damped system will oscillate for a long time before coming to rest. The frequency of force-free oscillation is called the natural frequency of the system.

When damping is made greater than critical, there is no overshoot but the time taken to reach the position of equilibrium is considerably longer. The types of response encountered with critical damping ($D = 1$) and damping less than critical are summarized in Fig. 14–11. With a step force applied or removed instantly, the response (a) is nonoscillatory for critical damping. With light damping ($D = 0.2$), the response (b) is partially oscillatory at a frequency less than the undamped resonant frequency of the system. Increasing the damping to 0.5 (c) results in an overshoot of approximately 15% followed by a heavily damped oscillation.

The time axis of Fig. 14–11 is plotted in percent of the undamped period T_0 (equal to the reciprocal of the resonant frequency with zero damping, i.e., the natural frequency). The resonant frequency with zero damping (f_0) is dependent on the relationship between the inertial component M or I and the stiffness K_2. It can easily be shown that

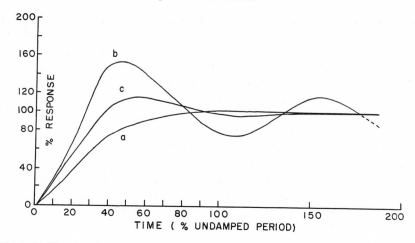

Figure 14–11. Transient response with various degrees of damping: (a) $D = 1.0$ (critical damping); (b) $D = 0.2$; (c) $D = 0.5$.

for the translational case
$$f_0 = \frac{1}{2\pi}\sqrt{\frac{K_2}{M}},$$

for the rotational case
$$f_0 = \frac{1}{2\pi}\sqrt{\frac{K_2}{I}},$$

for the electrical case
$$f_0 = \frac{1}{2\pi}\sqrt{\frac{1/C}{L}}.$$

Thus specifying the system constants permits calculation of values for the abscissa of Fig. 14–11. It is to be noted that, as the damping is decreased, the time for the system to rise from 0 to 100% becomes shorter and the overshoot is greater. Accordingly, the price of elimination of transient overshoot is prolongation of rise time. Therefore, in order to obtain more rapid response without excessive overshoot, it is necessary to use a stiffer or lighter system, that is, one with a higher resonant frequency. Thus, the undamped resonant frequency of a system, along with the coefficient of damping, determines the rise time.

Intimately associated with the response to a step input is the behavior of such systems when subjected to sinusoidal forces. Figure 14–12a illustrates the normalized response A_f/A_k when tested with a constant-amplitude variable-frequency sine wave of force A_k. With critical damping ($D = 1$), the frequency-response curve has a characteristic form, falling progressively as the frequency is increased. With zero damping the amplitude of motion increases and becomes larger and larger as the resonant frequency is approached. At the resonant frequency f_0, the amplitude theoretically approaches infinity. With driving frequencies above the resonant frequency, the amplitude is reduced; as the frequency is increased, the amplitude soon becomes immeasurably small. This condition, shown dotted in Fig. 14–12a, represents a limiting condition under which all operating characteristics are to be found.

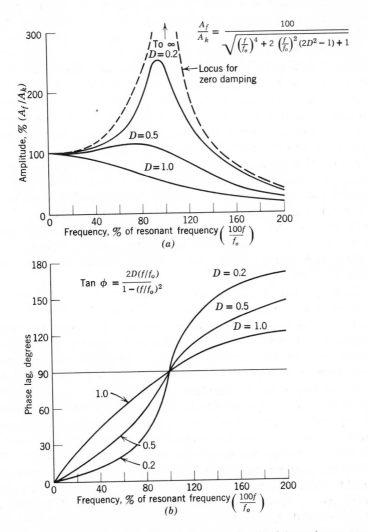

Figure 14–12. Sinusoidal frequency (a) and phase response (b) of damped resonant systems.

If the same procedure is carried out with various degrees of damping between zero and approximately 0.7, the amplitude increases slightly at first, rising to a peak and then falling rapidly as the frequency increases. The cases of $D = 0.2$ and $D = 0.5$ illustrate this point. The interesting behavior when $D = 0.7$ will be discussed later.

From Fig. 14–12 it is apparent that with critical damping the system can respond fully only to sine-wave frequencies up to a few percent of the resonant frequency. With light damping (0.2) there is a pronounced rise in the frequency response curve at approximately 95% of the undamped natural resonant frequency. When the damping is increased to 0.5, the frequency response curve is more uniform and exhibits less of a resonant rise. The frequency at a resonant rise is less than that for the undamped condition. In both cases as the frequency is increased beyond the maximum response, the amplitude falls progressively. The foregoing discussion shows that by assigning various values to the damping coefficient a family of amplitude-versus-frequency curves is determined. Those of most interest fall between zero and critical damping and assume a contour appropriate for their proximity to either of these curves.

When a periodic sine wave of force is presented to such systems, there is a time lag between the displacement of the mass and the applied force. This time lag is expressed in terms of degrees of a full cycle and is designated as phase shift. Damping has a pronounced effect on the phase characteristic of such systems. This relationship is shown in Fig. 14–12b. It is apparent from inspection of this figure that with some damping, between 0.5 and 1.0, phase shift can be nearly linear with frequency up to the natural resonant frequency f_0.

In deciding what degree of damping should be specified to obtain the best phase characteristic, it is useful to recall the three criteria for the faithful reproduction of an event: (a) linearity of amplitude, (b) adequate bandwidth of sine-wave frequency response, and (c) linearity of phase shift. Because amplitude linearity is usually easy to achieve, the following discussion will deal with the effect of damping on the sine-wave frequency and phase response.

Figure 14–13 shows the amplitude of the resonant rise in the sine-wave frequency response curve as damping is increased. On the basis of uniform sine-wave frequency response a damping of 0.7 results in no resonant peak in the curve. Although not shown in Fig. 14–13, but certainly indicated by Fig. 14–12b, it can be stated that this degree of damping provides a linear phase shift up to and slightly beyond the undamped resonant frequency. It is logical then to conclude that this degree of damping fulfills the requirements for faithful reproduction of an event. Although this is true, it must be remembered that the reproduction of a step input by a system having

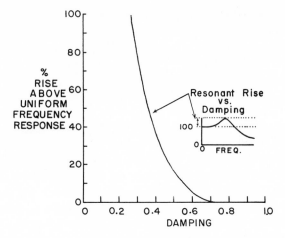

Figure 14-13. The effect of damping on the uniformity of the sine wave frequency response.

these constants is slightly compromised. Under these conditions the rise time (0 to 100%) is approximately half of the undamped period. Moreover a 5% overshoot is present. It is to be recalled that decreasing the damping shortens the rise time at the expense of overshoot. Since with 0.7 damping some overshoot must exist, it is logical to investigate the improvement in rise time as damping is further decreased to obtain a more rapid response from the system. Just what degree of damping is to be specified usually depends on the penalty that can be paid in terms of overshoot and rise time for a step function, along with the loss produced in the sine-wave frequency response.

From Fig. 14-14, which relates rise time and overshoot to the various degrees of damping, it is seen that if the damping is reduced from 0.7 to 0.65, the response time shortens by about 3% to 47% of the undamped period, while the overshoot increases by 2%, giving a total overshoot of 7%. Under these conditions sine-wave characteristics are not excessively compromised, since for 0.65 damping the resonant rise in the frequency response curve is slightly more than 1% and the phase error is approximately 4 degrees.

If a larger overshoot to the step function can be tolerated, a further decrease in rise time can be attained. At 0.6 damping the rise time is shortened to approximately 45% of the undamped period, but the overshoot is increased to about 10%. Under these conditions the resonant rise in the sine-wave curve is approximately 5%.

Thus it is apparent that, with devices in which resonance can occur, a shorter response time can be attained if a small degree of overshoot

RESPONSE TO STEP FUNCTION

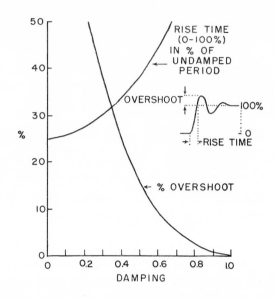

Figure 14–14. The effect of damping on rise time and overshoot in terms of the response to a step function.

can be tolerated when a step input is applied. The improvement in rise time simulates to some extent the characteristics of a stiffer system, that is, one with a higher natural frequency. With knowledge of the undamped resonant frequency and the degree of damping the entire behavior of a system having one degree of freedom can be predicted. When the response to a step function (rise time and overshoot) is known, the sine-wave frequency and phase characteristics can be deduced. Conversely, knowledge of the sine-wave frequency and phase response characteristics makes it possible to predict the response to a step function or a square wave.

In actual practice, to obtain a good compromise between all of the factors discussed, the damping of dynamic systems is usually adjusted to about 0.65. The characteristics of a system with one degree of freedom and this damping coefficient are shown in Table 14–2.

14–5. CONCLUSION

It is apparent that, for a system to reproduce a complex wave faithfully, consideration must be given to its harmonic spectrum. Then the sine-wave frequency and phase characteristics of the reproducing system must be

**Table 14-2   Characteristics of a Resonant System
with 0.65 Damping**

Undamped resonant frequency $= f_0$

Step Function	$\dfrac{1}{2.1\,f_0}$ seconds
Rise time (0 to 100% of terminal amplitude:)	
Overshoot (% over terminal amplitude)	7%
Sine Wave	
Bandwidth (to 70% of uniform amplitude response)	(0 to 108%)f_0
Resonant peak (above uniform response)	1.3%
Maximum phase error over (0 to 100%) f_0 range	4%

examined for their suitability for reproduction of all of the components of the complex wave. From such an investigation it is possible to determine the degree of fidelity of reproduction that can be expected.

REFERENCES

Geddes, L. A. 1951. A note on phase distortion. *EEG Clin. Neurophysiol.* 3:517–8.

Hansen, A. T. 1949. *Pressure Measurement in the Human Organism.* Copenhagen; Technisk Forlag.

Saunders, M. G., and R. M. Jell, 1959. Time distortion in electroencephalograph amplifiers. *EEG Clin. Neurophysiol.* 11:814–6.

Terman, F. E. 1943. *Radio Engineers Handbook.* New York; McGraw Hill Book Co.

Valley, G. E., and H. Wallman, 1948. *Vacuum Tube Amplifiers.* New York: McGraw Hill Book Co.

Index